PHOSPHATE AND MINERAL METABOLISM

ADVANCES IN EXPERIMENTAL MEDICINE AND BIOLOGY

Recent Volumes in this Series

Volume 171
GLUCOCORTICOID EFFECTS AND THEIR BIOLOGICAL CONSEQUENCES
Edited by Louis V. Avioli, Carlo Gennari, and Bruno Imbimbo

Volume 172
EUKARYOTIC CELL CULTURES: Basics and Applications
Edited by Ronald T. Acton and J. Daniel Lynn

Volume 173
MOLECULAR BIOLOGY AND PATHOGENESIS OF CORONAVIRUSES
Edited by P. J. M. Rottier, B. A. M. van der Zeijst, W. J. M. Spaan, and M. C. Horzinek

Volume 174
GANGLIOSIDE STRUCTURE, FUNCTION AND BIOMEDICAL POTENTIAL
Edited by Robert W. Ledeen, Robert K. Yu, Maurice M. Rapport, and Kunihiko Suzuki

Volume 175
NEUROTRANSMITTER RECEPTORS: Mechanisms of Action and Regulation
Edited by Shozo Kito, Tomio Segawa, Kinya Kuriyama, Henry I. Yamamura, and Richard W. Olsen

Volume 176
HUMAN TROPHOBLAST NEOPLASMS
Edited by Roland A. Pattillo and Robert O. Hussa

Volume 177
NUTRITIONAL AND TOXICOLOGICAL ASPECTS OF FOOD SAFETY
Edited by Mendel Friedman

Volume 178
PHOSPHATE AND MINERAL METABOLISM
Edited by Shaul G. Massry, Giuseppe Maschio, and Eberhard Ritz

---

PHOSPHATE AND MINERAL METABOLISM

Edited by
Shaul G. Massry
University of Southern California
Los Angeles, California
Giuseppe Maschio
University of Verona
Verona, Italy
and
Eberhard Ritz
University of Heidelberg
Heidelberg, Federal Republic of Germany

PLENUM PRESS • NEW YORK AND LONDON

Library of Congress Cataloging in Publication Data

International Workshop on Phosphate and Other Minerals (6th: 1983: Verona, Italy)
Phosphate and mineral metabolism.

(Advances in experimental medicine and biology; v. 178)
"Proceedings of the Sixth International Workshop on Phosphate and Other Minerals, held June 24-26, 1983, in Verona, Italy"—T.p. verso.
Bibliography: p.
Includes index.
1. Mineral metabolism—Congresses. 2. Phosphates—Metabolism—Congresses. 3. Mineral metabolism—Disorders—Congresses. I. Massry, Shaul G. II. Maschio, Giuseppe. III. Ritz, Eberhard. IV. Title. V. Series.
QP533.I58 1983 599′.0133 84-13450

DOI 10.1007/978-1-4684-4808-5

Proceedings of the Sixth International Workshop on Phosphate and other Minerals, held June 24-26, 1983, in Verona, Italy

MyCopy version of the original edition 1984
A Division of Plenum Publishing Corporation
233 Spring Street, New York, N.Y. 10013

TO OUR WIVES

Meira Massry
Emilia Maschio
Christina Ritz

AND TO OUR CHILDREN

PREFACE

We are pleased to present to our readers the Proceedings of the Sixth International Workshop on Phosphate and Other Minerals which was held in Verona, Italy, during June 24-26, 1983. It was hosted by Professor Giuseppe Maschio, Professor of Medicine and Chief, Department of Nephrology at the University of Verona.

The Sixth Workshop maintained the tradition of the previous ones. It provided a unique and outstanding opportunity for close interaction between scientist involved in the research of the overall field of Mineral Metabolism. The current Workshop was attended by 250 scientists from 15 countries including Austria, Canada, Denmark, England, France, Germany, Holland, Israel, Italy, Japan, Spain, Sweden, Switzerland, and the United States of America. The topics discussed included the renal handling of phosphate, transport of other minerals, intestinal absorption of calcium and phosphate and phosphate homeostasis in health and disease. Two symposia dealing with the recent developments of the interactions between minerals, parathyroid hormone, and blood pressure and between minerals and myopathies were included. In addition to the 15 State-of-the-Art Lectures, there were 43 oral and 63 poster presentations selected from over 200 abstracts submitted to the Program Committee.

The Seventh International Workshop on Phosphate and Other Minerals will be held during September, 1985, in Marseille, France. It will be hosted by Professor Michel Olmer, Chief of the Department of Nephrology at the University of Marseille. The theme of this coming Workshop will focus on the pathophysiology of phosphate homeostasis and the metabolism of other minerals.

We would like to express our thanks and appreciation for all those who have stimulated, encouraged, and supported us to hold the Sixth International Workshop in Verona. The meeting could not have been possible without the generous financial support of the City of Verona and Cassa Di Respamio Di Verona, Italy, Hoffman La Roche (USA), Plenum Publishing Company (USA), Procter and Gamble (USA), Sandoz (Italy), Veneto Regional Government (Italy), and the University of Verona (Italy). We would like to thank Ms. Joann Little for her secretarial help and Mrs. Haidy Samouha for her contributions in the organization of the Workshop.

Shaul G. Massry
Giuseppe Maschio
Eberhard Ritz

CONTENTS

RENAL HANDLING OF PHOSPHATE

CALCIUM AND MAGNESIUM TRANSPORT

INTESTINAL ABSORPTION OF PHOSPHATE AND CALCIUM

TOPICS ON BONE

MINERALS AND MYOPATHIES

CLINICAL TOPICS

MISCELLANEOUS

NUCLEAR MAGNETIC RESONANCE

RENAL HANDLING OF PHOSPHATE

THE BIOCHEMICAL MODIFICATIONS OF THE BRUSH BORDER MEMBRANE INDUCED BY VITAMIN D AND PARATHYROID HORMONE IN THEIR ACTIONS ON PHOSPHATE TRANSPORT

Keith Hruska, Brenda Kurnik and Masaharu Tsutsumi

Renal Division
Jewish Hospital/Washington University
St. Louis, MO

Supported by N.I.H. PPG AM09976 and PPG AM32087

Dr. Hruska is an Established Investigator of the American Heart Association

Since the development of techniques for the preparation and isolation of brush border membrane vesicles (BBMV),[1,2] from the luminal cell membrane of renal tubular epthelial cells considerable progress has been made in our understanding of renal tubular cell phosphate transport. A sodium dependent co-transport system capable of moving phosphate uphill against an electrochemical gradient has been characterized in BBMV. The stoichiometry of the carrier mechanism remains controversial. According to one report, it is either $2Na^{+}:HPO_4^{-2}$ or $Na^{+}:H_2PO_4^{-}$, dependent upon the charge of the phosphate species present in the bathing fluid, and phosphate transfer is electroneutral.[3] However, others have reported that at pH 6 the stoichiometry is $2Na:H_2PO_4^{-}$ and the carrier may be electrogenic at low pH.[4,5] Carrier activity increases as the pH of the medium is increased in the range of 6.0-8.5.[3-5] Thus, a mechanism of secondary active phosphate transport in the renal tubular brush border membrane (BBM) has been partially characterized.

The next major question is whether the active step of phosphate transport is the site at which the cellular movement of phosphate is regulated. This question remains unresolved. One of the major reasons to suggest that the sodium dependent phosphate carrier is the regulator of cellular phosphate transport has been the strong association between changes in carrier activity in vitro and adaptative changes in phosphate reabsorption in vivo. In experimental settings with increased or decreased phosphate reabsorption, similar changes in the activity of the sodium dependent carrier mechanism have been demonstrated. Thus, in the adaptation of phosphate transport to changes in phosphate load,[6,7] parathyroid hormone (PTH),[8,9] growth hormone,[9] and many other substances,[10] the activity of the sodium dependent phosphate carrier has exhibited the same change in activity as whole kidney phosphate reabsorption. An exception to this principle is the disparity between the resistance to the action of PTH observed in vivo during phosphate depletion and its continued effect on the Na^+-dependent carrier mechanism in BBMV from phosphate depleted dogs in vitro.[7]

The presence of the sodium dependent phosphate carrier mechanism in the isolated BBMV also has provided an opportunity for an investigation of the mechanisms by which carrier activity is controlled. To evaluate the mechanism of action of PTH on phosphate transport, we designed a set of experiments to examine the role of membrane phosphorylation in the control of phosphate carrier activity.[11] The hypothesis is schematically represented in Figure 1. It states that PTH, following binding to its receptors on the antiluminal membrane of renal tubular epithelial cells, stimulates a membrane bound enzyme, adenylate cyclase, stimulating the production of 3'5'-cyclic adenosine monophosphate (cAMP) from adenosine triphosphate (ATP). Cyclic AMP then serves as an intracellular "second messenger" determining the effects of PTH. One of the effects of cAMP is to stimulate the activity of a cAMP dependent protein kinase. This enzyme, shown in the diagram as being either a cytosolic or a BBM bound enzyme, is comprised of a regulatory and a catalytic unit. The catalytic unit separates from the regulatory unit following binding of cAMP to the regulatory unit. This binding and separation is affected in part by phosphorylation of the regulatory unit. The catalytic unit of cAMP dependent protein kinase then stimulates phosphorylation of a specific membrane protein related to the activity of phosphate transport. Phosphorylation of the protein would be associated with a decrease in phosphate transport and this effect of PTH would be reversed by dephosphorylation of the protein returning the activity of phosphate transport to the basal level. Dephosphorylation of the phosphorylated substrate would be accomplished by an enzyme, protein phosphatase. The other purported "second messenger" for the action of PTH, calcium (Ca^{2+}), is shown exhibiting a negative influence on adenylate cyclase and a possible role in the action of cAMP dependent protein kinase activity.

We have recently reported the results of experiments designed to test this hypothesis.[12] In these experiments, BBMV prepared from canine kidneys were utilized to detect the presence of cAMP dependent protein phosphorylation and relate this to changes in the activity of the sodium dependent phosphate carrier mechanism. As shown in Figure 2, exposure of BBMV to hypotonic solutions

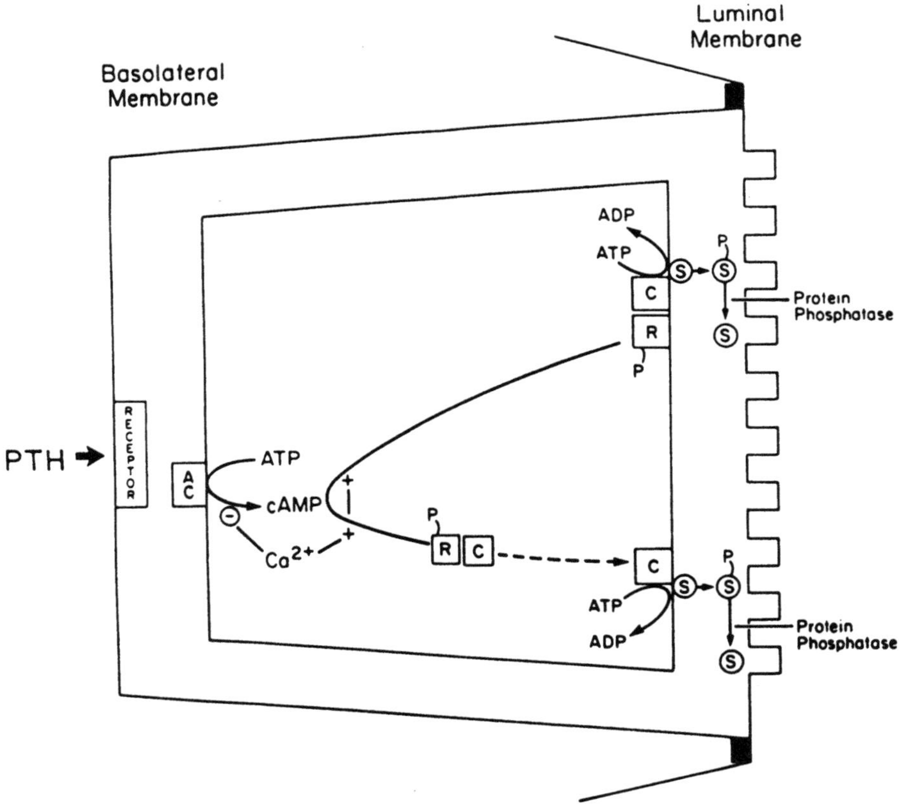

Figure 1 Schematic representation of the metabolic steps in cAMP dependent modulation of transport stimulated by PTH. AC, adenylate cyclase; ATP, adenosine triphosphate; cAMP, 3'5' cyclic adenosine monophosphate; R and C together are the regulatory and catalytic units of cAMP dependent protein kinase which is autophosphorylated on the regulatory unit stimulating separation of the catalytic unit which then serves to phosphorylate acceptor proteins, S. The phosphorylated acceptor proteins, S~P, are dephosphorylated by the activity of protein phosphatases.

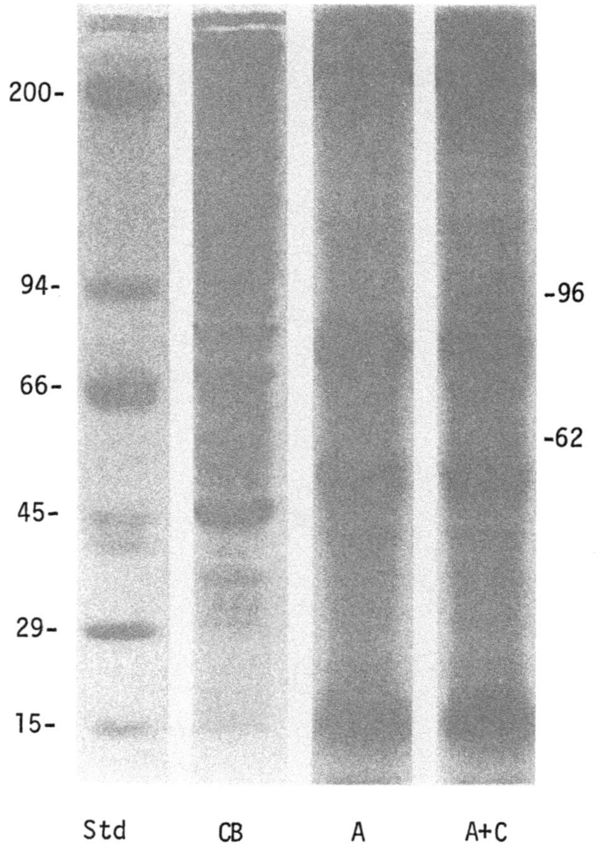

Figure 2 SDS polyacrylamide gel electrophoresis and autoradiography of BBM proteins. Canine BBMV, prepared in 10 mM $MgCl_2$, 10 mM KCL, 240 mM mannitol, and 5 mM Mes-Tris, pH 6.5, were exposed to solutions containing 10 mM $MgCl_2$, 10 mM KCL, 5 mM Mes-Tris, pH 6.5, and 10 µM ATP with [γ^{32}Pi]-ATP (5-20 µCi) with or without 10^{-6} M cAMP for 1 minute at 30°C. The reaction was terminated with 60 mM Tris HCL, pH 6.8, 12% sodium dodecylsulfate (w/v), and 30% glycerol (w/v). Samples of approximately 100 µG of protein were added to acrylamide slab gels (7.5%) and electrophoresis was performed as reported (12). Gels were stained with Commasie blue and exposed to radiographic film which was developed after 7 days of exposure. Lane STD, calibration for molecular weight. CB, BBM proteins stained with Commasie blue; A, autoradiogram of the CB sample which had been exposed to 10 µg [γ^{32}Pi]-ATP; and A+C, phosphorylation of BBMV as in lane A with the addition of 10^{-6} M cAMP. Cyclic AMP stimulated phosphorylation of two BBMV proteins with molecular sizes estimated at 96,000 and 62,000 in several experiments.

containing 10 µM ATP and 10^{-6} M cAMP resulted in cAMP dependent phosphorylation of two membrane proteins with the molecular weights of 96,000 (band V) and 62,000 (band IX). The cAMP dependent protein phosphorylation was shown to be dependent upon the hypotonicity of the solutions used in exposing the membrane to the test substances. This is in agreement with the right side out orientation of BBMV.[12,13] Since the cAMP dependent protein kinase is located in the cytoplasmic side of the membrane, a technique designed to afford access of ATP and cAMP to the kinase was required. We have shown that exposure of BBMV to hypotonic solutions causes a release of substances trapped in BBMV, and an incorporation of substances normally excluded from permeation into BBMV.[12,14] Also, following exposure to hypotonic solutions, BBMV rectify and maintain the capacity for concentrative transport of glucose and phosphate.[12,14] Addition of ATP and cAMP in an isotonic solution failed to produce cAMP dependent phosphorylation. As shown in Table I, sodium gradient dependent phosphate transport was decreased in membrane vesicles exposed to ATP and cAMP as compared to phosphate transport in vesicles exposed to ATP alone.[12] The additions were again made in hypotonic solutions. Phosphate transport was not affected by the addition of ATP and cAMP in an isotonic solution. Thus, the activity of cAMP dependent protein kinase and the detection of substrate proteins for the kinase activity in canine BBM was associated with a decrease in the activity of the sodium dependent phosphate carrier mechanism.

Table 1. Phosphate Uptake in Phosphorylated Membrane Vesicles

Uptakes of 25 µM ^{32}Pi were measured in membrane vesicles which had been phosphorylated in the presence of 10 µM ATP without (-) or with (+) 10^{-6} M cAMP under conditions of initial 100 mM NaCl or 100 mM KCl gradients (extravesicular > intravesicular). Data are presented as mean ± S.E. of at least 3 experiments (3 dogs) each performed in triplicate.

Solute (conditions)	Uptake			
	15 s		90 min	
	−cAMP	+cAMP	−cAMP	+cAMP
	pmol solute/mg protein			
(NaCl gradient)	227 ± 5.8	192 ± 5.2[a]	142 ± 7.8	135 ± 7.1
(KCl gradient)	7.5 + 0.3	7.5 + 1.3	58 + 2.1	67 + 2.5

[a] Uptake + cAMP < uptake − cAMP; $p < 0.0005$.

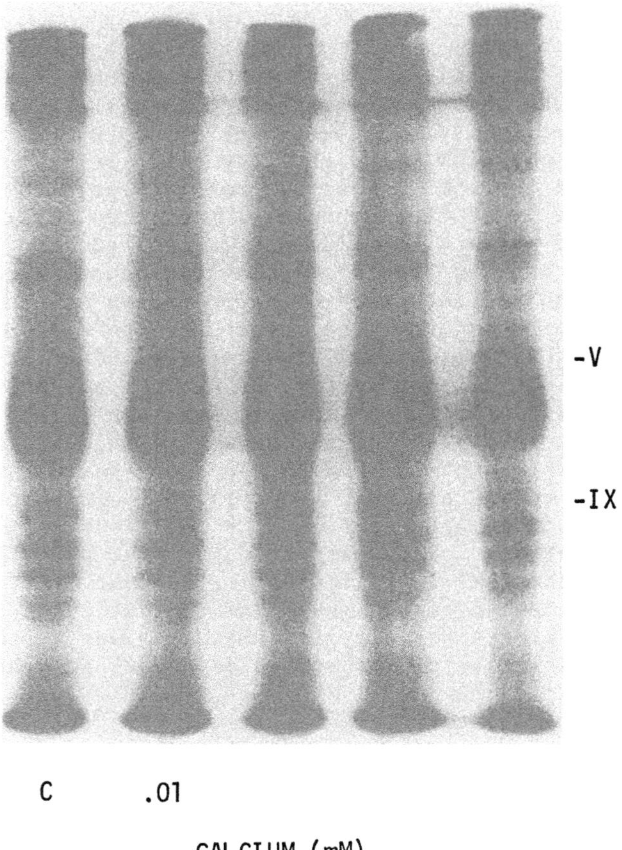

Figure 3 BBMV prepared as described in reference 12 and the legend to Figure 2 were exposed to hypotonic solutions containing 10 μM [γ^{32}Pi]-ATP and 10^{-6} M cAMP with variable concentrations of added calcium as shown. The protein substrates of cAMP dependent protein kinase are marked as band V and IX. Calcium failed to affect cAMP stimulation of ^{32}Pi incorporation into the acceptor proteins compared to zero added calcium, (C).

An interesting characteristic of the canine BBMV prepared by divalent cation (Mg^{2+}) induced precipitation of cortical homogenates and differential centrifugation was the lack of effect of added calcium on membrane phosphorylation. As shown in Figure 3, increasing concentrations of calcium in the solutions containing ATP and cAMP failed to affect the cAMP dependent protein phosphorylation. Since cAMP dependent protein kinase is a calcium dependent enzyme in some systems, this may indicate sufficient calcium bound to canine

BBMV following preparation for the support of protein kinase activity, or alternatively, it may indicate that the canine cAMP dependent protein kinase of the renal BBM is calcium independent. This result, as discussed below, differs from the cAMP dependent protein kinase activity of BBMV isolated from rat kidney.

We were able to demonstrate that the activity of the cAMP dependent protein kinase in canine BBMV was regulated by PTH.[12] The strategy employed in these experiments was to compare the activity of the cAMP dependent protein kinase as assessed by phosphorylation of the specific acceptor proteins in the PTH replete state to the activity of the kinase in the absence of PTH induced by a parathyroidectomy. In the presence of PTH, phosphorylation of the substrate proteins endogenously might be expected to inhibit further phosphorylation in vitro by cAMP. Whereas in the absence of PTH, endogenous phosphorylation of the substrate proteins would be expected to be less, and thus, the stimulation of phosphorylation by cAMP in vitro might be greater. These predictions were found to be true.[12] In addition, the decrease in phosphate transport induced by cAMP dependent protein phosphorylation was less in BBMV isolated from PTH replete dogs. The effect of cAMP on phosphate transport was greater in BBMV prepared from parathyroidectomized dogs, and it was reduced by administration of PTH in vivo to parathyroidectomized dogs. Thus, PTH appears to modulate the activity of the cAMP dependent protein kinase and the phosphorylation of BBM substrate proteins (S, in Figure 1) in the same manner it modulates phosphate transport. Taken together, these data support the hypothesis represented schematically in Figure 1. They do not address the question as to whether the cAMP dependent protein kinase in the isolated BBMV and the cytosolic cAMP dependent protein kinase are the same system,[15] nor the possibility that effect of PTH may be to increase the incorporation of the kinase into the BBM.

Additional studies demonstrated that the cAMP dependent protein phosphorylation was rapid (peaking within 1 min.) and that dephosphorylation occurred through the activity of a specific phosphatase. This latter point was assessed by the much more rapid dephosphorylation of the 62,000 M_r phosphorylated protein (band IX) than dephosphorylation of the other proteins of the BBMV. Hammerman et al,[16] have subsequently shown that dephosphorylation of the band IX protein is associated with a reversal of the effects of cAMP on phosphate transport in vitro. PTH appeared not to regulate the activity of the specific protein phosphatase since no effect on the rate of dephosphorylation of the band IX protein was induced by manipulation of PTH levels.

Effect of vitamin D on phosphate transport in rodent BBMV

We have recently begun a series of investigations designed to extend the analysis of membrane phosphorylation to the question of the mechanisms of action of vitamin D on phosphate transport. In order to begin these studies, we found it was first necessary to attempt to clarify the issues regarding the effects of vitamin D on renal phosphate transport. The confusion regarding this issue has been contributed to by the use of pharmacologic doses of vitamin D in acute studies, by administration of vitamin D to replete animals, and by the lack of attention to the metabolic complications associated with the production of rachitic vitamin D deficient animals. Most rachitogenic diets are relatively low in calcium and phosphorus. Animals on these diets become hypocalcemic and hypophosphatemic producing a state of secondary hyperparathyroidism, and resistance to the action of PTH administration induced by changes in PTH receptor function at the level of renal tubular cells.[17-18] As a result of these technical problems in experimental design, vitamin D has variously been reported to inhibit[19-21] or stimulate[22-24] phosphate transport.

We first attempted to design a model of vitamin D deficiency with normocalcemia, normophosphatemia, and normal levels of PTH.[25] To this end, weanling Sprague-Dawley rats were fed vitamin D deficient diets containing 1.8% calcium and 1.2% phosphorus for 5-6 weeks. Vitamin D deficient rats had plasma calciums of 2.63 $\pm$ 0.4 mM compared to 2.67 $\pm$ 0.3 mM for normal control rats. The plasma phosphorus was 2.42 $\pm$ 0.4 mM in vitamin D deficient animals compared to 2.43 $\pm$ 0.04 mM in normal control rats. 25(OH)D levels were undetectable in rats that were fed the vitamin D deficient diet and 1,25-di(OH)D_3 levels were 66 $\pm$ 20 picograms/ml compared to 130 $\pm$ 10 picograms/ml in the normal control rats. PTH levels were within the normal range in the vitamin D deficient rats at 180 $\pm$ 47 pmol equiv/L (normal range 103-220).

Administration of 60 pmol/100 g b.w. of 1,25$(OH)_2D_3$ to vitamin D deficient rats 48 hrs and 24 hrs prior to study produced significant hypercalcemia (2.8 $\pm$ 0.4 mM) and hyperphosphatemia (2.83 $\pm$ 0.1 mM) in rats who were continued during the 48 hr of vitamin D therapy on the 1.8% calcium/1.2% phosphorus diet. In rats who had a decrease in their dietary calcium and phosphorus intake into the low normal range, the elevation of plasma calcium and phosphorus were prevented.

BBMV prepared from vitamin D deficient and vitamin D repleted animals exhibited the same enrichments for alkaline phosphatase, the same decrease in Na^+, K^+-, ATPase activity, and the same initial rates of sodium gradient dependent glucose uptake indicating that the BBMV preparations in the vitamin D deficient and vitamin D repleted animals were similar. Sodium gradient dependent phosphate uptake, as shown in Figure 4, was significantly stimulated in the vitamin D repleted animals given the dietary adjustment compared to vitamin D deficient animals. Vitamin D repleted animals who did not

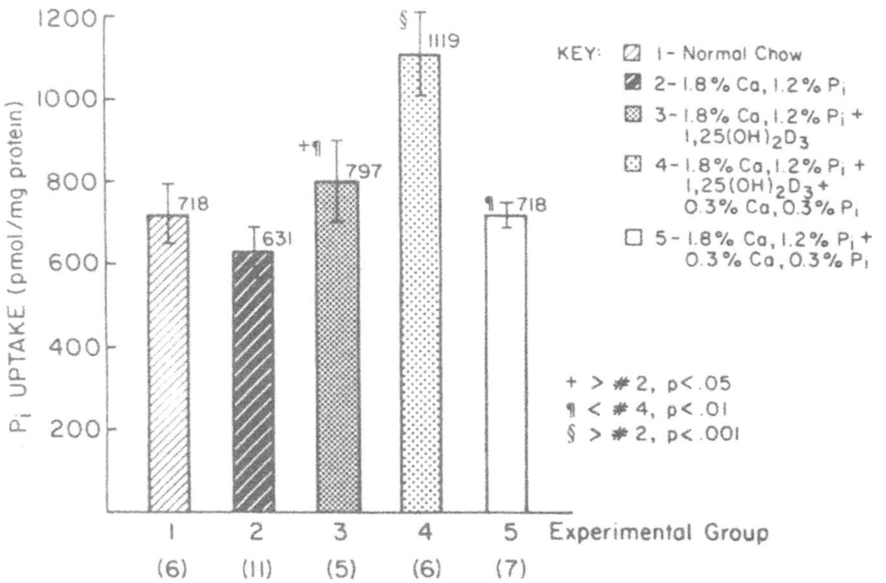

(6) (11) (5) (6) (7)

Figure 4 Effect of 1,25$(OH)_2D_3$ on phosphate uptake in BBMV from vitamin D deficient rats.[25] Rats were fed either normal diets or vitamin D deficient diets containing 1.8% calcium/1.2% phosphorus (see text). 1,25$(OH)_2D_3$, 60 pmol/100 g b.w., was administered 48 hr and 24 hr prior to study in Groups 3 and 4. The diets of Groups 4 and 5 were changed to 0.3% calcium/0.3% phosphorus during the 48 hrs prior to study. BBMV were prepared and exposed to hypotonic solutions as described in the legend to Figure 2. Phosphate uptake was initiated by the addition of 4 volumes of solution containing 54 mM NaCL, 5 mM Mes-Tris pH 6.5, and 25 µM ^{32}Pi KH_2PO_4 all in final concentrations. After incubation for 15 sec uptake was stopped by addition of 16 volumes of ice-cold 54 mM NaCL, 5 mM Na arsenate and rapid millipore filtration (0.65 micron filter). The filters were placed in 10 ml liquid scintillation counting fluid. Results are expressed as ± SE. Analysis of variance was utilized to examine the differences in phosphate uptake between experimental groups, and significance was determined for samples of unequal size as described by Snedecor.[34]

receive a change in diet also exhibited a significant increase in phosphorus uptake compared to BBMV from vitamin D deficient rats although the hyperphosphatemia and increase in phosphate load appeared to blunt the stimulatory effects of vitamin D on phosphate transport. The vitamin D deficient animals in which the diet was changed from 1.8% calcium and 1.2% phosphorus to 0.3% calcium and 0.3% phosphorus did not exhibit a change in phosphate uptake.

Cyclic AMP dependent protein phosphorylation of rodent BBMV

Phosphorylation of BBMV prepared from vitamin D deficient and vitamin D repleted rats treated as above was performed according to the protocol utilized for phosphorylation of canine BBMV described in the legend to Figure 2. As shown in Figure 5, phosphorylation of

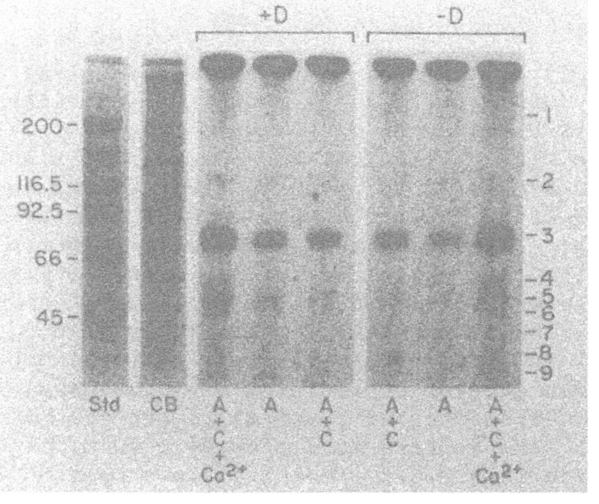

Figure 5 Cyclic AMP dependent protein phosphorylation of BBMV from rat kidneys. BBMV were isolated and exposed to solutions containing ATP or ATP and cAMP as described in the legend to Figure 2. Lanes labeled STD, molecular weight standards; CB, Commaise blue stained polyacrylamide gels of rat BBMV proteins; +D, BBMV prepared from vitamin D deficient rats treated with 60 pmol/100 g b.w. of $1,25(OH)_2D_3$ 48 and 24 hrs prior to study; A, 10 μM [$\gamma^{32}Pi$]-ATP; C, 10^{-6} M cAMP; and Ca^{2+}, 0.1 μM added calcium. The band 4 protein, a cAMP dependent ^{32}Pi acceptor protein, with a molecular weight of 62,000 is similar to the band IX protein phosphorylated by cAMP dependent protein kinase in canine BBMV. See text for further discussion.

BBMV of proteins in vitro following exposure to [γ^{32}Pi]-ATP was significantly different from the phosphorylation of canine BBMV. Generally, about 9 phosphorylated protein bands were detectable in rodent BBMV compared to approximately 16 bands usually detected in the canine BBMV. Cyclic AMP dependent phosphorylation of a protein with a molecular weight of 62,000 similar to that of the band IX of canine BBMV was demonstrable. However, this phosphorylation was generally faint and was significantly stimulated by the addition of 0.1 µM calcium. The stimulation of the cAMP dependent phosphorylation by the addition of calcium differs from the results in canine BBMVs, and it may indicate that insufficient calcium remains in the membrane during the preparative process of rodent BBMV compared to canine BBMV or it may indicate an intrinsic difference in the cAMP dependent kinases between the two species. The lack of difference in the cAMP dependent phosphorylation between BBMV from vitamin D deficient rats and BBMV from rats treated with 1,25$(OH)_2D_3$ is also shown in Figure 5. Furthermore, the addition of cAMP and ATP in vitro failed to reveal differential effects on phosphate transport between BBMV prepared from vitamin D deficient rats and rats treated with 1,25$(OH)_2D_3$. Deficient production of cAMP following stimulation of adenylate cyclase by PTH has been reported by Forte et al,[17,18] in vitamin D deficient rats. A 30% decrease in the activity of cAMP dependent protein kinase has been reported in vitamin D deficient chicks[26]. This effect on cAMP dependent protein kinase was not accounted for by the increase in the inhibitor of cAMP dependent protein kinase induced by vitamin D deficiency. The present studies indicate that vitamin D deficiency does not induce a decrease in the capacity of cAMP dependent protein kinase to phosphorylate the 62,000 molecular weight substrate protein of the BBMV.

We have also attempted to further extend the studies of dephosphorylation of the cAMP dependent substrate proteins[12,16] to the rodent BBMV. First we demonstrated that rapid dephosphorylation of the 62,000 molecular weight protein occurred with the process being complete within 5 min similar to the results previously reported in canine BBMV. Recent studies by Yusufi et al,[27] have suggested that incubation of BBM with phosphatidylinositol specific phospholipase-C (PI-PLC) results in a release of membrane alkaline phosphatase from the membrane. We were interested to test whether this decrease in alkaline phosphatase activity could be related to the protein phosphatase activity serving to dephosphorylate the cAMP dependent substrate proteins. As shown in Figure 6, incubation of BBMV isolated from normal rats or normal rat kidneys resulted in a significant prolongation of the cAMP dependent stimulation of phosphorylation of two proteins with molecular weights of 62,000 and 96,000. The 96,000 molecular weight substrate protein is similar to the band V protein reported in canine BBMV but is not routinely detected in rodent BBMV. Whether incubation with the PI-PLC

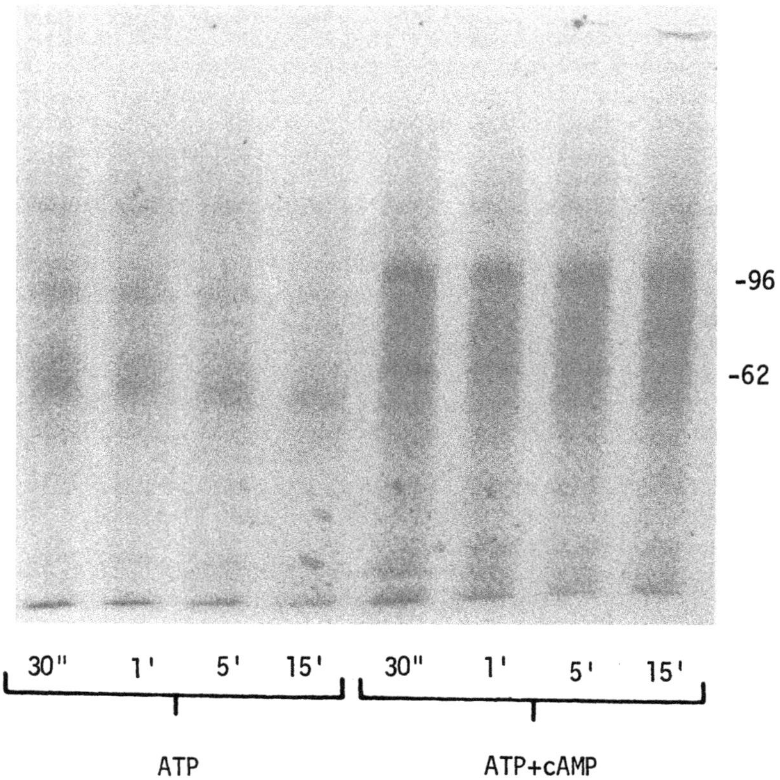

Figure 6 Cyclic AMP independent (ATP) and cAMP dependent (ATP + cAMP) protein phosphorylation of rat BBMV exposed to phosphatidyl-inositol specific phospholipase-C (Bacillus/Cerus). BBMV were prepared as described in the legend to Figure 2. BBMV were then exposed to 4 volumes of hypotonic solution containing 200 ng of phospholipase-C/mg protein (specific activity of phospholipase-C, 200 U/mg) for 10 min at 22°C. BBMV were then recentrifuged at 35,000 x g for 20 min. Following resuspension, phosphorylation was carried out as in the legend to Figure 2.

enhanced phosphorylation of this substrate protein or modified a membrane protein and increased its cAMP dependent phosphorylation remains unclear. Also, as shown in Figure 7, incubation of BBMV with PI-PLC decreased the phosphorylation of a group of proteins with molecular weights between 80-90,000 previously identified by DeJonge et al and Biber et al[28,29] as the phosphorylated intermediate of the calcium stimulated ATPase and alkaline phosphatase. In addition, incubation of BBMV with PI-PLC had dramatic effects on the phosphorylated phospholipids of the BBMV

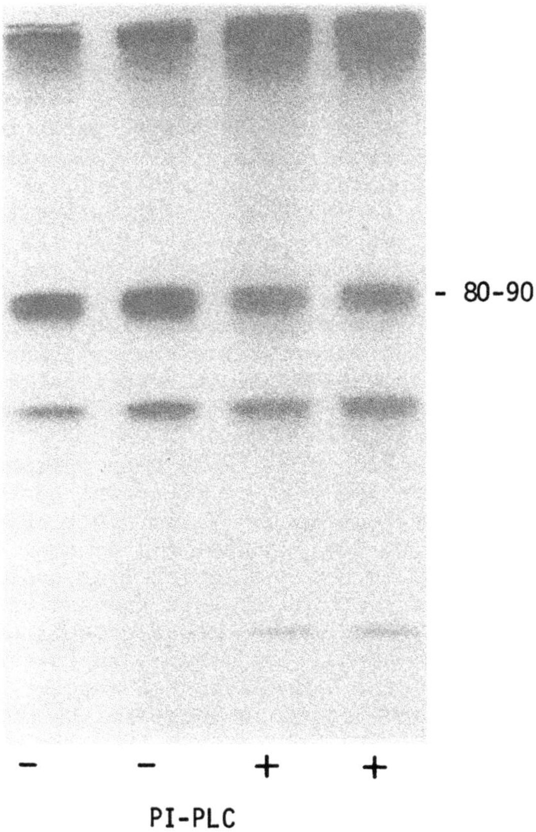

Figure 7 Effect of incubation of BBMV with PI-PLC on phosphorylation of membrane proteins. Incubation of rat BBMV with PI-PLC as in the legend to Figure 6. Phosphorylation, as described in the legend to Figure 2 and 6, after incubation with PI-PLC (+) was compared to phosphorylation of BBMV in its absence (-).

whose relationship to phosphate transport will be discussed below. These results indicate that the effects of incubating BBMV with PI-PLC are multiple with many of the effects having potential relationship to phosphate transport. These include, besides removal of alkaline phosphatase activity, partial removal of the phosphorylated intermediate of the calcium stimulated ATPase, decreased protein phosphatase activity related to the cAMP dependent phosphorylated substrate proteins and alteration of membrane phospholipids. These results make interpretation of the effects of

PI-PLC on phosphate transport extremely difficult to interpret.[27]

During the course of the studies on cAMP dependent protein phosphorylation, specific phosphorylation of membrane phospholipid was also discovered.[14] The phosphorylated products of phospholipid phosphorylation are phosphatidylinositol 4' monophosphate, phosphatidylinositol 4'5' triphosphate, and phosphatidic acid. The substrate for stimulation of phospholipid phosphorylation by ATP is phosphatidylinositol, and substrate levels in the BBMV decrease with phosphorylation, producing an increase in the membrane content of the phosphorylated products. Phosphorylation of these phospholipids is cAMP independent,[12] but stimulated by PTH.[30] Phospholipid phosphorylation does not detectably affect phosphate transport in either canine or rodent BBMV while it dramatically affects calcium uptake.[12,14]

The mechanism of action of vitamin D on phosphate transport in the enterocyte has been the subject of recent controversy. One laboratory[31-33] has suggested that vitamin D's effects are mediated through an alteration of BBM phospholipid content. $1,25(OH)_2D_3$ stimulates an increase in phosphatidylcholine content of the BBM, and an increase in the arachidonic acid content of the fatty acid component of phosphatidylcholine. These effects on the cell membrane phospholipid composition produce an increase in the "fluidity" of the membrane decreasing the barrier activity of membranes. This has been shown to increase the permeability of calcium and the possibility exists that this lipid effect also affects phosphate transport.

Our approach to this question has been to analyze the effect of $1,25(OH)_2D_3$ on renal phospholipid composition. Preliminary experiments to date suggest that phosphatidylcholine levels of renal BBM are in fact increased by $1,25(OH)_2D_3$. The relationship of this effect to phosphate transport remains to be tested.

In summary, studies from our laboratory demonstrate that both vitamin D and PTH have important biochemical effects on the renal BBM. PTH stimulates both protein and phospholipid phosphorylation. Phosphorylation of a specific substrate protein of cAMP dependent protein kinase with a molecular weight of 62,000 is regulated by PTH and associated with phosphate transport. Cylic AMP independent phosphorylation of BBM phospholipids appears to have important effects on cell membrane calcium content.

Vitamin D does not detectably affect cAMP dependent protein phosphorylation in a model of vitamin D deficiency without secondary hyperparathyroidism, where defective phosphate homeostasis occurs which is corrected by $1,25(OH)_2D_3$. The mechanism through which vitamin D exerts its effect on phosphate transport remains a matter of investigation, but an effect exerted through a change in cell membrane phospholipid composition must be considered.

References

1. A. G. Booth and A. J. Kenny, A rapid method for the purification of microvilli from rabbit kidney, Biochem. J. 142: 575, (1974).
2. C. Evers, W. Haase, H. Murer and R. Kinne, Properties of brush border vesicles isolated from rat kidney cortex by calcium precipitation, J. Memb. Biochem. 1:203 (1978).
3. L. Cheng and B. Sacktor, Sodium gradient-dependent phosphate transport in renal brush border membrane vesicles, J. Biol. Chem. 256:1556 (1981).
4. N. Hoffmann, M. Thees and R. Kinne, Phosphate transport by isolated renal brush border vesicles, Pflugers Arch. 362:147 (1976).
5. G. Burckhardt, H. Stern and H. Murer, The influence of pH on phosphate transport into rat renal brush border membrane vesicles, Pflugers Arch 390:191 (1981).
6. R. Stoll, R. Kinne and H. Murer, Effect of dietary phosphate intake on phosphate transport by isolated rat renal brush-border vesicles, Biochem. J. 180:465 (1979).
7. K. A. Hruska and M. R. Hammerman, Parathyroid hormone inhibition of phosphate transport in renal brush border vesicles from phosphate depleted dogs, Biochim. Biophys. Acta 645:351 (1981).
8. H. Murer, C. Evers, R. Stoll and R. Kinne, The effect of parathyroid hormone (PTH) and dietary phosphate on the sodium-dependent phosphate transport system located in the rat renal brush border membrane, in: "Current Problems in Clinical Biochemistry," W. G. Guder and W. Schmidt, eds., Hans Hubor Publishers, Bern (1979).
9. M. R. Hammerman, I. E. Karl and K. A. Hruska, Regulation of canine renal vesicle Pi transport by growth hormone and parathyroid hormone, Biochim. Biophys. Acta 603:322 (1980).
10. T. P. Dousa and S. A. Kempson, Regulation of renal brush border membrane transport of phosphate, Mineral Electrolyte Metab. 7:113 (1982).
11. R. Kinne and I. L. Schwartz, Isolated membrane vesicles in the evaluation of the nature, localization, and regulation of renal transport processes, Kidney Int. 14:547 (1978).
12. M. R. Hammerman and K. A. Hruska, Cyclic AMP-dependent protein phosphorylation in canine renal brush-border membrane vesicles is associated with decreased phosphate transport, J. Biol. Chem. 257:992 (1982).
13. W. Haase, A. Schafer, H. Murer and R. Kinne, Studies on the orientation of brush border membrane vesicles, Biochem. J. 172:57 (1978).

14. K. A. Hruska, S. C. Mills, S. Khalifa and M. R. Hammerman, Phosphorylation of renal brush-border membrane vesicles. Effect on calcium uptake and membrane content of polyphosphoinositides, J. Biol. Chem. 258:2501 (1983).
15. T. A. Noland, Jr. and H. L. Henry, Parathyroid hormone, vitamin D and the regulation of protein phosphorylation in chick kidney cells, in: "Vitamin D. Chemical, Biochemical and Clinical Endocrinology of Calcium Metabolism," A. W. Norman, K. Schaefer, D. V. Herrath and H.-G. Grigoleit, eds., Walter de Gruyter & Co., Berlin (1982).
16. M. R. Hammerman, V. A. Hansen and J. J. Morrissey, Cyclic AMP-dependent protein phosphorylation and dephosphorylation alter phosphate transport in canine renal brush border vesicles, Biochim. Biophys. Acta 755:10 (1983).
17. L. R. Forte, G. A. Nickols and C. S. Anast, Renal adenylate cyclase and the interrelationship between parrathyroid hormone and vitamin D in the regulation of urinary phosphate and adenosine cyclic 3',5'-monophosphate excretion, J. Clin. Invest. 57:559 (1976).
18. L. R. Forte, S. G. Langeluttig, R. E. Poelling and M. L. Thomas, Renal parathyroid hormone receptors in the chick: downregulation in secondary hyperparathyroid animal models, Am. J. Physiol. 242:E154 (1982).
19. J-P. Bonjour, C. Preston and H. Fleisch, Effect of 1,25-dihydroxyvitamin D_3 on the renal handling of Pi in thyroparathyroidectomized rats, J. Clin. Invest. 60:1419 (1977).
20. R. C. Muhlbauer, J-P. Bonjour and H. Fleisch, Tubular handling of Pi localization of effects of $1,25(OH)_2D_3$ and dietary Pi in TPTX rats, Am. J. Physiol. 241:F123 (1981).
21. R. Stoll, R. Kinne, H. Murer, H. Fleisch and J-P. Bonjour, Phosphate transport by rat renal brush border membrane vesicles: Influence of dietary phosphate thyroparathyroidectomy, and 1,25-Dihydroxyvitamin D_3, Pflugers Arch. 380:47 (1979).
22. C. T. Liang, J. Barnes, L. Cheng, R. Balakir and B. Sacktor, Effects of $1,25-(OH)_2D_3$ administered in vivo on phosphate uptake by isolated chick renal cells, Am. J. Physiol. 242:C312 (1982).
23. C. T. Liang, J. Barnes, R. Balakir, L. Cheng and B. Sacktor, In vitro stimulation of phosphate uptake in isolated chick renal cells by 1,25-dihydroxycholecalciferol, Proc. Natl. Acad. Sci. 79:3532 (1982).
24. H. Georgaki and J. B. Puschett, Acute effects of a "physiological" dose of 1,25-dihydroxy vitamin D_3 on renal phosphate transport, Endocrine Res. Comm. 9:135 (1982).
25. B. Kurnik and K. A. Hruska, Effects of $1,25(OH)_2D_3$ on phosphate transport in a normocalcemic normophosphatemic rat model of vitamin D deficiency, (Submitted for publication).
26. D. Rudack-Garcia and H. L. Henry, Effect of vitamin D status on cyclic AMP-dependent protein kinase activity and its heat-stable inhibitor in chick kidney, J. Biol. Chem. 256:10781 (1981).

27. A. N. K. Yusufi, M. G. Low, S. T. Turner and T. P. Dousa, Selective removal of alkaline phosphatase from renal brush-border membrane and sodium-dependent brush-border membrane transport, J. Biol. Chem. 258:5695 (1983).
28. H. R. De Jonge, W. E. J. M. Ghijsen and C. H. Van Os, Phosphorylated intermediates of Ca^{2+}-ATPase and alkaline phosphatase in plasma membranes from rat duodenal epithelium, Biochim. Biophys. Acta 647:140 (1981).
29. J. Biber, V. Scalera and H. Murer, Protein phosphorylation in proximal tubular brush-border membranes, Adv. Exp. Med. & Biol. 151:47 (1982).
30. S. Khalifa, S. Mills and K. A. Hruska, Stimulation of calcium uptake by parathyroid hormone in renal brush border membrane vesicles: relationship to membrane phosphorylation, J. Biol. Chem. (submitted for publication).
31. O. Fontaine, T. Matsumoto, D. B. P. Goodman and H. Rasmussen, Liponomic control of Ca^{2+} transport: Relationship to mechanism of action of 1,25-dihydroxyvitamin D_3, Proc. Natl. Acad. Sci. 78:1751 (1981).
32. T. Matsumoto, O. Fontaine and H. Rasmussen, Effect of 1,25-dihydroxyvitamin D_3 on phospholipid metabolism in chick duodenal mucosal cell, J. Biol. Chem. 256:3354 (1981).
33. D. Kreutter, T. Matsumoto, R. Peckham, K. Zawalich, W. H. Wen, D. T. Zolock and H. Rasmussen, The effect of essential fatty acid deficiency on the stimulation of intestinal calcium transport by 1,25-dihydroxyvitamin D_3, J. Biol. Chem. 258:4977 (1983).
34. G. W. Snedecor and W. G. Cochran, Statistical Methods, The Iowa State University Press, Ames (1967).

INTRACELLULAR PROCESSES THAT AFFECT RENAL PHOSPHATE TRANSPORT

Vincent W. Dennis and Peter C. Brazy

Duke University Medical Center
Department of Medicine
Durham, North Carolina 27710

Studies of phosphate transport in the proximal renal tubule have focused recently on interactions with intracellular processes, especially oxidative metabolism and gluconeogenesis. Intracellular inorganic phosphate is essential for oxidative phosphorylation and participates in mitochondrial respiration. Gluconeogenesis liberates phosphate. This review will summarize our recent observations on changes in phosphate transport with metabolic inhibitors, metabolic substrates and changes in gluconeogenesis.

METHODS

All studies were performed in isolated proximal tubules from the rabbit kidney. For these studies, rabbits were maintained on a normal diet. Transport rates for fluid and phosphate were determined in single perfused tubules using radioisotopes as described previously (1). Metabolic studies were performed in suspensions of rabbit cortical tubules incubated at 37°C in media that closely resembled the fluids used for measurements of transport rates. Oxygen consumption rates were measured with a Clark electrode. Glucose production rates were estimated from the accumulation of glucose measured chemically in media that were initially glucose-free. Lactate and alanine were the major substrates (1).

RESULTS

Metabolic Inhibitors

In a series of observations (1), we determined that one of

the most potent and useful metabolic inhibitors is rotenone which inhibits mitochondrial respiration at the NAD dehydrogenase. The addition of rotenone to suspensions of cortical tubules reduced QO_2 in a dose-dependent manner. The maximal inhibition of QO_2 was 88.1 $\pm$ 1.1 percent with half-maximal inhibition at a rotenone concentration of 1.61 $\pm$ 0.03 x 10^{-7}M in the absence of albumin. Rotenone inhibited cellular ATP content with a Ki of 2.1 $\pm$ 0.3 x 10^{-7}M. Consistent with its proposed mechanism of action, rotenone increased mitochondrial NADH measured fluorometrically (3).

In related studies during which transport rates were measured, rotenone at concentrations that maximally inhibit mitochondrial respiration (10^{-6}M) reduced net fluid absorption from 1.29 $\pm$ 0.14 to 0.0 $\pm$ 0.07 nl/mm.min. Phosphate transport from lumen to bath was reduced from 6.38 $\pm$ 2.74 to 0.41 $\pm$ 0.20 pmol/mm.min, indicating the elimination of net phosphate transport.

At submaximal concentrations, 10^{-7}M rotenone reduced fluid absorption from 1.42 to 0.84 nl/mm.min. In contrast to this partial inhibition, 10^{-7}M rotenone reduced phosphate transport from 2.68 to 0.34 pmol/mm.min indicating that phosphate transport is more sensitive to mitochondrial inhibition. A similar pattern had been noted previously with arsenate (2).

Mitochondrial Substrates

Mitochondrial substrates such as succinate and butyrate enhanced phosphate transport without detectable changes in glucose or net sodium transport. When added to the bathing medium to a final concentration of 1 mM, succinate or butyrate increased phosphate transport by 52 or 39 percent respectively. These observations represent the converse of those with mitochondrial inhibitors in that they indicate greater sensitivity of phosphate transport to changes in cellular metabolism. Similar observations were observed with short-chain fatty acids such as valerate which stimulated phosphate transport by 108 percent.

Phosphate Transport and Gluconeogenesis

In considering possible mechanisms by which these substrates might increase phosphate transport, we were influenced by our awareness of their associated actions on cellular metabolism, especially gluconeogenesis. Accordingly, we examined the effects of these substrates on glucose production by suspensions of rabbit proximal tubules. The addition of 1 mM valerate, butyrate or succinate increased glucose production to 56.0, 52 or 68 nmol/mm.protein.30 min, respectively, relative to control values of 22 nmol/mg protein·30 min when lactate and alanine served as substrates. To assess whether these increases in gluconeogenesis were causally related to the increases in phosphate transport, we used 3-mercaptopicolinic acid (3-MPA) to inhibit glucose production at phosphoenopyruvate carboxykinase. The addition of 3-MPA to tubules incubated with lactate and alanine reduced gluconeogenesis by 74 percent but had no effect on phosphate transport rates. Moreover, the addition of valerate to tubules incubated with 1 mM 3-MPA caused no increase in gluconeogenesis despite the greater than two-fold increase in glucose production that occurred in the absence of 3-MPA. In studies that measured transport rates, in the presence of 1 mM 3-MPA, the addition of valerate still stimulated phosphate transport from 2.55 to 5.16 pmol/mm.min. These studies indicate that the action of valerate to increase phosphate transport is not dependent on changes in gluconeogenesis.

DISCUSSION

These studies emphasize the special sensitivity of phosphate transport to changes in mitochondrial function; they fail to support any major relationship between phosphate transport and gluconeogenesis. As we had shown previously for the mitochondrial uncouplers arsenate and CCCP (2), submaximal concentrations of rotenone, an inhibitor of mitochondrial respiration, reduced phosphate transport more dramatically than fluid absorption rates despite their common dependence on sodium transport. The basis for this variation in sensitivity of fluid absorption and phosphate transport to partial inhibition of mitochondrial function may be related to several factors. First, sodium and phosphate may respond to different extents to the changes in electrical and chemical gradients that may result from partial inhibition of mitochondrial oxidative phosphorylation. Second, in addition to changes in intracellular solute concentrations, shifts in the intracellular compartmentation of sodium and phosphate may occur. Third, alterations in cellular metabolism may lead to changes in intracellular co-factors that may in turn regulate transport at the plasma membrane.

In this regard, the studies that correlate changes in phosphate transport with changes in gluconeogenesis seem to eliminate gluconeogenesis as a major regulatory process affecting phosphate transport in the proximal tubule. Specifically, although changes in phosphate transport may be accompanied by changes in gluconeogenesis, the relationship is not causal since the changes in phosphate transport still occur in the presence of 3-MPA that blocks the stimulation of gluconeogenesis. Furthermore, agents such as succinate, butyrate and valerate increase both gluconeogenesis and phosphate transport although PTH stimulates gluconeogenesis and <u>inhibits</u> phosphate transport (4).

Phosphate transport by the proximal convoluted tubules involves entry across the luminal brush border via a sodium:phosphate co-transport process, probably with a stoichiometry of two sodium ions to one divalent phosphate (5). Luminal entry represents the major energy barrier but may not necessarily represent the rate-limiting, kinetic barrier. Intracellularly, the activity of inorganic phosphate is affected not only by the luminal uptake but also by metabolic processes such as glycolysis, gluconeogenesis and oxidative phosphorylation. At least in vitro, the cellular requirement for inorganic phosphate is not met by the availability of phosphate in only the bath but depends in part on facilitated entry at the luminal surface (6). Accordingly, opportunities to regulate phosphate transport exists not only at the plasma membrane but also at interfaces with cellular metabolism, especially mitochondrial activities. If the exit step for phosphate is rate-limiting, changes in the cytosolic activity of inorganic phosphate may be expected to affect the absorption rate. These changes in cytosolic activity may occur in response to increases or decreases in the organification of phosphate or from shifts between cytosolic and mitochondrial compartments. In evaluating possible mechanisms that may regulate phosphate transport by the proximal tubule, it is therefore necessary to consider not only changes in the bulk phases but also changes in the intracellular environment brought about by redistribution of inorganic phosphate among metabolic pools.

REFERENCES

1. Gullans, S. R., Brazy, P. C., Dennis, V. W., and Mandel, L. J., 1982, Metabolic inhibitors: Effects on metabolism and transport in the proximal tubule, Am. J. Physiol. 243: F133-F140.
2. Brazy, P. C., Balaban, R. S., Gullans, S. R., Mandel, L. J., and Dennis, V. W., 1980, Inhibition of metabolism: relative effects of arsenate on sodium phosphate and glucose transport by the rabbit proximal tubule, J. Clin. Invest. 66:1211-1221.
3. Balaban, R. S., Dennis, V. W., and Mandel, L. J., 1981, Microfluorometric monitoring of NAD redox state in isolated perfused renal tubules. Am. J. Physiol. 240:F337-F342.
4. Nagata, N., and Rasmussen, 1970, Parathyroid hormone, 3'5' AMP, CA++, and renal gluconeogenesis, Proc. Natl. Acad. Sci., 65:368-374.
5. Cheng, L., and Sacktor, B., 1981, Sodium gradient-dependent phosphate transport in renal brush border membrane vesicles, J. Biol. Chem. 256:1556-1564.
6. Brazy, P. C., Gullans, S. R., Mandel, L. J. and Dennis, V. W., 1982, Metabolic requirement for inorganic phosphate by the rabbit proximal tubule: evidence for a Crabtree effect, J. Clin. Invest. 70:53-62, 1982.

Effect of Serum Calcium on Phosphate Transport

Wadi N. Suki

Baylor College of Medicine and The Methodist Hospital

Houston, Texas

An effect of serum calcium on renal phosphate excretion has been invoked by a number of investigators both in experimental animals and in man. These effects are complex and may be attributable to changes in the filtered load of phosphate or in the tubular handling of phosphate. These effects will be discussed separately.

Effects of Calcium on Filtered Phosphate: The excretion of phosphate may be altered when the serum phosphate, the GFR, or both are changed by virtue of a change in the filtered load of phosphate. Alterations in the serum calcium can induce changes in both serum phosphate and in the GFR.

1. Changes in serum phosphate: Raising the serum calcium has been shown to increase the serum phosphate concentration[1-8]. The source of the phosphate added to plasma may be the red blood cells,[3] and this effect of calcium may be observed even in the absence of the thyroid and parathyroid glands[4,5,9-11]. While raising the serum calcium raises the serum phosphate concentration, it depresses the ultrafiltrability of phosphate by the formation of calcium-phosphate-proteinate complexes which are not filterable[12,13]. The net result of these opposing changes may be only a small increase in ultrafiltrable phosphate.

2. Change in GFR: Acute elevations in the serum calcium to fairly high levels reduce GFR[3,8,14,15]. This fall in GFR appears to be due in part to the decrease in RBF and in another part to a decrease in the ultrafiltration coefficient of the renal glomerulus[16]. Similar falls in GFR have been shown to cause increase tubular phosphate absorption[17].

Effects of Calcium on Tubular Absorption of Phosphate: Studies in man and in experimental animals have yielded conflicting results on the effects of elevation or lowering of the serum calcium on renal phosphate absorption. Clearly, in order to obviate the problem presented by secondary hormonal changes studies of greatest interest are those carried out on thyroparathyroidectomized humans or experimental animals.

1. Effects of raising serum calcium: In hypoparathyroid patients raising the serum calcium may yield variable results[8] or an increase in phosphate excretion[4,5,7,9,18]. The increase in phosphate excretion, which can be attributed to increased filtered load, was observed in one study despite a fall of serum phosphate when calcium was infused for a prolonged period[18]. In experimental animals hypercalcemia has been shown to blunt the phosphaturia of volume expansion[19], and the infusion of calcium into the renal artery causes unilateral decreases in phosphate excretion[14]. In other studies, however, calcium infusion has been shown to increase phosphate excretion[20], or to have no effect on tubular capacity for phosphate absorption[21,22]. Micropuncture studies are no less conflicting with one study showing increased absorption in the proximal tubular, loop of Henle and distal tubule[23], while three others showing decreased absorption in the proximal tubule[24-26].

2. Effects of lowering serum calcium: In hypoparathyroid patients EDTA lowered phosphate excretion[27]. A more specific chelator of calcium, EGTA, however, increased phosphate excretion in TPTX rats and dogs[28,29]. Also, in rats infused with phosphate there is a progressive decline in the tubular reabsorption of phosphate that is reversed by raising the falling serum calcium[30]. In another study in dogs, however, EGTA had no effect on phosphate excretion[31].

3. Studies of tubular absorption of phosphate in vitro: In order to more directly examine the effects of calcium on phosphate absorption, we studied rabbit renal tubules isolated and perfused in vitro[32]. We found that high ambient calcium stimulates phosphate efflux in the proximal convoluted tubule, while low ambient calcium depresses it. These studies provide direct evidence for an effect of calcium on tubular handling of phosphate.

In summary, studies in man and in experimental animals yield conflicting information on the effect of calcium on phosphate absorption by the kidney. In vitro studies, however, demonstrate clearly that calcium stimulates phosphate absorption in the proximal convoluted tubule.

REFERENCES

1. H.A. Salvesen, A.B. Hastings, and J.F. McIntosh, The effect of the admnistration of calcium salts on the inorganic composition of the blood, J. Biol. Chem. 60:327 (1924).

2. C.H. Baylor, H.E. Van Alstine, E.H. Keutman, and S.H. Bassett, The fate of intravenously administered calcium. Effect on urinary calcium and phosphorus, fecal calcium and calcium-phosphorus balance, J. Clin. Invest. 29:1167 (1950).
3. P.S. Chen, Jr., and W.F. Neuman, Renal excretion of calcium by the dog, Am. J. Physiol. 180:623 (1955).
4. H.H. Hiatt, and D.D. Thompson, Some effects of intravenously administered calcium on inorganic phosphate metabolism, J. Clin. Invest. 36:573 (1957).
5. J.E. Howard, T.R. Hopkins, and T.B. Connor, On certain physiologic responses to intravenous injection of calcium salts into normal, hyperparathyroid and hypoparathyroid persons, J. Clin. Endocrinol. 13:1 (1953).
6. L.H. Kyle, M. Schaaf, and L.A. Erdman, The metabolic effects of intravenous administration of calcium, J. Lab. Clin. Med. 43:123 (1954).
7. B.E. Nordin, and R. Fraser, The effect of intravenous calcium on phosphate excretion, Clin. Sci. 13:477, (1954).
8. S. Wallach, and A.C. Carter, Metabolic and renal effects of acute hypercalcemia in dogs, Am. J. Physiol. 200:359 (1961).
9. R. Goldman, and S.H. Bassett, Effect of intravenous calcium gluconate upon the excretion of calcium and phosphorus in patients with idiopathic hypoparathyroidism, J. Clin. Endocrinol. 14:278 (1954).
10. E. Hausmann, Change in plasma phosphate concentration on infusion of calcium gluconate or Na_2 EDTA, Proc. Soc. Exp. Biol. 134:182 (1970).
11. J.B.B. Anderson, and R.V. Talmage, The effect of calcium infusion and calcitonin on plasma phosphate in sham-operated and thyroparathyroidectomized dogs, Endocrinology 93:1222 (1973).
12. A. Grollman, The condition of the inorganic phosphorus of the blood with special reference to the calcium concentration, J. Biol. Chem. 72:565 (1927).
13. T. Hopkins, J.E. Howard, and E. Eisenberg, Ultrafiltration studies on calcium and phosphorus in human serum, Bull. Johns Hopkins Hosp. 91:1 (1952).
14. A.R. Lavender, and T.N. Pullman, Changes in inorganic phosphate excretion induced by renal arterial infusion of calcium, Am. J. Physiol. 205:1025 (1963).
15. B. Chomdej, P.D. Bell, and L.G. Navar, Renal hemodynamics and autoregulatory responses to acute hypercalcemia, Am. J. Physiol. 232:490 (1977).
16. H.D. Humes, I. Ichikawa, J.L. Troy, and B.M. Brenner, Evidence for a parathyroid hormone dependent influence of calcium on the glomerular ultrafiltration coefficient, J. Clin. Invest. 61:32 (1978).
17. J.B. Puschett, Z.S. Agus, D. Senesky, and M. Goldberg, Effects of saline loading and aortic obstruction on proximal phosphate transport, Am. J. Physiol. 223:851 (1972).
18. E. Eisenberg, Effects of serum calcium level and parathyroid extracts on phosphate and calcium excretion in hypoparathyroid patients, J. Clin. Invest. 44:942 (1965).

19. M.M. Popovtzer, J.B. Robinette, K.M. McDonald, and C.K. Kuruvila, Effect of Ca^{++} on renal handling of PO_4^{3-} : Evidence for two reabsorptive mechanisms, Am. J. Physiol. 229:901.
20. J.L. Cuche, C.E. Ott, G.R. Marchand, J.A. Diaz-Buxo, and F.G. Knox, Intrarenal calcium and phosphate handling, Am. J. Physiol. 230:790 (1967a).
21. R.A. Peraino, and W.N. Suki, Influence of calcium on renal handling of phosphate, in: "Renal Handling of Phosphate", S.G. Massry and H. Fleisch, eds., Plenum, New York (1980).
22. T. Hostetter, E. Ghafary, D. Rouse, W.N. Suki, and G. Eknoyan, Effect of caclium infusion on renal phosphate reabsorption in the acutely and chronically thyroparathyroidectomized dog, in: "Phosphate Metabolism. Kidney and Bone", L. Avioli, P. Bordier, H. Fleisch, S. Massry, and E. Slatopolsky, eds., Armour Montagu, Paris (1976).
23. C. Amiel, H. Kuntziger, S. Couette, C. Coureau, and N. Bergounioux, Evidence for a parathyroid hormone-independent calcium modulation of phosphate transport along the nephron, J. Clin. Invest. 57:256 (1976).
24. G.F. DiBona, Effect of hypercalcemia on renal tubular sodium handling in the rat, Am. J. Physiol. 220:49 (1971).
25. B.R. Edwards, R.A.L. Sutton, and J.H. Dirks, Effect of calcium infusion on renal tubular reabsorption in the dog, Am. J. Physiol. 227:13 (1974).
26. S. Goldfarb, P. Bosanac, M. Goldberg, and Z.S. Agus, Effects of calcium on renal tubular phosphate reabsorption, Am. J. Physiol. 234:22 (1978).
27. H.L. Estep, C.T. Gardner, Jr., J.P. Taylor, A. Minott, and H. St. G. Tucker, Jr., Phosphate excretion patterns following intravenous injection of ethylenediaminetetraacetate (EDTA), J. Clin. Endocrinol. Metab. 25:1385 (1965).
28. H. Rasmussen, C. Anast, and C. Arnaud, Thyrocalcitonin, EGTA, and urinary electrolyte excretion, J. Clin. Invest. 46:746 (1967).
29. D. Rouse, S. Sessoms, B.J. Stinebaugh, and W.N. Suki, The effect of hypocalcemia on renal bicarbonate absorption, Min. Electr. Metab. (In Press) (1983).
30. A. Frick, and I. Durasin, Maximal reabsorption capacity for inorganic phosphate (TM_{Pi}) in the absence of parathyroid hormone in the rat: decrease of the TMPi during prolonged administration of phosphate and the role of calcium, Pflugers Arch. 377:9 (1978).
31. J.L. Cuche, C.E. Ott, G.R. Marchand, and F.G. Knox, Lack of effect of hypocalcemia on renal phosphate handling, J. Lab. Clin. Med. 88:271, 1976b).
32. D. Rouse, and W.N. Suki, The influence of calcium (Ca) on phosphate (PO_4) transport in proximal convoluted (PCT) and straight (PST) tubule segments of the rabbit nephron perfused in vitro, Abstracts of the 15th Annual Meeting, The American Society of Nephrology, p. 17A (1982).

INFLUENCE OF TEMPERATURE ON PHOSPHATE UPTAKE BY RENAL BRUSH BORDER MEMBRANE VESICLES

Michèle G. Brunette and Richard Béliveau

Department of Pediatrics, University of Montreal

Montreal, Quebec, Canada

INTRODUCTION

Most of the kinetic studies of phosphate (PO_4) uptake through renal brush border membrane (BBM) vesicles are performed at 20 to 25°C. In vivo, environment of these membrane is 37°C.

The only study regarding the effect of temperature on phosphate uptake was performed in a steady state situation i.e., in the absence of sodium and phosphate gradient (100 mM Na and 0.1 mM phosphate inside and outside the vesicles) (1). Therefore, the effect of temperature on Na gradient-dependent phosphate uptake remains unknown.

In this paper, we studied the kinetics of PO_4 uptake at various temperatures, and with a wide range of substrate concentrations. The results indicate that temperature of incubation alters the Vmax and the apparent Km. Moreover, at temperature above 25°C, a break in the Lineweaver-Burk and the Eadie-Hofstee plots are observed, suggesting a double mechanism system of transport.

MATERIALS AND METHODS

Experiments were performed in normal male Sprague Dawley rats fed usual Purina chow. BBM were prepared by Mg precipitation according to the technique initially described by Booth and Kenny (2). The uptake of PO_4 was measured using the filtration technique (Millipore filters 0.45 μm).

Following previous studies concerning the effect of temperature on PO_4 uptake profile vs time, a 10-sec incubation was chosen for all experiments in order to approach the optimal unidirectional influx. Na gradient-dependent uptake was calculated by subtracting passive uptake (no sodium in the incubation medium) from the total uptake.

RESULTS

At 35°C, the Lineweaver-Burk plot of PO_4 uptake by 7 rats BBM vesicles, shows a break at a substrate concentration of approximately 0.3 mM. The Vmax are 4.62 ± 0.04 nmol/mg/10 sec for low substrate concentrations, and 5.16 ± 0.05 nmol/mg/10 sec for high substrate concentrations. Fig 1 represents the corresponding Eadie-Hofstee plot. The two slopes yield two Km of 100 μM and 240 μM for the low and high substrate concentrations respectively.

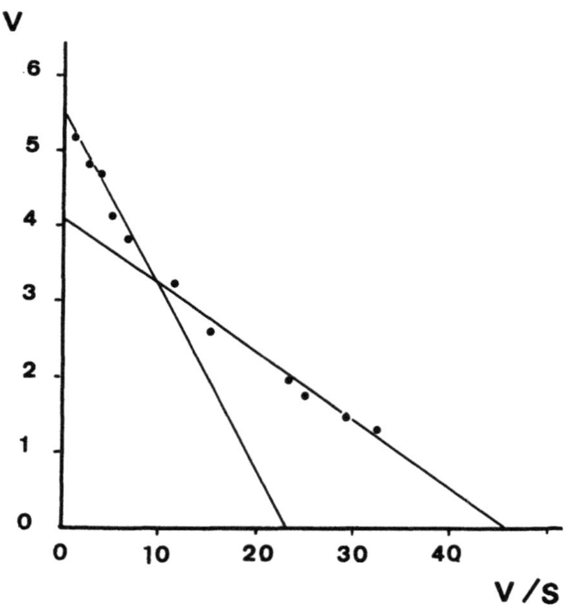

FIGURE 1: Eadie-Hofstee plot of PO_4 uptake at 35°C

The variations of Vmax and Km with temperature are presented on Table I. At temperature below 30, the Lineweaver-Burk plots were linear. The data presented in this table correspond to the low substrate concentrations only (0.04 to 0.3 mM PO_4). Temperature considerably influences both Vmax and apparent Km. From 5°C to 40°C the Vmax progressively increases, despite the fact that the uptake at low substrate concentrations slightly decreases above 30°C. The Arrhenius plot (Ln Vmax vs $1/T_k$) shows an abrupt break point at 23°C.

Finally the apparent Km continuously increases with temperature, to reach 135 µM at 40°C.

Table I

Effect of temperature on the apparent Km and Vmax of PO_4 uptake by BBM vesicles

T°C	Km (µM)	Vmax/nmol/mg
7	54 ± 0	0.56 ± 0.03
10	63 ± 5	0.99 ± 0.02
15	80 ± 6	2.08 ± 0.03
20	73 ± 7	2.71 ± 0.07
25	89 ± 1	3.86 ± 0.17
30	91 ± 7	4.09 ± 0.05
35	112 ± 5	4.74 ± 0.18
40	135 ± 15	4.90 ± 0.21

DISCUSSION

The break in the Eadie-Hofstee plot, observed at 35°C was not evident at 20° and 25°C. This is probably the reason why such a break was never reported before. It probably reflects a double system of PO_4 uptake, with low and high affinity respectively. Phosphate concentration in the rat plasma and then in glomerular filtrate is 2.5 mM. This concentration decreases along the proximal tubule to reach approximately 1.5 mM at the entry of the pars recta (3, 4, 5). Therefore, the highest concentrations of substrate utilized in our experiments better correspond to the tubular fluid composition than the lowest values, which in turn are those used in experiments reported in literature. If we attempt to separate the two systems of transport, by subtracting the uptake due to the high affinity system from the total uptake measured with high substrate concentrations, the new Km obtained for the low affinity system is 17 mM, which is very high. Indeed it would appear logical to hypothesize a transport system whose Km remains within the range of natural concentrations of substrate in tubular fluid.

Temperature modifies membrane fluidity and enzyme activity. It is normal therefore that uptake velocity varies with temperature. Le Grimellec (6) reported a break in the Arrhenius plot of alkaline phosphatase activity in BBM at 26°C. The break point of Vmax, in our experiments was 23°C which is close to the above temperature. This correspondence may result from a change of the physical state of the membrane, which affects both the enzyme activity and the PO_4 uptake. It may also suggest a more direct link between these two parameters.

In conclusion:

Temperature modifies both Vmax and Km in the kinetics of PO_4 uptake by rat BBM. At temperature above 30°C, our data suggest a dual mechanism of PO_4 uptake, one with low affinity and high velocity, evident at substrate concentrations above 300 µM, and the other with high affinity (Km 100 µM) and low velocity.

REFERENCES

1. De Smedt H, Kinne R: Temperature dependence of solute transport and enzyme activities in dog renal brush border membrane vesicles. Bioch Biophys Acta 648: 247-253, 1981.

2. Booth A, Kenny AJ: A rapid method for the preparation of microvilli from rabbit kidney. Biochem J 142: 575-581, 1974.

3. Strickler JC, Thompson DD, Klose RM, Giebisch G: Mircopuncture study of inorganic phosphate excretion in the rat. J Clin Invest 43: 1596-1607, 1964.

4. Gekle D: Der EinfluB von Parathormon auf die NierenfunKtion. Pflügers Arch 323: 96-120, 1971.

5. Brunette MG, Taleb L, Carrière S: The effect of parathyroid hormone on phosphate reabsorption along the nephron of the rat. Am J Physiol 225: 1076-1081, 1973.

6. Le Grimellec C, Giocondi MC, Carrière B, Carrière S, Cardinal J: Membrane fluidity and enzyme activities in brush border and basolateral membrane on the dog. Am J Physiol 242: F246-F253, 1982.

PARATHYROID HORMONE (PTH) STATUS AND PHOSPHATE (Pi) TRANSPORT IN PROXIMAL BRUSH BORDER MEMBRANE VESICLES (BBMV) AND WHOLE KIDNEY

J. Caverzasio and J.P. Bonjour

Department of Pathophysiology, University of Berne and Division of Pathophysiology, Department of Medicine, University of Geneva Switzerland

PTH and dietary Pi are independent factors which influence the tubular Pi reabsorptive capacity as assessed by determining the maximal tubular reabsorption of Pi per volume of glomerular filtrate (max. TRPi/ml GF) (1). Both factors can also alter the Na^+-dependent Pi transport system located in the luminal membrane of the proximal tubule (2, 3). In the situation of Pi restriction, plasma PTH level is markedly decreased as compared to normal Pi feeding (4).
To what extent the change in the PTH status which occurs during Pi restriction affects the response of Pi transport in whole kidney and brush border membrane vesicles (BBMV) is not known. In order to study this question we have compared the time-course of the response of the Pi transport in whole kidney and BBMV isolated from renal cortical slices in sham-operated (SHAM) and chronically thyroparathyroïdectomized (TPTX) rats.

In a first study SHAM and TPTX rats were switched from normal (0,8 g %) to low diet (0,2 g %). Max. TRPi/ml GF and the initial (3, 6 and 9 sec.) Na^+-dependent Pi uptake by BBMV were determined before and after 1, 2, 3 and 8 days of Pi restriction.
In a second study we have explored whether a change of the Na^+-dependent Pi transport system in the BBMV could be detected as early as two hours after a first exposure to a low Pi diet.

The results of the first series of experiments indicate that before Pi restriction max TRPi/ml GF ($\bar{x} \pm$ SEM) was 1.94 $\pm$ 0.04 and 4.03 $\pm$ 0,14 μmol/ml GF in SHAM and TPTX rats respectively. The corresponding initial rate of the Na^+-dependent Pi uptake at 3 sec. was 137 $\pm$ 23 in SHAM and 272 $\pm$ 41 pmol/mg protein in TPTX rats. During Pi restriction the initial difference in max TRPi/ml GF remained constant throughout the time course study (1, 2, 3 and 8 days). At 8 days, max. TRPi/ml GF was in SHAM 3.08 $\pm$ 0.09 and in TPTX 5.04 $\pm$ 0,18 μmol/ml GF. In sharp contrast, in BBMV the initial difference between SHAM and TPTX diminish with time to be completely abolished 8 days after starting the Pi restriction (SHAM: 425 $\pm$ 69; TPTX: 434 $\pm$ 40 pmol/mg prot. at 3 sec.).

The results of the second study indicate that after the first exposure to a low Pi diet, a stimulation of the Na^+-dependent Pi uptake by BBMV can be observed already after 2 hours. Indeed, the initial Na^+-dependent Pi uptake determined at 3 sec. incubation time was stimulated by 70 % after 2 hours and by more than 100 % 4 hours after the first low Pi meal as compare to the values measured in BBMV from animals maintained under a normal Pi diet. This phenomenon was associated with a concommitant decrease in plasma Pi concentration and the disappearance of Pi in the urine.

In conclusion, the overall tubular Pi transport capacity and the Na^+-dependent Pi transport system appear to be quite differently affected by changes in the PTH status during Pi restriction. Only, under HPD but not under LPD the effect of thyroparathyroïdectomy observed in the whole kidney is expressed at the level of BBMV. This dissociation suggests that modulation of the Na^+-dependent Pi transport system in the luminal membrane of the proximal tubule is not responsible for the response of the overall tubular Pi transport to removal of the parathyroid glands.

Finally the Na^+-dependent Pi transport system localized in the luminal membrane of proximal tubule is able to react quite rapidly, ie within two hours, to variations in Pi intake.

REFERENCES

1. Troehler, U., Bonjour J.P., and Fleisch, H., 1976, Inorganic phosphate homeostasis: Renal adaptation to the dietary intake in intact and thyroparathyroidectomized rats, J.Clin.Invest. 57: 264.

2. Stoll, R., Kinne, R., Murer, H., Fleisch, H., and Bonjour, J.P., 1979, Phosphate transport by rat renal brush border membrane vesicles: Influence of dietary phosphate, thyroparathyroidectomy and 1,25 dihydroxyvitamin D3, Pflügers Arch. 380: 47-52.

3. Evers, C., Murer, H., and Kinne, R., 1978, Effect of parathyrin on the transport properties of isolated renal brush border vesicles. Biochem. J. 172: 49-56

4. Freudiger, H., Caverzasio, J., Fischer, J., Trechsel, U. and Bonjour, J.P., Urinary cyclic AMP and parathyroid hormone status in rats with intact and reduced renal mass. Manuscript in preparation.

ACKNOWLEDGMENTS

This work has been supported by the Swiss National Science Foundation (3.824.79 and 3.806.0.82), the Procter and Gamble Company, Cincinnati, USA, and the Ausbildungs- und Förderungsfonds der Arbeitsgemeinschaft für Osteosynthese (AO), Chur, Switzerland.

RENAL BRUSH BORDER MEMBRANES IN X-LINKED HYPOPHOSPHATEMIC MICE: A STUDY OF THE PROTEIN KINASE ACTIVITY

Michèle G. Brunette and Richard Béliveau

Department of Pediatrics, University of Montreal

Montreal, Quebec, Canada

INTRODUCTION

A few years ago Tenenhouse et al. (1), reported that phosphate (PO_4) uptake by renal brush border membrane (BBM) vesicles from hypophosphatemic mice (Hyp) was half that of normal. Thus, the defect in uptake observed in vitro reflects the defect of PO_4 reabsorption in vivo (2, 3). This modification of the BBM responsible for the decreased uptake of PO_4 does not interfere with its adaptation to PO_4 deprivation (4), although this adaptation remains incomplete (5), nor does it with the normal response to parathyroidectomy (3).

In a previous study, we reported that the adenylate cyclase response of microdissected proximal tubules to parathyroid hormone was abnormally low (6). This abnormal response may be due to a hyperparathyroidism state, which has never been proven with certainty. It may also result from an abnormal protein kinase activity of the brush border membrane, which could secondarily affect the regulation of adenylate cyclase.

In this study we present data concerning the protein phosphorylation of BBM from normal (N) and Hyp mice. Incubation of membranes with $y^{32}P$-ATP resulted in phosphorylation of 11 proteins. An additional protein (85 000 app mol wt) appears when cAMP is added to the incubation medium. In Hyp mice, the phosphorylation showed a tendency to be decreased for all of the 11 proteins; but no abnormality could be detected with regard to the cAMP dependent phosphorylation of protein 85 000.

METHODS

Experiments were performed in male Hyp mice bred in our laboratory. The BBM were prepared according to the method initially described by Booth and Kenny (7). The membranes freshly prepared were incubated 2 min at 20°C in 50 mM MES pH 6.5 containing 25 μM γ^{32}P-ATP. Proteins were precipitated in TCA and dissolved in SDS. Electrophoresis was performed on exponential gradients of polyacrylamide gel. The phosphorylated bands were localized in the gel by autoradiography and subsequent scanning of the autoradiogram.

RESULTS

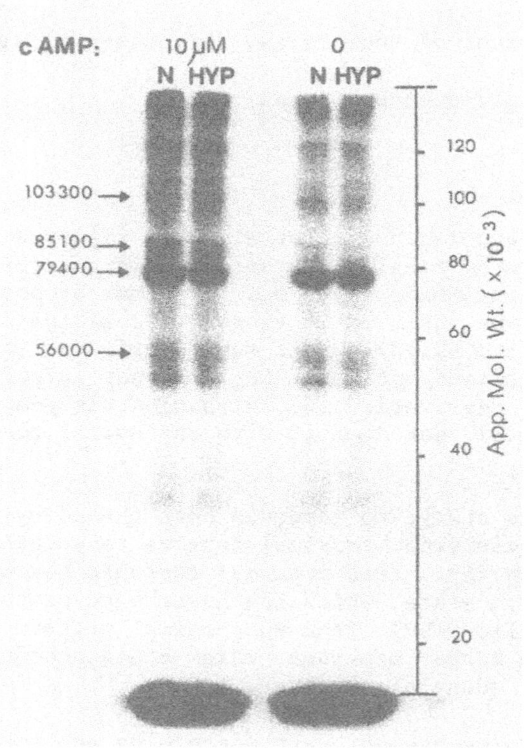

Fig 1 : Autoradiogram of phosphorylated BBM from N and Hyp mice and without cAMP

Fig 1 illustrates an autoradiogram of four electrophoresis, corresponding to the BBM proteins from normal and Hyp mice, with (left side) and without (right side) the addition of cAMP in the incubation medium. In normal mice 11 proteins are phosphorylated. The highest radioactivity appears with an apparent molecular weight of 79 000. This protein was shown in the rat to be the same molecule which binds inorganic PO_4 (8) and to correspond to the monomer of alkaline phosphatase (9). When 10 μM cAMP is added to the incubation medium, a strong supplementary band appears immediately above the alkaline phosphatase monomer, with an apparent molecular weight of 85 000. The maximal enhancement of this phosphorylation is obtained at pH between 7 and 9 and the dose response curve shows a maximal phosphorylation with 10 μM cAMP.

In Hyp mice, a uniform tendency to present a lower phosphorylation of the 11 proteins was observed. However, due to variations from one experiment to the other, this difference between N and Hyp mice was not significant. As illustrated in Fig 1, the cAMP dependent phosphorylation of protein 85 000 is well preserved, and a quantitative estimate of this phosphorylation did not show any abnormality.

DISCUSSION

Protein phosphorylation of BBM has never been reported in mice. Dog BBM show two proteins whose phosphorylation is cAMP dependent (10). Their apparent molecular weights are 96 000 and 62 000. Because protein 96 000 in the dog is situated immediately above the darkest band which is probably the monomer of alkaline phosphatase, we believe that it corresponds to the protein 85 000 of mouse BBM.

Our attempt to detect a cAMP dependent phosphorylation abnormality in Hyp BBM failed. These results suggest an integrity of the intrinsic protein kinase activity, and of the capacity of protein 85 000 to be phosphorylated under the influence of cAMP. Opinions concerning the parathyroid activity in Hyp mice are divergent. A recent study reported slightly elevated levels of the circulating hormone (11). Our experiments of phosphorylation in vitro are probably too crude to provide new arguments for or against a chronic status of hyperparathyroidism in these animals. However, they eliminate a gross abnormality of membrane protein phosphorylation as a cause of the phosphaturia, which is the principal trait of the disease.

REFERENCES

1. Tenenhouse HS, Scriver CR, McInnes RR, Glorieux F: Renal handling of phosphate in vivo and in vitro by the X-linked hypophosphatemic male mouse: evidence for a defect in the brush border. Kidney Int 14: 236-244, 1978.

2. Giasson SD, Brunette MG, Danan G, Vigneault N, Carrière S: Micropuncture study of renal phosphorus transport in hypophosphatemic vitamin D-resistant rickets mice. Pflugers Arch Eur J 371: 33-38, 1977.

3. Cowgill LD, Goldfarb S, Lau K, Slatopowsky E, Agus ZS: Evidence for an intrinsic renal tubular defect in mice with genetic hypophosphatemic rickets. J Clin Invest 63: 1203-1210, 1979.

4. Tenenhouse HS, Scriver CR: Renal adaptation to phosphate deprivation in Hyp mouse with X-linked hypophosphatemia. Can J Biochem 57: 938-944, 1979.

5. Muhlbauer RC, Bonjour JP, Fleish H: Abnormal tubular adaptation to dietary Pi restriction in X-linked hypophosphatemic mice. Am J Physiol 242: F353-F359, 1982.

6. Brunette MG, Chabardes D, Imbert-Teboul M, Clique A, Montegut M, Morel F: Hormone sensitive adenylate cyclase along the nephron of genetically hypophosphatemic mice. Kidney Int 15: 357-369, 1979.

7. Booth A, Kenny AJ: A rapid method for the preparation of microvilli from rabbit kidney. Biochem J 142: 575-581, 1974.

8. Béliveau R: Characterization of phosphate binding by alkaline phosphatase in rat kidney brush border membrane. Pflugers Arch Eur J. In press.

9. Booth AG, Kenny AJ: Proteins of the kidney microvillus membrane. Identification of subunits after sodium dodecyl sulfate polyacrylamide gel electrophoresis. Biochem J 159: 395-407, 1976.

10. Hammerman HR, Hruska KA: Cyclic AMP dependent protein phosphorylation in canine renal brush border membrane vesicles is associated with decreased phosphate transport. J Biol Chem 257: 992-999, 1982.

11. Kiebzak GM, Ross BA, Meyer RA: Secondary hyperparathyroidism in X-linked hypophosphatemic mice. Endocrinology 11: 650-652, 1982.

BIOCHEMICAL STUDIES OF THE CONTROL OF RENAL TUBULAR PHOSPHATE REABSORPTION

Michael F. Grahn, Riffat Parveen & Peter J. Butterworth

Department of Biochemistry, Chelsea College
University of London
Manresa Road, London SW3 6LX UK

Introduction

The proximal tubule of the kidney is the site of several important physiological processes including the reabsorbtion of inorganic phosphate from the glomerular filtrate and the production of glucose from intermediate metabolites. The phosphate reabsorption performed by the kidney seems to be the major controlling factor in maintaining overall phosphate homeostasis.

Kidney phosphate transport activity is under elaborate physiological control; parathyroid hormone induces a phosphaturia in normal animals whereas a low phosphate diet leads to a diminution of phosphate excretion that is resistant to stimulation by parathyroid hormone [1,2]. The infusion of vitamin D_3 in the presence of parathyroid hormone to phosphate-replete animals increases the kidney phosphate reabsorbtion, as does the addition of 1,25-dihydroxycholecalciferol to isolated chick kidney tubule cells [3].

The mechanisms by which these changes are brought about are not clear. Parathyroid hormone stimulates the production of cyclic AMP throughout both proximal and distal tubule segments [4], but micropuncture studies have not produced agreement on the sites at which parathyroid hormone decreases the rate of phosphate reabsorbtion. The early portion of the proximal convoluted tubule has shown conflicting responses of phosphate reabsorbtion to parathyroid hormone (see the review by Jacobson, [2]).

The rate of gluconeogenesis depends on the availability of substrates, the most important of which are probably glycerol and amino acids [3,4], and can be stimulated by several hormones including the catecholamines and parathyroid hormone [5].

The proximal tubule cell functions of phosphate reabsorbtion and gluconeogenesis have recently been linked in an attempt to explain the mode of action of parathyroid hormone on phosphate reabsorbtion. Dousa and co-workers have proposed that release of cyclic AMP, stimulated by parathyroid hormone results in an increased rate of gluconeogenesis. This leads to an increase in the concentration of free NAD^+ in the cell which inhibits phosphate transport by interacting directly with the membrane carrier [6,7,8].

In earlier studies [9] utilising isolated chick kidney tubule cells we found that the addition of metabolic substrates which lead to greater glucose production did not lead to a reduced rate of phosphate accumulation, as would be predicted by this hypothesis, but conversely led to a stimulation of phosphate transport. We now report further studies aimed at clarifying the nature of the link between gluconeogenesis and phosphate accumulation.

Methods and Materials

Isolated kidney tubule cells were prepared from 2-4 week old male Light Sussex/Rhode Island Red crossbred chicks as described in Grahn and Butterworth [9]. Briefly, kidneys were removed, diced, and incubated in buffer containing collagenase and hyaluronidase (0.8 mg/ml and 0.5mg/ml respectivly) for 30 minutes. The cells were then separated and washed in a phosphate-free medium by repeated gentle centrifugation. The final suspension contains predominantly 3-30 cell fragments of proximal tubule with the smaller units predominating. Electron microscopy together with the high alkaline phosphatase acivity and low hexokinase activity allow the cells to be identified as originating from the proximal tubule. Initial rates of phosphate accumulation were determined by rapid separation of the cells from incubation medium containing [^{32}P] Pi followed by the determination of the radioactivity in the cell portion [9].

Brush border membrane vesicles were produced from whole kidney homogenates by the calcium precipitation method of Beck and Sacktor [10].

Glucose was assayed in the incubation media after separation and removal of the cells by the glucose oxidase assay [11]. For experiments in which 3-mercaptopicolinate was employed glucose was determined by the Nelson method [12] as the mercapto compound interfered with the glucose oxidase procedure.

Oxygen uptake was followed in a Rank oxygen electrode assembly at 37°C and protein was determined by the method of Lowry et al [13] using bovine serum albumin as standard.

3-Mercaptopicolinic Acid was a gift from Smith, Kline and French Laboratories Ltd., Welwyn Garden City, Herts., U.K.

Results

The actions of a range of metabolic substrates on the initial rate of phosphate accumulation are shown in table 1. Both of the gluconeogenic substrates pyruvate and lactate stimulate the rate of phosphate accumulation within 2 minutes of incubation. The uptake of phosphate in the absence of Na^+ is small [14] and was unaffected by pyruvate. Glycerol, although considered to be an important gluconeogenic substrate in the kidney [4], did not markedly stimulate phosphate accumulation, even when present at relatively high concentrations.

Table 1 also shows the amount of glucose produced by tubule cell incubations over a one hour period in the presence of the various substrates tested. Although the degree of stimulation of gluconeogenesis varied considerably between different cell preparations, the relative effectiveness of the substrates was always the same. Pyruvate stimulated most glucose production whereas succinate and glycerol were approximately half as effective. In order to reach this level of gluconeogenesis from glycerol however, a relatively high concentration of this substrate was required. With the exception of glycerol it appears that the degree of stimulation of phosphate accumulation is related to the degree of stimulation of gluconeogenesis (Figure 1).

Table 1 The Actions of Metabolic Substrates on Phosphate Accumulation and Gluconeogenesis

Substrate	Concn. (mM)	Pi Accumulation (% of Control)		Glucose Production (pmol/min/mg protein)	
None	—	100	(n=2)	38±1	(n=8)
Glucose	1	90	(n=2)	——	
Pyruvate	1	153±5	(n=6)	1162±132	(n=16)
Lactate	1	146	(n=2)	——	
Glycerol	10	107±6	(n=6)	504±72	(n=16)
Succinate	1	125	(n=2)	558±66	(n=16)

Kidney tubule cells were prepared in the absence of metabolic substrates and incubated at 37°C with gentle shaking. Metabolic substrates were added after a 10 minute equilibration period.

The basal rate of phosphate uptake was 324 ± 37 pmol/minute/mg of protein (n=18). The phosphate accumulation for each experiment is expressed as the mean±s.e.m of the percentage of the control rate. Values within an experiment are the means of 2 duplicate incubations.

Glucose production was measured over a 1 hour incubation period during which the gas phase above the cell suspension was purged with 5% CO_2/95% O_2 in order to maintain aerobiosis. The values are the mean±s.e.m. of n incubations.

In order to distinguish between a direct action of the substrates and one resulting from the flux of metabolites to glucose, 3-mercaptopicolinic acid, was added to inhibit phosphoenolpyruvate carboxykinase. In the presence of the inhibitor, glucose production from pyruvate and succinate was decreased by 51% and 30% respectively (significant at the p=0.001 level). Gluconeogenesis from glycerol however, was decreased by only 15%. The relative insensitivity of glycerol to this inhibitor is not unexpected since glycerol enters the pathway after the phosphoenolpyruvate stage. Figure 1 shows that 3-mercaptopicolinate, which has no effect on phosphate accumulation in the absence of gluconeogenic substrate or in the presence of glycerol, does inhibit the phosphate accumulation stimulated by pyruvate and perhaps succinate.

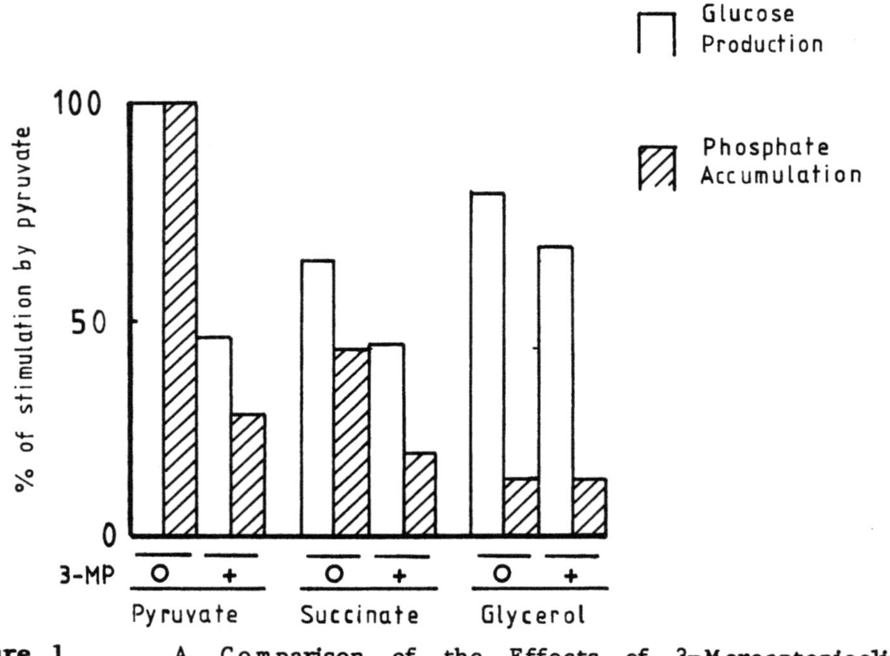

Figure 1 A Comparison of the Effects of 3-Mercaptopicolinate on Gluconeogenesis and Phosphate Accumulation

The figure shows the increments, relative to substrate-free controls, of glucose production and phosphate accumulation produced by the substrates pyruvate (1 mM), lactate (1 mM) and glycerol (10 mM) in the presence and absence of 0.1 mM 3-mercaptopicolinate after 2 minutes incubation. The bars show the means of 3 experiments relative to the effect of pyruvate (100%).

In one experiment the accumulation of radio-labelled glucose (1.3 µM) was determined in addition to that of phosphate by dual-label scintillation counting. The basal uptake was 92 pmol/minute/mg of protein and this was increased to 117 pmol/minute/mg of protein on addition of pyruvate (127% of control). The inclusion of 3-mercaptopicolinate slightly lowered the rate of glucose accumulation seen in the presence of pyruvate to 109 pmol/minute/mg of protein (119% of control). This change was probably not significant and so these results demonstrate that the effect of metabolites is largely specific to phosphate transport, even though glucose transport in this tissue is also dependent upon the sodium gradient [15].

Another experimental approach to differentiate between a direct action of pyruvate on the phosphate carrier and an action mediated by pyruvate metabolism was to examine the effects of pyruvate on phosphate accumulation into a brush-border membrane vesicle preparation. In a brush border membrane vesicle preparation the presence of pyruvate (1 mM) in the uptake medium slightly decreased (by 5%) the rate of phosphate accumulation, measured over the first 20 s. of incubation, perhaps by competition for the Na^+ gradient (16). It is clear that pyruvate has no direct stimulatory action on the phosphate carrier.

The metabolic consequences of substrate addition were further investigated by measuring the rate of oxygen consumption of tubule cell suspensions (Table 2). The rate of oxidative phosphorylation is closely linked to active transport processes including that of phosphate [17]. The basal rate of oxygen consumption of a tubule cell suspension was increased only slightly on addition of glycerol (10 mM) or pyruvate (1 mM). The addition of succinate (1 mM) caused the rate of oxygen consumption to double. This rate was close to the maximum cellular oxygen consumption capacity, since addition of dinitrophenol (25 µM) could not further increase the rate of oxygen consumption.

Table 2 Tubule Cell Oxygen Uptake

Substrate	Concn. (mM)	Oxygen Uptake (nmol/min./mg protein)		% of Basal
None		2.18 ± 0.09	(n=15)	100
Glycerol	10	2.84 ± 0.11	(n=4)	130
Pyruvate	1	2.90 ± 0.14	(n=5)	133
Succinate	1	5.08 ± 0.24	(n=4)	233
DNP	0.025	5.18 ± 0.25	(n=15)	238

Isolated kidney tubule cells were incubated in buffer containing 10 mM glucose in an oxygen electrode at 37°C. The uncoupler 2,4-dinitrophenol (DNP) was finally added to all incubations and the uncoupled rate of respiration determined. The values are the mean±s.e.m of n incubations.

Discussion

These results clearly cannot support the hypothesis that an increased rate of gluconeogenesis is a step in the process which inhibits phosphate uptake in proximal tubule cells. The addition of the substrates pyruvate and succinate, which stimulate glucose production, results in a considerable increase in the rate of phosphate accumulation.

The increased phosphate uptake appears not to derive from a direct action on the carrier but to result from the metabolism of the substrates by the cell since pyruvate has no effect on phosphate transport into brush border membrane vesicles which possess the transport system, but none of the cellular metabolic apparatus. The rapidity of the action of pyruvate would seem to rule out any action that is dependent on protein synthesis.

The added substrates may be metabolised either by the Krebs cycle, leading to oxidative phosphorylation or by the gluconeogenic pathway, resulting in glucose production. Because of the low hexokinase activity of these cells [18] the addition of substrates that normally arise by the metabolism of glucose-6-phosphate is likely to enhance oxidative phosphorylation relative to that when glucose is the only respiratory fuel. The measurements of oxygen utilisation show that this is so particualy for succinate. An increased production of ATP is likely to result in an enhanced electrochemical gradient of Na^+ across the cell because of an increased activity of the Na^+-K^+ ATPase situated in the basolateral membrane. Therefore those transport processes requiring Na^+ co-transport would be activated. Na^+-dependent glucose transport is activated by pyruvate, but not to the same extent as is phosphate uptake. Thus the stimulation of phosphate uptake by pyruvate cannot wholly be ascribed to the effects of an increased Na^+ gradient. In addition, if ATP availability were the major effector of increased phosphate transport then succinate, which stimulates most oxidative metabolism, would be expected to stimulate phosphate accumulation to the greatest extent. The experiments show this to be untrue.

These conclusions are re-inforced by the experiments using 3-mercaptopicolinate, a potent specific inhibitor of phosphoenol-pyruvate carboxykinase [19] which is essential for gluconeogenesis from pyruvate. 3-mercaptopicolinate has no effect on the production of glucose from glycerol (which does not require phosphoenolpyruvate carboxykinase activity) or on the uptake of phosphate in the presence of glycerol.

The main point requiring clarification is how the flux of metabolite from phosphoenolpyruvate to triose phosphate can influence the rate of entry of phosphate into the cell. It is of interest that changes in kidney cell phospholipid concentrations have been associated with parathyroid hormone action leading to a decrease in phosphate transport [20] and perliminary results obtained by us indicate that a stimulation of phosphate incorporation into phospholipid accompanies the generalised increase in phosphate accumulation caused by gluconeogenic substrates.

Acknowledgements

We thank the National Kidney Research Fund for their support for this project and the Government of Pakistan and the British Council for a grant supporting RP. P.J.B. thanks the Wellcome Trust for a travel grant.

References

1. Dennis, V. W., Stead. W. W., & Myers, J. L., Renal handling of phosphate and calcium, Annu. Rev. Physiol. 41:257-271 (1979)
2. Jacobson, H. R., Functional segmentation of the mammalian nephron, Am. J. Physiol. 241:F203-218 (1981)
3. Watford, M., Hod, Y., Chiao, Y-B., Utter, M. F. & Hanson, R. W., The unique role of the kidney in gluconeogensesis in the chicken, J. Biol. Chem. 256:10023-10027 (1981)
4. Wirthensohn, G., Vandewalle, A. & Guder, W. G., Renal glycerol metabolism and the distribution of glycerol kinase in rabbit nephron, Biochem. J. 198:543-549 (1981)
5. Guder, W. G. & Rupprecht, A., Metabolism of isolated kidney tubules. Independent actions of catecholamines on renal cyclic adenosine 3'-5'-monophosphate levels and gluconeogenesis, Eur. J. Biochem. 52:283-290 (1975)
6. Kempson, S. A., Colon-Otero, G., LiseOu, S-Y., Turner, S. T. & Dousa, T. P., Possible role of nicotinamide adenine dinucleotide as an intracellular regulator of renal transport of phosphate in the rat, J. Clin. Invest. 67:1347-1360 (1981)
7. Berndt, T. J., Knox, F. G., Kempson, S. A. & Dousa, T. P., Nicotinamide adenine dinucleotide and renal response to parathyroid hormone, Endocrinology 108:2005-2007 (1981)
8. Turner, S. T., Kiebzak, G. M. & Dousa, T. P., Mechanism of glucocorticoid effect on renal transport of phosphate, Am. J. Physiol. 243:C227-C236 (1982)
9. Grahn, M. F. & Butterworth, P. J., Modulation of phosphate accumulation in isolated chick kidney cells by gluconeogenic substrates, Bioscience Rep. 2:661-666 (1982)
10. Beck, J. C. & Sacktor, B., The sodium electrochemical potential-mediated uphill transport of D-glucose in renal brush border membrane vesicles, J. Biol. Chem. 253:5531-5535 (1978)
11. Bergmeyer, H. U. & Bernt, E., Glucose determination with glucose oxidase and peroxidase, in: "Methods of Enzymatic Analysis", Bergmeyer, H. U., ed., Academic Press, N.Y. (1974)

12. Nelson, N., A photometric adaptation of the Somogyi method for the determination of glucose, J. Biol. Chem. 153:375-380 (1944)

13. Lowry, O. H., Rosebrough, N. J., Farr, A. L. & Randall, R. J., Protein measurement with Folin phenol reagent, J. Biol. Chem. 193:265-275 (1951)

14. Grahn, M. F. & Butterworth, P. J., Phosphate uptake by proximal tubule cells isolated from chick kidney, Biochem. Soc. Trans. 9:465-466 (1981)

15. Barrett, P. Q. & Aronson, P. S., Glucose and alanine inhibition of phosphate transport in renal microvillus membrane vesicles, Am. J. Physiol. 242:F126-F131 (1982)

16. Browne, J. L., Sanford, P. A. & Smyth, D. H., Transfer and metabolism of citrate, succinate, α-keto-glutarate and pyruvate by hamster small intestine, Proc. R.S.(Lond.)[B] 200:117-135 (1978)

17. Gullans, S. R., Brazy, P. C., Soltoff, S. P., Dennis, V. W. & Mandel, L. J. Metabolic inhibitors: effects on metabolism and transport in the proximal tubule, Am. J. Physiol. 243:F133-F140 (1982)

18. Vandewalle, A., Wirthensohn, G., Heidrich, H-G. & Guder, W. G., Distribution of hexokinase and phosphoenolpyruvate carboxykinase along the rabbit nephron, Am. J. Physiol. 240:F492-F500 (1981)

19. Robinson, B. H. & Oei, J., 3-Mercaptopicolinic acid; a preferential inhibitor of the cytosolic phosphoenolpyruvate carboxykinase, FEBS Lett. 58:12-15 (1975)

20. Farese, R. V., Bidot-Lopez, P., Sabir, M. A., & Larson, R. E. The phosphatidate-polyphosphoinositide cycle: activation by parathyroid hormone and dibutyryl cyclic AMP in rabbit kidney cortex, Ann. N. Y. Acad. Sci. 372:539-551 (1981)

ROLE OF c-AMP AND NAD IN THE REGULATION OF Na^+-DEPENDENT PHOSPHATE TRANSPORT ACROSS RAT RENAL BRUSH BORDER MEMBRANES

Jürg Biber, Piotr Gmaj, Kerstin Malmström and Heini Murer

Institute of Physiology, University of Zürich
Zürich, Switzerland

The activity of the sodium-dependent P_i-transport system in the brush border membrane changes in concordance with the tubular phosphate reabsorption under a variety of physiological conditions (Dousa and Kempson, 1982). Two mechanisms were postulated to be involved in these adaptations: a cyclic-AMP dependent phosphorylation of brush border membrane protein(s) (Hammerman and Hruska, 1982) and a direct interaction of NAD with the membrane (Kempson et al., 1981), apparently via a ADP-ribosylation of certain membrane proteins (Hammerman et al., 1982).

The investigation of the effects of ATP and NAD on P_i-transport in vitro is, however, complicated by the high hydrolytic activity of the isolated brush border membranes, which results in a rapid liberation of variable amounts of P_i from the nucleotides and consequently isotope dilution, trans-stimulation and cis-inhibition effects (Tennenhouse and Chu, 1982; Angielski et al., 1982).

In the present study we investigated the effects of ATP, c-AMP and NAD - introduced into the intravesicular space by osmotic shock - on the Na^+-dependent P_i-transport, protein phosphorylation and ADP-ribosylation in isolated rat kidney brush border membrane vesicles. These studies - performed under conditions which reduced or eliminated the non-specific isotope dilution effects - suggest that neither protein phosphorylation nor NAD has a specific effect on the Na^+-dependent transport of phosphate.

METHODS

Brush border membrane vesicles (BBMV) were isolated from kidneys of Sprague Dawley rats by a magnesium precipitation method (Biber et al., 1981). The membranes were incubated for 2 hrs at 20° C in 600 mM mannitol, 5 mM $MgCl_2$, 20 mM Hepes-Tris, pH 7.2, and were then diluted 1:16 into a medium containing 5 mM $MgCl_2$, 20 mM Hepes-Tris, pH 7.2 and given concentrations of ATP, c-AMP or NAD (osmotic shock).

Phosphorylation by 20 µM ATP (or γ-^{32}P-ATP) was performed either in the presence or in the absence of c-AMP for 20 sec at 25° C as described by Biber et al. (1983). For the ribosylation studies, BBMV were diluted into the hypotonic medium containing 10 mM NAD (or ^{32}P-NAD). For further analysis of the NAD-effect, BBMV were either used directly or passed first through an anion exchanger column (Dowex 1X2) to remove extravesicular NAD and its hydrolysis products. The phosphorylated respectively ribosylated BBMV's were used for the following analysis. When indicated, the membranes were incubated for 30 min at 25° C prior to the analysis. (i) Transport of solutes was initiated by transferring the osmotically shocked vesicles to an incubation medium to obtain the final concentrations of 100 mM NaCl and 0.1 mM $K_2H^{32}PO_4$ or 0.1 mM (^{3}H)D-glucose. Transport was measured by a rapid filtration technique (Burckhardt et al., 1981). (ii) SDS-polyacrylamide gel-electrophoresis was performed according to Laemmli [1970) on 8.4 % gels. Prior to electrophoresis, aliquots of the treated BBMV's were denaturated in 2 % SDS (2 min at 95° C) either in the presence (phosphorylated samples) or in the absence of β-mercatoethanol (ribosylated samples). (iii) After deproteinization with perchloric acid (10 %, final), NAD was determined enzymatically using L-lactate and lactate-dehydrogenase. (iv) For thin layer chromatography, BBMV were solubilized with formic acid in methanol (0.3 M final concentration). The samples were applied to cellulose acetate plates (Merck, F254) which were developed in butanol: ethanol: 0.5 M ammonium formate: 0.5 M HCl = 6 : 5 : 6 : 3 (v/v).

Autoradiography of the dried gels and the thin layer plates was performed with Kodak X-ray films (SO 282) at -70° C. All radiochemicals were obtained from NEN (Boston).

RESULTS

Opening of brush border membrane vesicles by osmotic shock

The protein phosphorylation pattern of BBMV osmotically shocked in the presence of γ-^{32}P-ATP is shown in Figure 1. Several polypeptides are phosphorylated in osmotically shocked vesicles, but only one peptide of a M_r of 78 kD (presumably alkaline phosphatase) is phosphorylated under isotonic conditions. When γ-^{32}P-ATP is added 1 min after the osmotic shock, an identical phosphorylation pattern as under isotonic conditions is observed (Figure 1, Lane 6). These results suggest that the BBMV are impermeable for ATP, but that the nucleotide can be trapped in the vesicles by an osmotic shock, whereupon the intravesicular proteins become available for posphorylation. The fact that no phosphorylation (except for the 78 kD band) occurs when γ-^{32}P-ATP is added after the osmotic shock suggest that the vesicles open only transiently during the dilution into the hypotonic medium, and that the reclosed vesicles are still of right-side out orientation.

The trapping of ATP, L-glucose and NAD in the osmotically shocked vesicles is shown in Table 1. If it is assumed that the intravesicular volume is 1 µl/mg protein, it can be calculated that more than 60 % of the vesicles have opened during the hypotonic treatment.

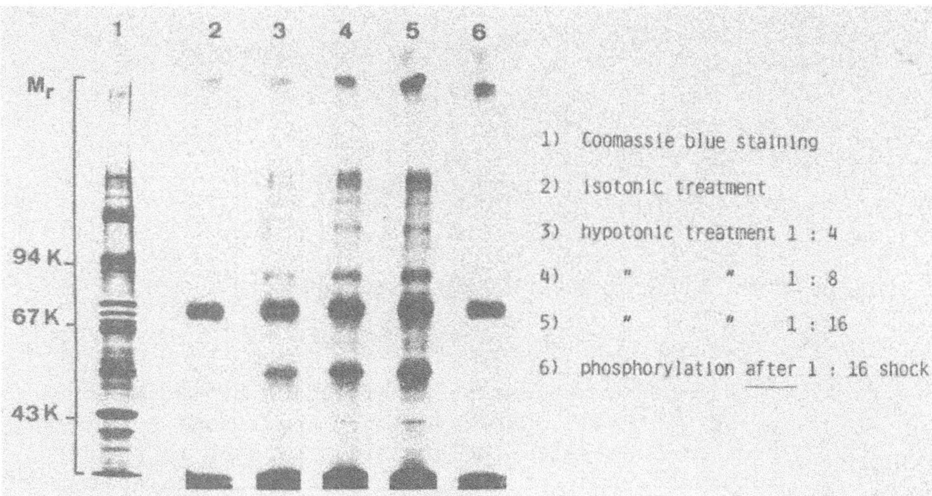

Figure 1. Phosphorylation of rat BBMV by 20 µM γ-^{32}P-ATP under isotonic and hypotonic conditions.

c-AMP dependent protein phosphorylation and solute transport

The effect of a simultaneous addition of various amounts of c-AMP to the hypotonic phosphorylation medium is illustrated in Figure 2. As indicated, ^{32}P-incorporation into various polypeptides is strongly influenced by c-AMP (e.g. 40 kD; 46 kD; 55 kD and various bands higher than 120 kD). The effect of c-AMP is near maximal at 10 µmoles/l c-AMP. Under isotonic conditions c-AMP does not affect the phosphorylation pattern (not shown).

Sodium dependent phosphate and D-glucose transport is analyzed with the same membrane vesicles as used for the gel-electrophoretic analysis (Figure 3). The presence of an overshoot of P_i- and D-glucose transport demonstrates that the membrane vesicle integrity is retained after osmotic rupture. When compared to control vesicles (osmotic shock in the absence of ATP and c-AMP), initial P_i-uptake is clearly inhibited (approx. 17 %, $p < 0.01$, paired Student's t-test) by ATP in the absence of c-AMP. Phosphorylation by ATP in the presence of 100 µM c-AMP results in no

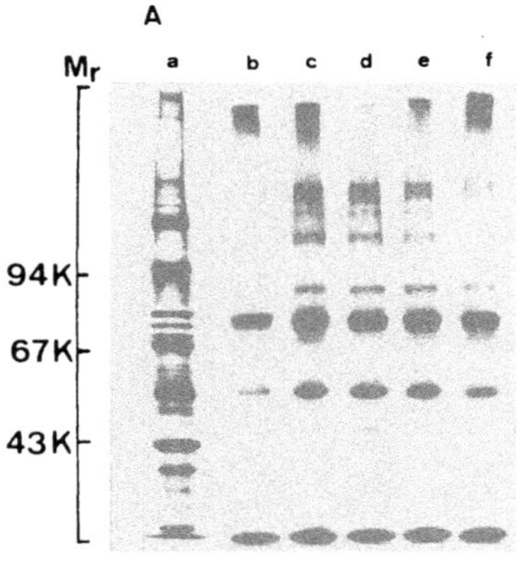

Figure 2. Cyclic-AMP dependent phosphorylation of rat BBMV by 20 µM γ-^{32}P-ATP under hypotonic conditions.
Lane a: Coomassie Blue staining. Lanes b to f show autoradiograms of a phosphorylation in the absence of c-AMP (b) or in the presence of c-AMP: 0.1 µM (f); 1 µM (e); 10 µM (d) and 100 µM (c).

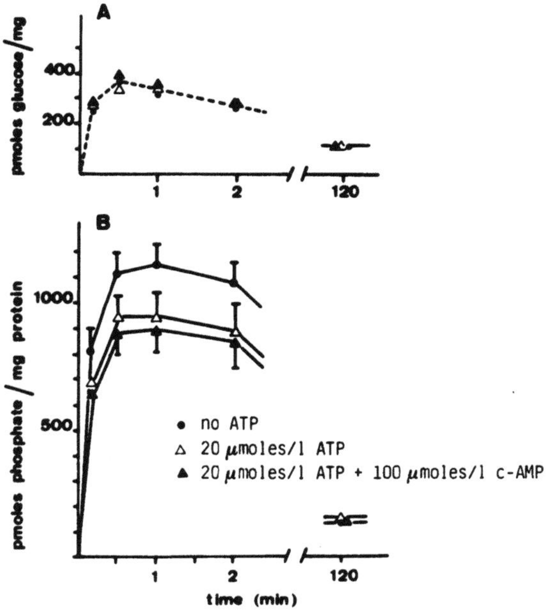

Figure 3. Time course of Na^+-dependent D-glucose (A) and phosphate transport (B) of BBMV phosphorylated by 20 µM ATP either in the presence or in the absence of 100 µM c-AMP.

Table 1. Opening of brush border membrane vesicles by osmotic shock

Addition	Intravesicular content nmoles/mg Control	Shocked	% of opening
10 mM NAD	0.2	6.7	65
20 µM (^3H)-ATP	0.03	0.05	100
100 µM (^3H)L-glucose	0.002	0.064	62

Extravesicular ATP and L-glucose were removed by millipore filtration. Extravesicular NAD was removed by passing the vesicles through Dowex 1X2 column.

further (statistically significant) inhibition of P_i-uptake (Figure 3B). As indicated in Figure 3A, the uptake of D-glucose is not changed by these treatments, indicating the absence of non-specific changes of the membrane permeability.

To exclude rapid dephosphorylation reactions as a possible reason for the lack of the c-AMP dependent phosphorylations with respect to the P_i-transport, γ-thio-ATP is used as phosphoryl donor instead of ATP. However, again no inhibition of P_i-transport is observed after a hypotonic treatment of the BBMV with γ-thio-ATP in the presence of c-AMP (not shown).

The results suggest that c-AMP dependent changes of the protein phosphorylation (Figure 2) are not involved in the regulation of P_i-transport in the isolated rat renal brush border membrane vesicles. The slight inhibitory effect of ATP is suggested to be non-specific. Evidence for such a non-specific effect is obtained by a hypotonic treatment of the BBMV in the presence of a number of other nucleotides (GTP, ITP, ADP). By all of these reagents a similar inhibition of P_i-uptake is observed as illustrated for ATP in Figure 3 (data not shown).

Effects of intravesicular NAD on $^{32}P_i$-transport

The Na-dependent $^{32}P_i$-uptake by the BBMV containing NAD in the intravesicular space is shown in Figure 4. In control vesicles NAD was added 2 min after osmotic shock, and both membranes were passed through Dowex 1X2 column to remove extravesicular NAD. The $^{32}P_i$-uptake is stimulated rather then inhibited by intravesicular NAD. The stimulation is enhanced when the NAD-containing vesicles are preincubated for 30 min at 25° C before the uptake measurements. The hydrolysis of intravesicular NAD is shown in Figure 5. In osmotically shocked vesicles a part of ^{32}P label is found in NAD and a part in vesicle-bound P_i. After 30 min incubation at 25° C the amount of label in NAD is decreased, but still a considerable amount of NAD is present in the intact form. In control vesicles to which NAD was added after osmotic shock no label was found in NAD, but some inorganic phosphate had been incorporated (not shown). These results provide evidence that although NAD is present in the intravesicular space, no inhibition of phosphate transport occurs as a result of its interaction with the cytoplasmic surface of the membrane. On the contrary, a significant stimulation is observed which can be attributed to partial hydrolysis of NAD and a trans-stimulation of $^{32}P_i$-uptake by intravesicularly liberated phosphate.

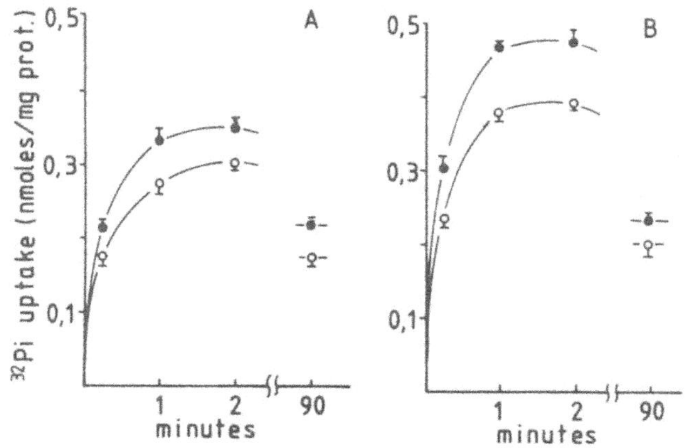

Figure 4. Effects of intravesicular NAD on Na^+-dependent P_i-uptake by the BBMV. Experimental vesicles were osmotically shocked in the presence of 10 mM NAD, the same amount of NAD was added to control vesicles 2 min after osmotic shock. Both samples were passed through Dowex 1X2 column to remove extravesicular NAD. The vesicles were preincubated at 25° C for either 1 min (A) or 30 min (B) before the uptake experiment. (o--o) control; (•--•) NAD in.

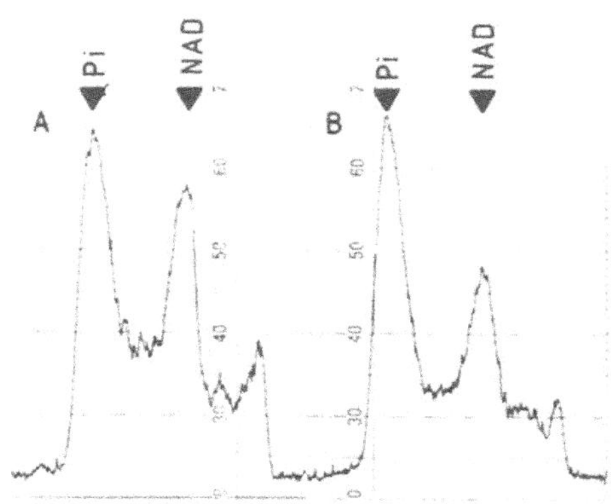

Figure 5. Hydrolysis of intravesicular NAD. The experimental conditions were as in Figure 4, except that 25 µCi/ml of ^{32}P-NAD was added. The traces show the scans of thin layer chromatograms of the extracts of vesicles incubated for 1 min (A) or 30 min (B) at 25° C.

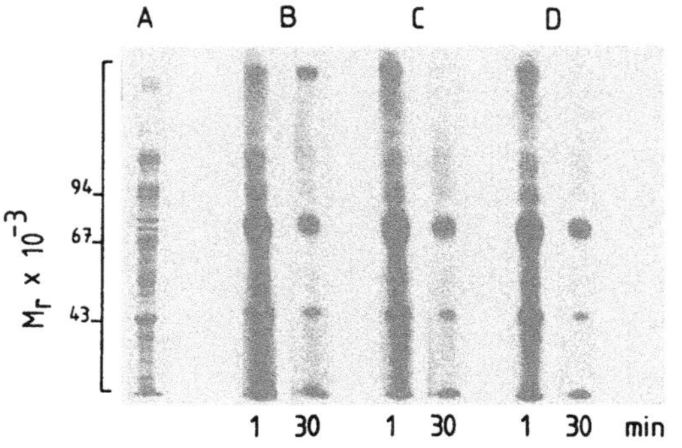

Figure 6. Incorporation of ^{32}P from ^{32}P-NAD into brush border membrane proteins. (A) Coomassie Blue staining; (B) osmotically shocked vesicles; (C) vesicles incubated in the presence of 0.1 % saponin; (D) vesicles under isotonic conditions.

Figure 5 shows that ^{32}P from NAD is rapidly incorporated into a number of brush border membrane proteins, but the incorporation is the same in osmotically shocked vesicles, in vesicles treated with saponin and in vesicles incubated under isotonic conditions. Thus, in contrast to protein phosphorylation, no change in ^{32}P-incorporation is seen when the inner surface of the vesicles is made accessible to NAD. The amount of protein labelling gradually decreases during prolonged incubation, but again no difference between osmotically shocked and non-shocked vesicles becomes apparent. These data indicate that ^{32}P is rapidly exchanged between NAD and the brush border membrane protein, but there is no specific $^{32}P_i$-incorporation at the cytoplasmic membrane surface. When (adenine-2.8-^3H)-NAD is used instead of ^{32}P-NAD in an identical labelling experiment, no incorporation of adenine moiety into brush border membrane proteins can be found (not shown). This negative result supports the conclusion that no ADP-ribosylation of the brush border membrane protein(s) occurs under conditions used in this study.

CONCLUSIONS

The data presented in this paper indicate that at least three (and probably more) brush border membrane proteins are phosphorylated in a c-AMP dependent manner. The phosphorylation, however, does not correlate with any changes of Na^+-dependent P_i-transport, since (i) the P_i-transport is not affected by c-AMP dependent phosphorylation by ATP or γ-thio-ATP and (ii) a small inhibition of P_i-uptake is observed in the presence of ATP, GTP, ITP and ADP;

the slight inhibitory effect of these nucleotides is therefore non-specific and might result from isotope dilution due to hydrolysis of the nucleotides.

ACKNOWLEDGMENTS

This work was supported by the Swiss National Science Foundation, Grant No. 3.226-083.

REFERENCES

Angielski, S., Zielkiewicz, J., and Dziezko, G., 1982, Metabolism of NAD by isolated rat renal brush border membranes, Pflügers Arch., 395:159.

Biber, J., Stieger, B., Haase, W., and Murer, H., 1981, A high yield preparation of rat kidney brush border membranes. Different behaviour of lysosomal markers, Biochim. Biophys. Acta, 647:169.

Biber, J., Malmström, K., Scalera, V., and Murer, H., 1983, Phosphorylation of rat kidney brush border membranes: Role of c-AMP dependent protein phosphorylation in the regulation of phosphate transport, Pflügers Arch., in press.

Bradford, M.M., 1976, A rapid and sensitive method for the quantitation of microgram quantities of protein utilizing the principle of protein dye binding, Anal. Biochem., 72:248.

Burckhardt, G., Stern, H., and Murer, H., 1981, The influence of pH on the phosphate transport into renal brush border membrane vesicles, Pflügers Arch., 390:191.

Dousa, T.P., and Kempson, S.A., 1982, Regulation of renal brush border membrane transport of phosphate. Mineral Electrolyte Metab., 7:113.

Hammerman, M.R., and Hruska, K.A., 1982, Cyclic AMP-dependent protein phosphorylation in canine renal brush border membrane vesicles is associated with decreased phosphate transport, J. Biol. Chem., 257:992.

Hammerman, M.R., Hauser, V.A., and Morrisey, J.J., 1982, ADP-ribosylation of canine renal brush border vesicle protein is associated with decreased phosphate transport, J. Biol. Chem., 257:12380.

Kempson, S.A., Colon-Otero, G., Ou, S.L., and Dousa, T.P., 1981, Possible role of nicotinamide-adenine dinucleotide (NAD) as an intracellular regulator of renal phosphate transport. J. Clin. Invest., 67:1347.

Laemmli, U.K., 1970, Cleavage of structural proteins during the assembly of the head of bacteriophage T_4, Nature, 227:680.

Tenenhouse, H.S., and Chu, Y.L., 1982, Hydrolysis of nicotinamide-adenine dinucleotide by purified renal brush border membranes, Biochem. J., 204:635.

GLUCONEOGENESIS, CYTOSOLIC REDOX POTENTIAL, AND PHOSPHATE AND FLUID TRANSPORT IN THE ISOLATED RABBIT PROXIMAL TUBULE

Norimoto **YANAGAWA**, Glenn T. **NAGAMI** and Kiyoshi **KUROKAWA**

Nephrology Divisions, Medical and Research Services Veterans Administration Sepulveda and Wadsworth Hospitals and Department of Medicine, University of California at Los Angeles (UCLA) School of Medicine Los Angeles, California 90073

INTRODUCTION

Gluconeogenesis (GNG) in the kidney represents an important metabolic activity localized to the proximal tubules (1). It has been suggested that renal GNG may play a key role in the regulation of renal ammoniagenesis in metabolic acidosis (2) and also may contribute to blood glucose concentrations (3). However, it is not known whether renal GNG serves any functional role in solute and fluid transport in the proximal nephron. Recent observations from several laboratories suggested that GNG may play some role in the regulation of fluid and inorganic phosphate (Pi) reabsorption in the proximal tubule. For example, Dousa and associates proposed that cytosolic concentrations of the oxidized form of nicotinamide adenine dinucleotide (NAD^+) may control proximal Pi reabsorption and as such GNG may modulate Pi transport through altering the cytosolic level of NAD^+ (4). Silva and colleagues, who studied isolated perfused rat kidney, suggested that GNG and sodium reabsorption may compete for the common energy source, resulting in reciprocal changes in the rates of GNG and fluid reabsorption in the proximal tubules (5,6).

The ratio of free cytosolic NAD^+ to NADH, which reflects the cytosolic redox potential, is directly proportional to the ratio of cytosolic pyruvate to lactate, thus pyruvate x NADH = K x lactate x NAD. As a result changes in cytosolic concentration of pyruvate and lactate may alter the cytosolic redox potential.

Since renal tubule membranes are not restrictive to a variety of substrates (8), changing the available substrate from lactate to pyruvate, or vice versa, will alter the cytosolic redox state in a predictable direction. Also, addition to the tubules of methylene blue, a proton acceptor which converts NADH to NAD^+ (9), should produce a more oxidized redox state.

In the present study we examined more directly the possible relationship between GNG, cytosolic redox potential, and proximal tubular transport functions using proximal S2-3 segments isolated from rabbit kidneys. The rates of GNG were altered by changing the substrate in the bath, by lowering bath pH to 7.0 or by addition of 3-mercaptopicolinate. Cytosolic redox potential was altered by changing the substrate in the bath medium from pyruvate to lactate and vice versa and by adding methylene blue to the bath medium.

MATERIALS AND METHODS

Rabbit proximal S2-3 segments of the superficial nephron were dissected and used for the present study. For studies determining glucose production, tubule segments were incubated in the presence of 1 mM acetate and 5 mM of a gluconeogenic substrate at 30°C for 30 or 60 min in Kreb-Ringer-bicarbonate buffer, pH 7.4, equilibrated with $95\% O_2/5\% CO_2$. The amount of glucose produced was measured in replicate samples of the incubation medium using a method described by Chick and Like (10).

Proximal S2-3 segments of superficial nephrons were perfused in vitro using conventional methods as reported previously in detail (11). Bath medium contained 1 mM Na-acetate and sodium salt of a gluconeogenic substrate, 5 mM, and was equilibrated with 95% $O_2/5\% CO_2$ at 37°C. In those experiments in which the substrate in the bath was changed or 3-mercaptopicolinate was added to the bath, a 30 minute equilibration time was placed between each period. Results are expressed as the mean of 4-5 timed collections of tubular fluid.

RESULTS

1. Effects of changes in cytosolic redox potential on Jp and Jv

i) Oxidation of redox potential: Oxidation of cytosolic redox potential, that is an increase in the ratio of free HAD^+ to NADH, was brought about either by changing the substrate in the bath from lactate to pyruvate or by addition of methylene blue to the bath. As shown in Figure 1, Jp did not change in response to both procedures nor did Jv (data not shown).

ii) Reduction of redox potential: Reduction of cytosolic redox potential, thus a decrease in cytosolic free NAD content, was brought about by changing the substrate in the bath from pyruvate to lactate. This maneuver had no significant effect on Jp (Figure 1) and Jv (0.55±0.11 vs. 0.59±0.19 nl/mm/min).

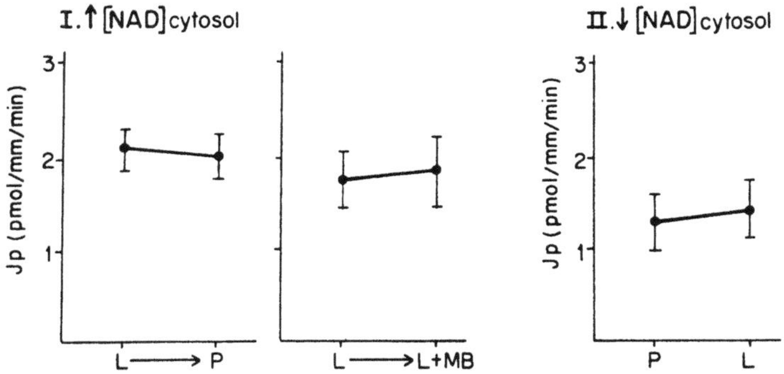

Figure 1: Jp in response to the change of substrate from lactate (L) to pyruvate (P) and P to L, and to the addition of methylene blue (MB) in the presence of lactate.

2. Gluconeogenesis and Jp and Jv

i) Glucose production from different substrates: The rates of glucose production varied significantly with different substrates. Glucose production from pyruvate was greater than that from either lactate or glutamate. Changing the substrate in the bath from glutamate to pyruvate, from glutamate to lactate, or from lactate to pyruvate had no effect on Jp as shown in Figure 2 nor on Jv (data not shown).

ii) Effect of 3-MP on GNG and on Jp and Jv: Addition of 3-MP, a specific inhibitor of a key enzyme of gluconeogenesis, phosphoenolpyruvate carboxykinase (PEPCK), inhibited glucose production by approximately 75%, but had no effect on either the Jp as shown in Figure 3 or on Jv (data not shown).

iii) Effects of acid pH and 3-MP on GNG and on Jp and Jv: The Jv and Jp were measured with normal (7.4) and acid (7.0) pH in the presence of a-ketoglutarate as substrate. As shown in Figure 4, lowering the pH of the incubation medium from 7.4 to 7.0 resulted

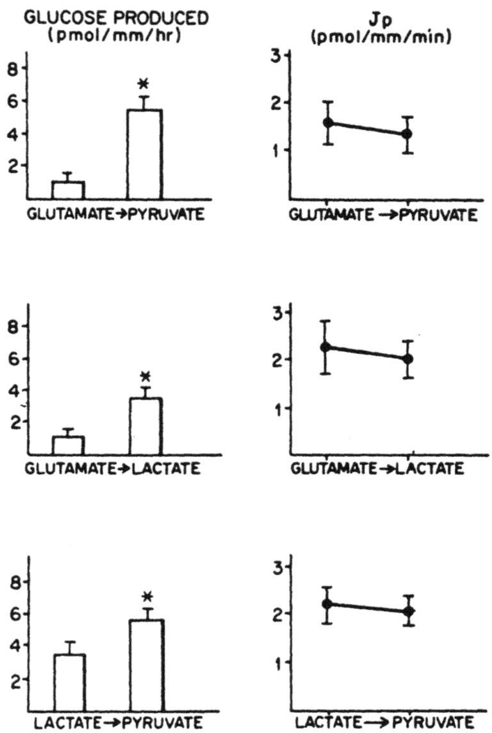

Figure 2: Effect of different substrates on glucose production and Jp. *=$p<0.05$.

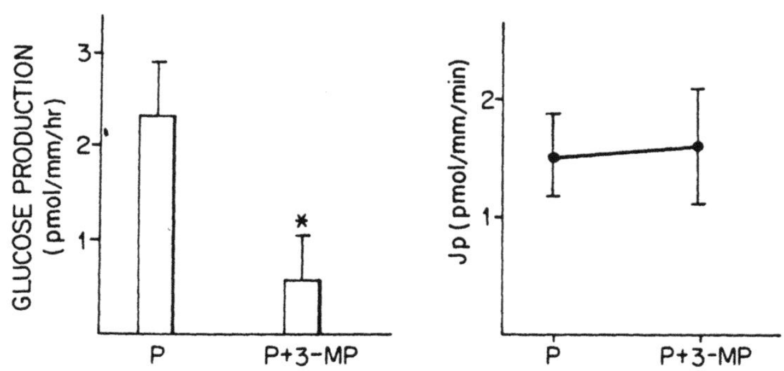

Figure 3: Effects of 3-mercaptopicolinate (3-MP) on glucose production from 5 mM pyruvate (P) and Jp. *=$p < 0.01$.

in a 33% increase in glucose production by the same tubules (8.74+0.52 to 11.90+0.62 pmol/mm/hr, p 0.01). Addition of 3-MP (1 mM), either before or after the change of the pH, abolished the stimulation of GNG by the acid pH (Figure 4). On the other hand, lowering the pH of the bath medium suppressed both Jv (from 0.31+0.10 to 0.08+0.09 nl/mm/min, p<0.01) and Jp (from 2.59+0.30 to 1.72+0.21 pmol/mm/min, p<0.01). Nonetheless, when 3-MP was added to the bath, either before or after the bath pH was changed, the inhibition of Jv and Jp by acid pH persisted (Figure 4).

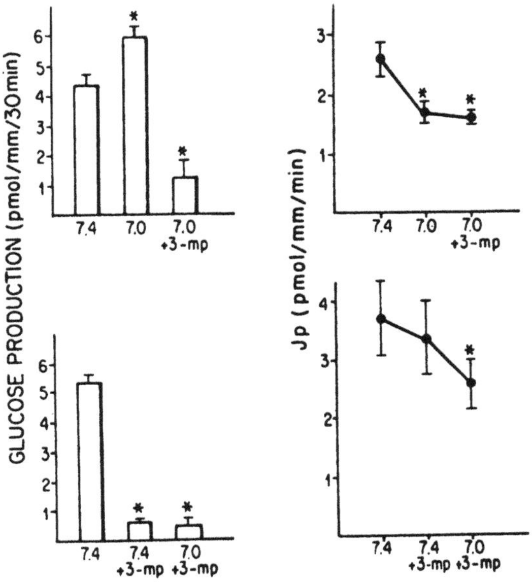

Figure 4: Effects of bath pH from 7.4 to 7.0 with and without 3-mercaptopicolinate (3-mp) on Jp and glucose production from a-ketoglutarate. *=p<0.01.

DISCUSSION

A number of metabolic and hormonal stimuli are known to affect renal GNG and tubular Pi reabsorption in opposite directions. For example, metabolic acidosis, fasting, parathyroid hormone, glucocorticoids are known to enhance GNG and inhibit Pi reabsorption and cause phosphaturia. When it was found that NAD^+ and NADH inhibit the uptake of Pi by brush border membrane vesicles of proximal tubules in vitro (4) and that a phosphaturic agent such as parathyroid hormone caused an increase in Pi excretion and renal tissue NAD^+/NADH ratio (12), Dousa et al proposed that changes in the concentrations of these pyridine nucleotides in the cell may affect and regulate Pi transport in the proximal tubule (4). Since the majority of NADH, but not NAD^+, in the cytosol is protein bound (7), it was suggested that the concentration in the cytosol of free NAD^+ may be sufficiently high to inhibit Pi transport in the brush border membranes and that changes in its concentration may be a factor regulating the Pi transport in the proximal tubules (4). Because changes in cytosolic redox potential are reflected by changes in the ratio of NAD^+ to NADH, it was suggested that changes in the cytosolic redox potential in proximal tubular cells may alter the rate of Pi transport so that a more oxidized redox state (higher NAD^+:NADH ratio) inhibits Pi reabsorption (12-14). Further, it has been assumed that the rate of renal gluconeogenesis may regulate the cytosolic redox state through reactions of the gluconeogenic pathway involving the conversion of NAD^+ to NADH, for example, the conversion of diphosphoglycerate to glyceraldehyde-phosphate catalyzed by glyceroaldehyde-3-phosphate dehydrogenase. Therefore, stimulation of gluconeogenesis would increase levels of NAD^+ and/or produce a more oxidized redox potential in the cytosol thereby inhibiting tubular Pi reabsorption. Studies by Dousa and associates seem to support such a hypothesis (12-16). They showed that perturbations known to stimulate gluconeogenesis and to cause phosphaturia such as metabolic acidosis, parathyroid hormone, glucocorticoids are associated with either an increase in renal tissue NAD^+ or an increase in the ratio of NAD^+/NADH.

Although the above model may explain the observed relationship between GNG and Pi transport by proximal tubules, other studies may not support this thesis. First, NAD^+ does not inhibit Pi uptake in brush border membrane vesicles in the same manner that phospaturic stimuli, such as PTH and metabolic acidosis inhibit Pi transport. NAD^+ inhibits Pi uptake in the brush border membrane vesicles by raising the Km for Pi transport (17) while PTH and metabolic acidosis inhibit Pi transport by the brush border membranes by lowering the Vmax (18, 19). Recent studies suggest that the inhibitory effects of NAD^+ on Pi uptake by brush border membranes may be due to liberation of Pi from the NAD^+ by hydrolysis leading to a dilution of radiolabeled Pi and an apparent reduction in Km (17, 20, 21).

Secondly, changes in the rate of GNG may not results in predictable changes in the cytosolic redox potential. Measurement of the cytosolic redox potential is extremely difficult with available techniques. In vivo measurements of redox potential in the rat kidney have shown that PTH causes reduction and calcitonin oxidation of the redox potential of the mitochondria of superficial proximal convoluted tubules (22). Indirect yet accurate estimates of the ratio of free cytosolic NAD^+ to NADH can be made by measuring intracellular concentrations of lactate and pyruvate (7). Available data show that the ratio of lactate to pyruvate in the kidney do not consistently change in response to acidosis or to PTH both of which stimulate GNG (7, 23-27). These data do not support the contention that phosphaturic stimuli are mediated through changes in NAD^+ concentration or oxidation of cytosolic redox potential brought about by changes in the rate of GNG.

Results of the present studies also do not support the view that cytosolic free NAD^+ concentration or the redox potential plays a regulatory role in Pi transport in renal proximal tubules. Although we did not measure the actual cytosolic free NAD^+ and NADH because of obvious technical reasons, it is reasonable to assume that changing the substrate in the bath medium between pyruvate and lactate will alter the ratio of cytosolic pyruvate to lactate resulting in a shift in redox potential in the cytosol to either a more oxidated or reduced state. Since the intracellular concentrations of pyruvate and lactate in the kidney are approximately 0.02-0.07 mM and 0.3-1.5 mM, respectively (23-26), the presence of 5 mM of either pyruvate or lactate would provide a sufficient concentration gradient of these substrates across the cell membrane to allow influx and to alter cytosolic redox potential. Changing the available substrate from lactate to pyruvate would result in a more oxidized cytosolic redox state (higher NAD^+/NADH), whereas changing the available substrate from pyruvate to lactate would result in a more reduced redox state. Our results indicate that such changes in substrate do not result in any significant change in Jp or Jv suggesting that cytosolic redox potential does not play an important role in the regulation of Pi transport in the proximal tubules. Raising the cytosolic NAD^+:NADH ratio by another means, namely, addition of methylene blue (9) did not affect Jv or Jp in isolated proximal tubules.

Although changes in substrate in the incubation medium resulted in significant differences in rates of GNG, such change in substrate did not alter Jp or Jv across the proximal tubule. These findings suggest that the alteration in GNG brought about by different substrates does not affect either the Jv or Jp of the proximal tubules. Furthermore, addition of 3-MP, an inhibitor of PEPCK, a key enzyme of gluconeogenesis, inhibited GNG from pyruvate by 75%, but did not affect Jv or Jp. These observations again suggest the absence of a link between GNG and Jp or Jv in the proximal tubules. A reduction in the pH of the incubation medium to 7.0 stimulated GNG and suppressed Jv and Jp as might be expected from previous reports by others (28). Addition of 3-MP abolished the stimulation of GNG by low pH but left unaltered the suppression of Jv and Jp by low pH. These data thus indicate that the effect of the acidic pH on the transport functions are independent of its effect to stimulate GNG.

Silva et al (5, 6) suggest that GNG and sodium transport may not be tightly coupled in basal conditions, but under stimulated conditions sodium transport prevails at the expense of GNG. The results of our present study demonstrate that Pi transport and fluid reabsorption in the proximal tubule are not tightly regulated by GNG. The dissociation of Pi and sodium transport, major active transport functions of the proximal tubule, from GNG, an energy-consuming pathway, indicates that the energy requirement for transport functions in the proximal tubule is maintained, under the condition studies, despite varying rates of GNG.

The present findings together with studies by others do not support the thesis that regulation of Jp or Jv is mediated directly by changes in the cytosolic redox potential or by changes in the rate of gluconeogenesis.

Acknowledgements: A portion of this study has appeared as abstracts in Kidney Intl 23: 114, 1983 and in Clin Research 31: 446A, 1983. This work was supported by the Veterans Administration and in part by USPHS grant AM-21351. Dr. Nagami was a research fellow supported by a NIH training grant T32-AM-07270 and is an Associate Investigator of Veterans Administration.

REFERENCES

1. Schmidt U, Guder WG: Sites of enzyme activity along the nephron. Kidney Intl 9:233-242, 1976

2. Cohen J, Kamm DE: Renal metabolism: relation to renal function, in: The Kidney, 2nd edition, edited by Brenner BM, Rector FC Jr, Philadelphia, Saunders, 1981, p. 144

3. Kida K, Nakajo S, Kamiya F, Toyama Y, Nishio T, Nakagawa H: Renal net glucose release in vivo and its contribution to blood glucose in rats. J Clin Invest 62:721-726, 1978

4. Kempson SA, Colon-Otero R, Ou SYL, Turner St, Dousa TP: Possible role of nicotinamide adenine dinucleotide as an intracellular regulator of renal transport of phosphate in the rat. J Clin Invest 67:1347-1360, 1981

5. Silva P, Ross B, Spokes K: Competition between sodium reabsorption and gluconeogenesis in kidneys of steroid-treated rats. Am J Physiol 238: F290-F295, 1980

6. Silva P, Hallac R, Spokes K, Epstein FH: Relationship among gluconeogenesis , Q_{O2} and Na^+ transport in the perfused rat kidney. Am J Physiol 242: F508-F513, 1982

7. Williamson DH, Lund P, Krebs HA: The redox state of free nicotinamide adenine dinucleotide in the cytoplasm and mitochondria of rat liver. Biochem J 103: 514-527, 1967

8. Krebs H: Gluconeogenesis. The Croonian Lecture 1963. Biol J 159: 545-564, 1963

9. Preuss HG, Weiss FR: Rate-limiting factor in rat kidney slice ammoniagenesis. Am J Physiol 221:458-464, 1971

10. Chick W, Like AA: Ultramicro method of determination of glycogen and glucose by enzymic labeling with adenosine triphosphate-r-^{32}P. Anal Biochem 32: 340-347, 1969

11. Yanagawa N, Nissenson RA, Edwards B, Yeung P, Trizna W, Fine LG: Functional profile of the isolated uremic nephrons. Intrinsic adaptation of phosphate transport in the rabbit proximal tubule. Kidney Intl 23: 674-683, 1983

12. Berndt TJ, Knox FG, Kempson SA, Dousa TP: Nicotinamide adenine dinucleotide and renal response to parathyroid hormone. Endocrinology 109:2005-2007. 1981

13. Kempson SA: Effect of metabolic acidosis on renal brush border membrane adaptation to low phosphate diet. Kidney Intl 22:225-233. 1982

14. Turner ST, Kiebzak GM, Dousa TP: Mechanism of glucocorticoid effect on renal transport of phosphate. Am J Physiol 243: C227-C236, 1982

15. Ou SYL, Kempson SA, Dousa TP: Relationship between gluconeogenesis and content of nicotinamide adenine dinucleotide in renal cortex. Life Sci 29:1195-1202, 1981

16. Berndt TJ, Pfeifer JD, Knox FG, Kempson SA, Dousa TP: nicotinamide restores phosphaturic effect of PTH and calcitonin in phosphate deprivation. Am J Physiol 242:F447-F452, 1982

17. Lang RP, Yanagawa N, Nord E, Fine LG: Nucleotides competitively inhibit Na-dependent phosphorus uptake by bruch border membrane of rabbit proximal tubules. Kidney Intl 23:103, 1983 (Abstract)

18. Murer H, Stern H, Burckhardt G, Storelli C, Kinne R: Sodium dependent transport of inorganic phosphate across the renal brush border membrane. Adv Expt Med Biol 128:11-23, 1980

19. Levine BS, Ho K, Kraut JA, Coburn JW, Kurokawa K: Effect of metabolic acidosis on phosphate transport by the renal brush border membrane. Biochim Biophys Acta 727: 7-12. 1983

20. Tenenhouse HS, Chu YL: Hydrolysis of NAD by purified renal brush border membranes. Biochem J 204:635-638, 1982

21. Angielski S, Zielkiewicz J, Dzierzko G: Metabolism of NAD by isolated rat renal brush border membranes. Pflugers Arch 395:159-161, 1982

22. Kimura S, Ogata E, Yoshitoshi Y, Nishiki K and Kobayashi S: Calcitonin, Ca++ and oxidation-reduction state of pyridine nucleotide in tubular cells, in Endocrinology 1973, edited by Taylor S, London, William Heinemann Medical Books, London, 1974, p. 153

23. Vinay P, Allignet E, Pichette C, Watford M, Lemieux G, Gougoux A: Changes in renal metabolic profile and ammoniagenesis during acute and chronic metabolic acidosis in dog and rat. Kidney Intl 17: 312-325, 1980

24. Alleyne GAO: Renal metabolic response to acid-base changes. II. The early effects of metabolic acidosis on renal metabolism in the rat. J Clin Invest 49:943-951, 1970

25. Nagata N, Rasmussen H: Parathyroid hormone and renal cell metabolism. Biochemistry 7:3728-3733, 1968

26. Hems DA, Brosnan JT: Effects of ischaemia on content of metabolites in rat liver and kidney in vivo. Biochem J 120: 105-111, 1970

27. Burch H, Lowry OH, Meinhardt L, Max P Jr, Chyu KJ: Effect of fructose, dihydroxyacetone, glycerol and glucose on metabolism and related compounds in liver and kidney. J Biol Chem 245: 2092-2102, 1970

28. Dennis VW, Woodhall PB, Robinson RR: Characteristics of phosphate transport in isolated proximal tubule. Am J Physiol 231:979-985, 1976

COMPARISON OF THE EFFECT OF NUCLEOTIDES ON PHOSPHATE TRANSPORT IN RENAL BRUSH BORDER MEMBRANE VESICLES AND INTACT PROXIMAL TUBULES

Leon G. Fine, Ronald Lang, Edward P. Nord,
and Norimoto Yanagawa

Divisions of Nephrology
UCLA Center for the Health Sciences and
Sepulveda Veterans Administration Hospital
University of California, Los Angeles
School of Medicine
Los Angeles, California, USA

It has been proposed that nicotinamide adenine dinucleotide (NAD) may be an important regulator of sodium-dependent phosphate (P) transport across the proximal tubular brush border membrane (BBM). NAD appears to cause inhibition of P uptake by BBM vesicles _in vitro_, and the _in vivo_ administration of nicotinamide leads to phosphaturia[1]. The NAD effect on P-transport has been linked to ADP-ribosylation of the BBM[2].

The present study attempted to determine a) whether the inhibitory effect of NAD on P transport is specific or whether other adenine and guanine nucleotides have a similar effect and b) whether the effects of nucleotides are comparable in isolated BBM vesicles and in intact proximal tubules perfused _in vitro_.

Our results indicate that a variety of nucleotides cause apparent inhibition of ^{32}P uptake by BBM vesicles. However, the apparent "competitive inhibition" is due to hydrolysis of the nucleotides by BBM with release of free P. When the specific activity of ^{32}P was corrected for this change in P concentration, no inhibition was observed. In contrast to these results, micromolar concentrations of the nucleotides inhibited lumen-to-bath flux of P across isolated perfused proximal tubules. Thus, the described inhibitory effect of NAD on isolated BBM P transport is an artifact that can be observed with other P-containing nucleotides. On the other hand, luminal application of nucleotides inhibits P uptake in intact proximal tubular cells by mechanisms which, presumably, are not due to direct interaction with the BBM. These results have been reported previously by us[3].

Rabbit proximal straight tubules were perfused in vitro using standard techniques. BBM vesicles from rabbit renal cortex were prepared by a calcium precipitation method. The following compounds were tested: NAD, ADP-ribose, 5'AMP, ATP, ADP, and GDP.

Application of nucleotides (10^{-5} M) to the lumen of isolated perfused proximal straight tubules inhibited lumen-to-bath flux of 3.0 mM P by approximately 50%. A dose-response for ADP-ribose is shown in Figure 1. Similar results were obtained with NAD, ADP, and 5'AMP.

The effects of nucleotides were tested on isolated BBM vesicles. Initial rates of Na-dependent P uptake were determined and the two second uptake used for kinetic determinations. Figure 2a illustrates the effect of 0.1 mM NAD, ADP-ribose, and ADP on the kinetics of P uptake in the presence of a 100 mM NaCl gradient. The BBM were exposed to the nucleotides for 30 minutes prior to the uptake determination. Control experiments yielded a K_m of 0.22 mM and V_{max} of 31 nmol/mg·min. All the nucleotides increased

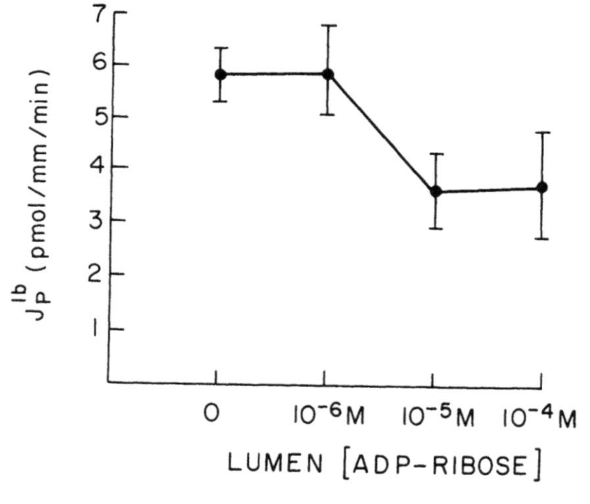

Figure 1. Effect of ADP-ribose in the perfusate on lumen-to-bath phosphate flux in isolated perfused proximal straight tubules (n = 5; mean ± SE).

K_m to 0.39 - 0.42 mM without altering V_{max}. This is consistent with "competitive inhibition." Similar effects were observed with ATP and GDP. In these experiments, the assumption was made by previous workers that the chemical phosphate concentration (and, hence, the specific activity of ^{32}P) remains constant throughout the experiment. When this was tested directly, however, it was found that a 30 minute incubation of BBM with nucleotides elevated the P concentration of the medium by 0.15 - 0.22 mM, indicating hydrolysis of the nucleotides. Similar results have been reported by Tenenhouse, et al.[4]. When the kinetics were recalculated using the corrected ^{32}P specific activity, no evidence for competitive inhibition could be found (Figure 2b).

Since BBM contains alkaline phosphatase, we examined whether the nucleotide hydrolysis was due to the activity of this enzyme. Alkaline phosphatase in BBM vesicles was inhibited 96% by 10 mM theophylline and ^{32}P uptake measured. The apparent inhibitory effects of NAD and ADP were still evident, suggesting that nucleotide hydrolysis proceeded even after inhibition of alkaline phos-

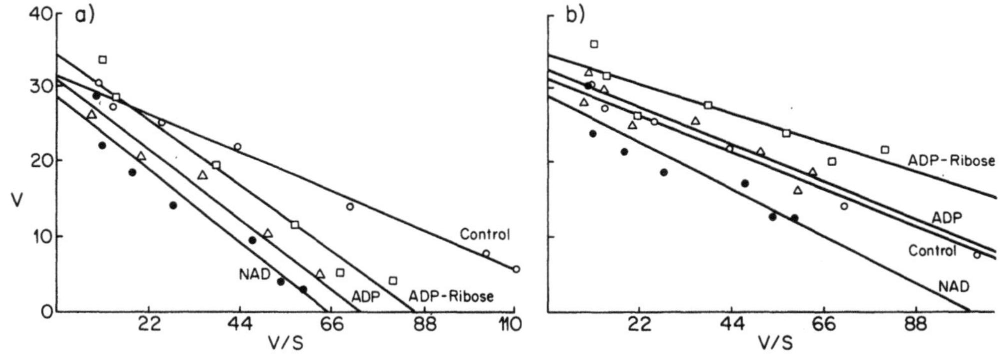

Figure 2. a) Eadie-Hofstee plot of P uptake at 2 seconds under control conditions and in the presence of 0.1 mM concentrations of NAD, ADP-ribose, and ADP. Studies were performed with a 100 mM NaCl gradient (out > in). Control:K_m 0.22 mM, V_{max} 31.2 nmol/mg·min; NAD:K_m 0.42 mM, V_{max} 27.7 nmol/mg·min; ADP-ribose:K_m 0.39 mM, V_{max} 34.1 nmol/mg·min; ADP:K_m 0.41 mM, V_{max} 30.6 nmol/mg·min. b) The same experiment after correction of ^{32}P specific activity for elevation in medium P concentration generated by nucleotides. NAD:K_m 0.28 mM, V_{max} 28.7 nmol/mg·min; ADP-ribose:K_m 0.18 mM, V_{max} 34.4 nmol/mg·min; ADP:K_m 0.23 mM, V_{max} 32.2 nmol/mg·min (mean values) (V = nmol/mg protein·min).

phatase activity. Thus, phosphatases other than alkaline phosphatase must be responsible for this process. The presence of non-specific phosphatase activity in the rabbit BBM has been described previously[5].

These studies indicate that a variety of nucleotides inhibit phosphate reabsorption by the proximal tubule when applied to the luminal surface. This is achieved at a concentration which is more than two orders of magnitude lower than the P concentration in the perfusate and, thus, is not consistent with simple competitive inhibition. Since studies on BBM indicate that inhibition does not occur by direct interaction of the nucleotides with the luminal membrane, some other mechanism must be sought. The fact that a wide variety of nucleotides exerts similar effects on P transport in the intact tubule minimizes the specific role which has been proposed for NAD as a regulator of P transport in the proximal tubule.

References

1. SA Kempson, G Colon-Otero, S-YL Ou, ST Turner, and T Dousa. Possible role of nicotinamide adenine dinucleotide as an intracellular regulator of renal transport of phosphate in the rat. J Clin Invest. 67:1347-1360 (1981).
2. MR Hammerman, VA Hansen, and JJ Morrisey. ADP-ribosylation of canine renal brush border membrane vesicle protein is associated with decreased phosphate transport. J Biol Chem. 257:12380-12386 (1982).
3. RP Lang, N Yanagawa, EP Nord, L Sakhrani, S Lee, and LG Fine. Nucleotide inhibition of phosphate transport in the renal proximal tubule. Am J Physiol. In Press (1983).
4. HS Tenenhouse and YL Chu. Hydrolysis of nicotinamide-adenine dinucleotide by purified renal brush border membranes. Biochem J. 204:635-638 (1982).
5. SG George and AJ Kenny. Studies on the enzymology of purified preparations of brush border from rabbit kidney. Biochem J. 134:43-57 (1973).

THE USEFULNESS OF ISOLATED RENAL CORTICAL CELLS TO STUDY PHOSPHATE TRANSPORT

Nicole Tessitore, Lakhi M. Sakhrani, and Shaul G. Massry

Division of Nephrology, University of Southern California, School of Medicine, Los Angeles, California

Much of the work on the metabolic support of transport in the kidney has utilized renal homogenates, renal slices and isolated renal tubules. However, these are not ideal systems because of their limited luminal access for transport and/or their anaerobic nature. Isolated perfused kidney and microperfused tubular segments have also been used for this purpose and do not have the above disadvantages. A useful additional tool is the use of isolated renal cells in suspension, in which access to luminal transporters and diffusion of oxygen would not be limiting.

Recently, it has been proposed that phosphate (P) transport in the kidney is metabolically regulated by gluconeogenesis (GNG) via cytosolic NAD^+ or $NAD^+/NADH$ ratio (1) and the isolated renal cells would allow a direct evaluation of this thesis.

Our study was undertaken with two aims in mind:
1) to evaluate the potential usefulness of the isolated cortical cells system by assessing its metabolic and functional viability;
2) to examine the role of GNG and cytosolic redox potential in regulating P transport.

Isolated cells were obtained from the rabbit kidney cortex, following the procedure by Heidrich and Dew (2-3). Briefly, New Zealand white male rabbits, 2 kg. were used. Kidney was perfused in situ with hypertonic Earle's solution supplemented with citrate, followed by perfusion with hypertonic Earle's solution with 2 mM $CaCl_2$. The kidney was then removed, the cortex was separated from medulla and minced. The mince was incubated for 5 minutes in hypertonic Earle's solution with calcium and then filtered sequentially through 250 μm and 60 μm meshes to get rid of tubules and debris. The filtrate was collected, washed and resuspended in the appropriate buffer. The resulting suspension consisted of cortical cells, 95% of which were single, with occasional clusters of 2-5 cells. The yield from two kidneys varied from 1 to 4 x 10^8 cells and from 8 to 14 mg. of protein. Glucose and ATP were measured with HK/G6PDH method (4). Protein was determined by the Comassie blue assay of Bradford (5), with bovine serum albumin as standard. Uptakes of ^{32}P-phosphate and ^{14}C-alpha-methylglucoside (AMG) were evaluated by a centrifugation method.

The criteria we used for the viability are summarized in Table I. The membrane of these cells are intact, as judged by the exclusion of trypan blue by more than 95% of these cells. ATP content is a useful measure of cell viability. Our values of 9.3± 0.7 nmole/mg protein are comparable to those reported in literature (6).

TABLE I: CRITERIA FOR VIABILITY OF THE ISOLATED RENAL CELLS

- Trypan blue exclusion 95%
- ATP content (n = 9): 9.3±0.7 nmole/mg protein
- Net glucose production with substrates
- Hormone responsiveness

The capacity for glucose production is an established property of the proximal tubule (7). Therefore, we tested the ability of these cells to make glucose with different substrates. Net glucose production rate with lactate, fumarate, succinate and pyruvate at 10 mM is 53.1±4.0, 87.4±4.3, 78.8±5.9 and 177.7±10.2 nmole/mg protein/hour respectively, values quantitatively similar to those reported in microdissected tubules (8) and isolated tubule suspension (9) from the rabbit.

The kidney is a target organ of many hormones and accordingly we evaluated the capacity of our cells to respond to various agonists. Isoproterenol (10^{-6}M), 1,34 bovine PTH (10 µ/ml) and DBcAMP (10^{-4} M) increased the glucose production with 10 mM lactate by 65%, 47% and 44% respectively, as has been described for the isolated cortical tubules (10-11).

The time courses of phosphate and AMG uptakes by these cells was also studied. The transport of both solutes is highly Na dependent and is linear up to 3-5 minutes. In the early time points, the Na-independent uptake accounts for less than 12% of the total uptake for phosphate and less than 6% for AMG. Similar data are obtained with AMG when 0.1 mM phlorizin is used.

Since both glucose and P are reabsorbed in the proximal tubule via a Na-coupled transport system located in the brush border membrane and since the uptakes across the basolateral membrane are Na-independent (12-13), our data show that the great bulk of P and AMG transport is across the luminal membrane of proximal cells.

The role of cytosolic redox potential as an intracellular regulator of P transport (1) was tentatively evaluated by clamping the cytosolic redox potential in the oxidized or reduced state induced by changing the extracellular pyruvate/lactate ratio, as has been done in the liver (14). No difference in P uptake was found in presence of 5 mM pyruvate and 5 mM lactate (3.9±-0.4 and 3.4± 0.3 nmole/mg protein/2 min respectively), suggesting that the transport of P is independent of changes in cytosolic redox potential.

In order to evaluate the role of GNG in regulating P transport, P uptake was evaluated in a situation in which either GNG was stimulated by 5 mM succinate or inhibited by 1 mM 3-mercaptopicolonic acid (3MPC), a specific inhibitor of PEPCK (15) (TABLE III). In these experimental conditions, P uptake was stimulated by 52% by succinate and the presence of 3MPC did not modify the effect of the substrate. To exclude an effect of 3MPC other than that on GNG, it should be noted that the inhibitor of GNG had no effect on P transport in substrate-free conditions.

Table II: EFFECT OF GLUCONEOGENESIS ON PHOSPHATE UPTAKE

	Net glucose production (nmole/mg protein/h)	P uptake (% of control)
Substrate Free	n.d.	100±14
Substrate Free + 3MPC	n.d.	100±12
Succinate 5 mM	17.2±1.4	152± 8
Succinate 5 mM + 3MPC	1.7±1.7	160± 5

Several conclusions can be drawn from this study:
1) Isolated cortical cells in suspension retain metabolic and functional viability, as assessed by a number of criteria. This provide a useful additional tool for studies of renal physiology.
2) The changes in cytosolic redox potential do not influence P transport.
3) No cause and effect relationship between GNG and P transport is shown.

REFERENCES

1. S.A. Kempson, A. Colon-Otero, S.L. Ou, T.P. Dousa, Possible role of nicotinamide-adenine dinucleotide (NAD) as an intracellular regulator of renal phosphate transport, J. Clin. Inv. 67:1347 (1981).
2. H.G. and M.E. Dew, Homogeneous cell population from rabbit kidney cortex, J. Cell. Biol. 74:780, 1977.
3. A. Vandewalle, B. Kopfer-Hobelsberger, H.G. Heidrich, Cortical cell populations from rabbit kidney isolated by free-flow electrophoresis: Characterization by measurement of hormone-sensitive adenylate cyclase, J. Cell. Biol. 92:505 (1982).
4. P.K. Maitra and R.W. Estabrook, A fluorometric method for the enzymic determination of glycolytic intermediates, Anal. Biochem. 7:472 (1964).

5. M.M. Bradford, A rapid and sensitive method for the quantitation of micrograms quantities of protein utilizing the principle of protein-dye binding, Anal. Chem. 72:248 (1976).
6. R.S. Balaban, S.P. Soltoff, J.M. Storey, L.J. Mandel, Improved renal cortical tubule suspension: Spectrophotometric study of O_2 delivery, Am. J. Physiol. 238:F50, (1980).
7. U. Schmidt and W.G. Guder, Sites of enzyme activity along the nephron, Kidney Int. 9:233 (1976).
8. A. Maleque, H. Endou, C. Koseki, F. Sakai, Nephron heterogeneity: Gluconeogenesis from pyruvate in rabbit nephron, Febs Lett. 116:154 (1980).
9. S.R. Gullans, P.C. Brazy, V.W. Dennis, L.J. Mandel, Interaction between gluconeogenesis and sodium transport in the proximal tubule, Kidney Int. 23:223 (1983).
10. W.G. Guder and O.H. Wieland, Metabolism of isolated kidney tubules. Additive effects of parathyroid hormone and free-fatty acids on renal gluconeogenesis, Eur. J. Biochem. 31: 69 (1972).
11. K. Kurokawa and S.G. Massry, Evidence for stimulation of renal gluconeogenesis by catecholamines, J. Clin. Inv. 52: 961 (1973).
12. R. Kinne, H. Murer, E. Kinne-Safran, M. Thees, G. Sachs, Sugar transport by renal plasma membrane vesicles. Characterization of the systems in the brush-broder microvilli and basal-lateral plasma membranes, J. Memb. Biol. 21:375 (1975).
13. N. Hoffman, M. Thees, R. Kinne, Phosphate transport by isolated renal brush border vesicles, Pflug. Arch. 362:147 (1976).
14. T. Bucher and H. Sies, Mitochondrial and cytosolic redox states in perfused rat liver: Methods and problems in metabolic compartmentation in "Use of isolated liver cells and kidney tubules in metabolic studies", Eds: J.M. Tager, H.D. Soling, J.R. Williamson. Amsterdam, p. 41 (1975).
15. N.W. Di Tullio, C.E. Berkoff, B. Blank, V. Kostos, E.J. Stack, H.L. Saunders, 3-Mercaptopicolinic acid, an inhibitor of gluconeogenesis, Biochem. J. 138:387 (1974).

CALCIUM (Ca) MEDIATED PHOSPHATE (PO4) TRANSPORT IN THE PROXIMAL CONVOLUTED TUBULE (PCT) OF THE RABBIT

Diane Rouse and Wadi N. Suki

Baylor College of Medicine and The Methodist Hospital

Houston, Texas

INTRODUCTION

Several clearance studies have suggested a direct effect of calcium (Ca) on phosphate (PO4) handling by the kidney. Micropuncture studies by Amiel and colleagues[1] have shown enhancement of fractional phosphate reabsorption in the proximal convoluted tubule when plasma calcium was raised from low towards normal values in parathyroidectomized rats. Conversely, Goldfarb et al [2] have shown a decline in fractional phosphate reabsorption in this portion of the nephron with the induction of mild hypercalcemia in thyroparathyroidectomized dogs. The divergence of these results may be due to species differences, the level of plasma phosphate or ionized calcium before and after calcium chloride administration, or the other various indirect effects of calcium on phosphate handling by the nephron.

The purpose of the present study was to examine the effect of calcium on phosphate reabsorption in proximal tubule segments using the isolated tubule microperfusion technique. In this way the indirect effects of calcium could be avoided.

METHODS

Segments of superficial (SF) and juxtamedullary (JM) proximal straight (S3) or convoluted (S2) tubule segments were isolated from New Zealand white female rabbits maintained on a normal phosphate diet. The tubules were mounted for perfusion by the method of Burg, et al [3] within 30 minutes of sacrifice of the animal. An artificial solution which mimicked ultrafiltrate of plasma was used to perfuse and bathe the tubule segments. The solutions were symmetrical except for the addition of ^{3}Hmethoxy inulin and ^{32}P to the perfusate for the measurement of fluid absorption (Jv) and lumen-to-bath phosphate flux, respectively. Fetal calf serum was added to the bath in the final concentration of 5% v/v. The pH and PCO_2 of all solutions was maintained by gassing and the temperature regulated to 38°C. Potential difference (PD) was measured using agarose-Ringer's bridges and calomel half cells.

Five groups of tubules were studied.

Group I: Lumen-to-bath PO4 flux was measured in SF and JM proximal straight tubule (PST) segments with normal bath and perfusate ionized Ca, 1.3 mM, and high bath and perfusate ionized Ca, 2.5mM.

Group II: The same protocol as in Group I was repeated in SF and JM proximal convoluted tubule (PCT) segments.

Group III: Lumen-to-bath PO4 flux was measured in SF and JM PCT segments with normal bath and perfusate ionized Ca, 1.3 mM, and low bath and perfusate ionized Ca, 0.2mM.

Group IV: Lumen-to-bath PO4 flux was measured in SF and JM PCT segments using normal ionized Ca in the bath and perfusate before and after the addition of the calcium ionophore A21394 to both solutions to the final concentration of 5×10^{-6} M.

Group V: The protocol in Group IV was repeated except trifluoperazine was added to the bath and perfusate in the concentration of 10^{-4} or 10^{-5} M.

Tubule segments were perfused at 19-25 nl/min.

RESULTS

Raising bath and perfusate ionized Ca had no effect on Jv, PD or lumen-to-bath PO4 flux in PST segments (Group I). In PCT segments (Group II) Jv and PD remained unchanged when bath and perfusate ionized Ca was raised, however lumen-to-bath PO4 flux significantly increased. When bath and perfusate ionized Ca was lowered from 1.3 to 0.2 mM (Group III) there was a significant increase in Jv, no change in PD and a significant decline in lumen-to-bath PO4 flux.

Increasing intracellular ionized Ca with the addition of ionophore (Group IV) caused a significant increase in Jv, fall in PD but no significant change in lumen-to-bath PO4 flux. Decreasing the intracellular Ca-calmodulin complex with trifluoperazine (Group V) caused a significant decline in Jv but no significant change in PD or lumen-to-bath PO4 flux.

CONCLUSIONS

The results of these studies demonstrate a direct effect of calcium on phosphate reabsorption in PCT segments. Increasing ambient ionized Ca enhances unidirectional efflux and lowering ambient ionized Ca inhibits the efflux. The level of calcium has no influence on unidirectional efflux in PST segments. The effect of calcium on phosphate transport in PCT segments does not appear to be mediated by changes in cytosolic ionized Ca alone although fluid absorption does appear to be influenced by cytosolic ionized Ca levels.

REFERENCES

1. C. Amiel, H. Kuntziger, S. Couette, C. Coureau, and N. Bergounioux, Evidence for a parathyroid hormone-induced calcium modulation of phosphate transport along the nephron, J. Clin. Invest. 57:256 (1976).
2. S. Goldfarb, P. Bosanac, M. Goldberg, and Z.S. Agus, Effects of calcium on renal tubular phosphate reabsorption, Am. J. Physiol. 234(1):F22 (1978).
3. M. Burg, J. Grantham, M. Abramow, and J. Orloff, Preparation and study of fragments of single rabbit nephrons. Am. J. Physiol. 210:1293 (1966).

GLUCOCORTICOID-INDUCED INHIBITION OF THE REABSORPTION OF INORGANIC PHOSPHATE IN THE PROXIMAL TUBULE IN THE ABSENCE OF PARATHYROID HORMONE

Anselm Frick, Ivan Durasin, and Mechtild Neuweg

Department of Physiology
University of Munich
Munich, Federal Republic of Germany

Roberts and Pitts (1) demonstrated a reduction of the maximal reabsorptive capacity for inorganic phosphate (Tm_{Pi}) due to cortisone administration in dogs. For different reasons we reexamined this effect in the rat (2) and confirmed the former observation both in the presence and the absence of parathyroid hormone. In order to localize this glucocorticoid effect in the nephron we employed the micropuncture techniques. Our results from proximal convolutions together with the data from the whole kidney suggest an important proximal locus of action of hydrocortisone in the Pi-transport.

Methods

Adult female Sprague-Dawley rats kept on a standard diet (Altromin; 0.90 g Ca and 0.80 g Pi/100 g diet) were anaesthetized with Inactin (Byk-Gulden, FRG) intraperitoneally and parathyroidectomized (PTX) by cauterisation under microscopic inspection 3 h before the micropuncture.

Two groups were studied: 1.) Control: PTX (n=12), and 2.) Experimental: PTX + Hydrocortisone (Hoechst, FRG) (n=10). The dose of hydrocortisone was 0.03 mg/min per rat and was begun 90 min before the micropuncture and was continued throughout the experiments. A similar pharmacological dose was also used by other investigators (3,4). Besides of the infusion of inulin, all animals were infused i.v. with a modified Ringer solution (Ringer phase). Subsequently the infusion solution was changed containing inorganic phosphate to achieve Tm_{Pi} values (Pi-Ringer phase). The infusion rate was 0.15 ml/min.

After the general surgery the left kidney was exposed through an abdominal incision and carefully placed in a Plexiglas cup (5) and prepared for the micropuncture. The rat temperature was maintained at 37°C with a heated animal board. The details of micropuncture techniques have been described previously (6,7). Tubular fluid samples were obtained from the end of the proximal convolution of superficial nephrons localized by the linear flow of lissamine green according to the method of Steinhausen (8) and Gertz (9). The microsamples were collected quantitatively. The volume of the microsamples was measured and the concentrations of inulin and inorganic phosphate were determined with the anthrone method (10) and the phosphomolybdate method (11), respectively. The details of the microdetermination were described previously (6).

Results and Discussion

In Tables 1 - 3 the results with hydrocortisone from the whole kidney and the proximal tubule are given. The glucocorticoid effect on the reabsorption of inorganic phosphate was seen during the Ringer and the Pi-Ringer phases. During normal concentrations of Pi in plasma (Table 2) and during elevated Pi levels (Table 1, 3) the inhibition of the reabsorption of Pi was documented. Both the absolute reabsorption of Pi/sngfr and the fractional reabsorption of Pi along the proximal convolution were decreased during hydrocortisone infusion. Thus in the absence of parathyroid hormone a glucocorticoid-induced inhibitory effect on the reabsorption of inorganic phosphate in the proximal tubule was found.

Table 1. Effects of Hydrocortisone In PTX Rats During Phosphate-Ringer (Clearance Data)

	Control (n=12)	Hydrocortisone (n=10)	P
b.w. (g)	244 ± 10	242 ± 8	n.s.
GFR (ml/min)	2.99 ± 0.51	2.89 ± 0.23	n.s.
V_{Ur} (ml/min)	0.09 ± 0.04	0.15 ± 0.03	< 0.005
$[Ca]_P$ (mEq/l)	2.32 ± 0.24	2.25 ± 0.23	n.s.
$[Pi]_P$ (mmol/l)	5.54 ± 0.30	4.70 ± 0.28	< 0.001
FE_{Pi} (%)	28.5 ± 8.2	42.3 ± 4.1	< 0.001

Abbreviations: b.w. = body weight; P = plasma; FE = fractional excretion. (Mean values ± S.D.)

Table 2. Effects of Hydrocortisone In PTX Rats During Ringer (Proximal Convolution)

	Control (n=12)	Hydrocortisone (n=10)	P
$(TF/P)_{In}$	1.83 ± 0.31	1.56 ± 0.36	< 0.05
sngfr (nl/min)	38.5 ± 10.9	43.5 ± 11.1	n.s.
$[Pi]_P$ (mmol/l)	2.28 ± 0.18	2.20 ± 0.25	n.s.
$(TF/P)_{Pi}$	0.10 ± 0.06	0.26 ± 0.13	< 0.001
$\frac{(TF/P)_{Pi}}{(TF/P)_{In}}$	0.05 ± 0.03	0.18 ± 0.11	< 0.001
Pi-reabs. (pmol/min)	87.3 ± 23.8	78.5 ± 26.1	n.s.
$\frac{\text{Pi-reabs.}}{\text{sngfr}}$ (pmol/nl)	2.19 ± 0.21	1.79 ± 0.32	< 0.001

Abbreviations: TF = tubular fluid collected from the end of proximal convolutions; P = plasma; sngfr = single nephron glomerular filtration rate; $(TF/P)_{Pi}/(TF/P)_{In}$ = fractional delivery of Pi to the loop of Henle. (Mean values ± S.D.)

From the analysis of these data obtained from the proximal tubule and the whole kidney we get indirect information regarding the distal nephron: In the Pi-Ringer phases (Table 1, 3) control animals showed a fractional reabsorption of Pi along the proximal convolution of 41% of the filtered load and an overall fractional reabsorption of 71%, yielding a fractional reabsorption of 30% for later segments. In the experimental animals the reabsorption of Pi along the proximal convolution was 29% and the overall fractional reabsorption was 58%; again a difference of 29% for later segments was found. Thus although we cannot exclude an effect of hydrocortisone on distal phosphate transport, our results suggest that the primary site of action is the proximal tubule.

A proximal locus of action is also supported by the results of Mishina et al. (12), who found a higher content of glucocorticoid receptors in the proximal than in the distal tubule. Furthermore, the studies of Freiberg et al. (13) and of Turner and coworkers (14) using dexamethasone and triamcinolone, respectively, demonstrated an inhibition of the Na dependent specific transport of phosphate (15) in the proximal brush border vesicles. Dousa

Table 3. Effects of Hydrocortisone In PTX Rats During Phosphate-Ringer (Proximal Convolution)

	Control (n=12)	Hydrocortisone (n=10)	P
$(TF/P)_{In}$	1.63 ± 0.22	1.51 ± 0.27	n.s.
sngfr (nl/min)	40.9 ± 7.1	43.8 ± 9.9	n.s.
$[Pi]_P$ (mmol/l)	5.54 ± 0.30	4.70 ± 0.28	< 0.001
$(TF/P)_{Pi}$	0.93 ± 0.13	1.03 ± 0.09	< 0.025
$\frac{(TF/P)_{Pi}}{(TF/P)_{In}}$	0.59 ± 0.09	0.71 ± 0.12	< 0.01
Pi-reabs. (pmol/min)	95.1 ± 29.5	59.7 ± 28.2	< 0.005
$\frac{\text{Pi-reabs.}}{\text{sngfr}}$ (pmol/nl)	2.34 ± 0.59	1.35 ± 0.54	< 0.001

Abbreviations: See Table 2. (Mean values ± S.D.)

suggests that the glucocorticoid-induced decrease of the luminal Pi uptake may correlate with an increase of the rate of the renal cytoplasmic gluconeogenesis and an elevated content of NAD^+ in renal cortical slices (14).

In summary, the present <u>in-vivo</u> experiments demonstrate that glucocorticoids can inhibit the renal Pi transport even in the absence of parathyroid hormone and provide evidence that the important nephron site for this effect is the proximal tubule.

Acknowledgement

This work was supported by a grant from the Deutsche Forschungsgemeinschaft (Fr. 239/8 and 239/9-1).

The authors gratefully acknowledge the expert technical assistance of Miss R. Kagerer and Miss E. Sereda. Dr. J.P. Briggs assisted with language editing and Mrs. K. Schaipp gave secretarial assistance.

References

1. K. E. Roberts and R. F. Pitts. The effects of cortisone and desoxycorticosterone on the renal tubular reabsorption of phosphate and the excretion of titrable acid and potassium in dogs. Endocrinology 52:324-330 (1953)
2. A. Frick, I. Durasin, and M. Neuweg. Phosphaturic response of hydrocortisone in the presence and the absence of parathyroid hormone. Pflügers Arch. 392:99-105 (1981)
3. G. Peters. Der Einfluß von Nebennierenrindenhormonen auf die renale Wasser- und Elektrolytausscheidung bei adrenalektomierten und normalen Ratten nach Gabe von Wasser oder isotonischer NaCl-Lösung und im Durst. Naunyn-Schmiedeberg's Arch.exp.Path.u.Pharmak. 235:155-184 (1959)
4. M. Wiederholt, H. Stolte, J. P. Brecht, and K. Hierholzer. Mikropunktionsuntersuchungen über den Einfluß von Aldosteron, Cortison und Dexamethason auf die renale Natriumresorption adrenalektomierter Ratten. Pflügers Arch. 292:316-333 (1966)
5. H. Wirz. Der osmotische Druck in den cortikalen Tubuli der Rattenniere. Helv.Physiol.Pharmacol.Acta 14:353 (1956)
6. A. Frick. Proximal tubular reabsorption of inorganic phosphate during saline infusion in the rat. Am.J.Physiol. 223:1034-1040 (1972)
7. A. Frick and I. Durasin. Proximal tubular reabsorption of inorganic phosphate in adrenalectomized rats. Pflügers Arch. 385:189-192 (1980)
8. M. Steinhausen. Eine Methode zur Differenzierung proximaler und distaler Tubuli der Nierenrinde von Ratten in vivo und ihre Anwendung zur Bestimmung tubulärer Strömungsgeschwindigkeiten. Arch.Ges.Physiol. 277:23-35 (1963)
9. K. H. Gertz, J. A. Mangos, G. Braun, and H. D. Pagel. On the glomerular tubular balance in the rat kidney. Arch.Ges. Physiol. 285:360-372 (1965)
10. H. H. Hilger, J. D. Klümper, and K. J. Ullrich. Wasserrückresorption und Ionentransport durch die Sammelrohrzellen der Säugetierniere. Arch.Ges.Physiol. 267:218-237 (1958)
11. P. S. Chen, Jr., T. Y. Toribara, and H. Warner. Microdetermination of phosphorus. Anal.Chem. 28:1756-1758 (1956)
12. T. Mishina, D. W. Scholer, and I. S. Edelman. Glucocorticoid receptors in rat kidney cortical tubules enriched in proximal and distal segments. Am.J.Physiol. 240:F 38-45 (1981)
13. J. M. Freiberg, J. Kinsella, and B. Sacktor. Glucocorticoids increase the Na^+-H^+ exchange and decrease the Na^+ gradient-dependent phosphate-uptake systems in renal brush border membrane vesicles. Proc.Natl.Acad.Sci.USA 79:4932-4936 (1982)

14. S. T. Turner, G. M. Kiebzak, and T. P. Dousa. Mechanism of glucocorticoid effect on renal transport of phosphate. Am.J.Physiol. 243:C227-C236 (1982)
15. N. Hoffmann, M. Thees, and R. Kinne. Phosphate transport by isolated renal brush border vesicles. Pflügers Arch. 362: 147-156 (1976)

EFFECT OF 1,25-DIHYDROXYCHOLECALCIFEROL ON THE EXTRARENAL HANDLING OF INORGANIC PHOSPHATE IN THYROPARATHYROIDECTOMIZED BUT NOT IN INTACT RATS

Ulrich Troehler, Jean-Philippe Bonjour* and Herbert Fleisch

Department of Pathophysiology, University of Bern, Murtenstrasse 35, CH - 3010 Bern, and
*Division of Pathophysiology, Dept. of Medicine Hôpital cantonal, CH - 1211 Geneva 4
Switzerland

1,25-dihydroxycholecalciferol ($1,25(OH)_2D_3$) and parathyroid hormone have been shown to act on fluxes of inorganic phosphate (Pi) in bone and gut levels[1-6] and directly or indirectly in the kidney. These effects influence the level of Pi in the extracellular space (ECS).

In the present paper we have investigated whether parathyroidectomy and $1,25(OH)_2D_3$ have also an effect on the retention of Pi outside the extracellular space, i.e. intracellularly and/or in bone mineral ($RICB_{Pi}$).

In order to assess such an effect on extrarenal handling of Pi, we have determined $RICB_{Pi}$ using acute intravenous infusions of Pi as follows:

In a first set of experiments, three groups of rats were studied, namely sham-operated (SHAM), thyroparathyroidectomized (TPTX) and TPTX rats treated with $1,25(OH)_2D_3$ (26 pmoles/day i.p. for one week; TPTX + $1,25(OH)_2D_3$). All TPTX rats were supplemented with thyroxin at a dose of 4 µg injected s.c. three times weekly. On the experimental day, rats were infused first either Pi (SHAM and TPTX + $1,25(OH)_2D_3$) or NaCl (TPTX) in order to adjust their endogenous $[Pi]_{Pl}$.

to levels of about 3.50 mM comparable between the experimental groups. They were then further infused known amounts of Pi designed to rise $[Pi]_{Pl.}$ by about .50 mM over 45 min, in all three groups. The amount of Pi excreted in the urine in excess of base line values and $[Pi]_{Pl.}$ before and after the two infusions were measured. Thus, $RICB_{Pi}$ could be calculated for a given $[Pi]_{Pl.}$ independently of any effect which the experimental manoeuvres have on the renal excretion of Pi: it results as the difference between the amount of Pi infused and the increased amount excreted in the urine due to Pi infusion minus the increased quantity retained in ECS due to the infusion ($RICB_{Pi} = Pi_{Inf} - \uparrow Pi_U - \uparrow Pi_{ECS}$). The exact setting of the conditions of $[Pi]_{Pl}$ was important in order to exclude any effect of $[Pi]_{Pl.}$ on $RICB_{Pi}$.

Results show that $RICB_{Pi}$ was markedly diminished in TPTX as compared to sham-operated rats. This decrease was corrected by $1,25(OH)_2D_3$ treatment. Since, as expected, endogenous plasma calcium concentration ($[Ca]_{Pl.}$) was markedly lower in TPTX rats than in both their sham-operated and TPTX counterparts treated with $1,25(OH)_2D_3$, the question arises whether this difference plays a role in the effects of parathyroidectomy and $1,25(OH)_2D_3$ on $RICB_{Pi}$.

In a second set of experiments we thus studied whether chronic alteration of $[Ca]_{Pl.}$, as achieved by varying dietary Ca intake, also influenced extrarenal handling of Pi. The studies were performed in TPTX rats supplemented with $1,25(OH)_2D_3$ (26 pmoles/day i.p. for 6 days). Despite this treatment, $[Ca]_{Pl.}$ remained significantly lower in the animals on a low Ca diet (0.1 %) for one week than in those fed a high Ca diet (1.20 %) and $RICB_{Pi}$ in the hypocalcemic group was about half the value observed in the normocalcemic rats.

Thus, it is possible that the effect of $1,25(OH)_2D_3$ in hypoparathyroid rats is due to the rise in calcemia brought about by the vitamin D metabolite. In order to further substantiate this possibility, we investigated in a third series of experiments the influence of $1,25(OH)_2D_3$ in a situation with normal PTH status and where $1,25(OH)_2D_3$ at the dose effective in TPTX rats had no effect on $[Ca]_{Pl.}$, i.e. in SHAM operated rats. Indeed, $1,25(OH)_2D_3$ did not significantly change $RICB_{Pi}$ in this condition.

Knowing the effects of parathyroidectomy and $1,25(OH)_2D_3$ as well as of plasma Ca level on renal tubular capacity to reabsorb Pi, it was interesting to put the present findings on extrarenal handling of Pi in parallel with our earlier observations on renal handling of Pi made in the same conditions[7,8]. This comparison yielded in fact an inverse relationship between the effects of parathryoidectomy, $1,25(OH)_2D_3$ and $[Ca]_{Pi}$ on $RICB_{Pi}$ and those on maximal tubular reabsorption of Pi (TmPi/ml GF). Furthermore, the non-effect of $1,25(OH)_2D_3$ on $RICB_{Pi}$ in SHAM rats was paralleled by no change in TmPi/ml GF[7]. With respect to this finding it is noteworthy that there seems to be no species difference since reports in the literature show that the decrease in TmPi/ml GF could only be observed in hypoparathyroid but not in euparathryoid patients[9-11].

In summary, parathyroidectomy decreases net retention of intravenously infused Pi outside the extracellular space, i.e. intracellularly and/or in bone mineral, wheras $1,25(OH)_2D_3$ and/or chronic rise in calcemia enhance $RICB_{Pi}$. The effect of $1,25(OH)_2D_3$ can be seen in TPTX but not SHAM rats. In our conditions the effect of the D-metabolite might well be mediated through its rising the plasma calcium concentration. There is, furthermore a relationship between the extrarenal and the renal tubular effects of parathyroidectomy, $1,25(OH)_2D_3$ and ($[Ca]_{Pl.}$). This relationship leads to the speculation that parathyroidectomy, $1,25(OH)_2D_3$ and/or $[Ca]_{Pl.}$ act on both extrarenal and renal targets in the same manner. Alternatively, there might be a causal relationship between the extrarenal and renal effects as suggested earlier[12,13]. These experiments show that much remains to be learned about the relation of extrarenal and renal handling of Pi.

REFERENCES

1. L. Castillo, Y. Tanaka, and H.F. DeLuca, The mobilization of bone mineral by 1,25-dihydroxyvitamin D_3 in hypophosphatemic rats, Endocrinology 97: 995-999 (1975).

2. D.B.N. Lee, M.W. Walling, U. Gafter, V. Silis, and J.W. Coburn, Calcium and inorganic phosphate transport in rat colon. Dissociated response to 1,25-dihydroxyvitamin D_3, J. Clin. Invest. 65: 1326-1331 (1980).

3.. R.R. Recker, S.G. Massry, J.R. Lau, and P.D. Saville, The hyperphosphatemic effect of disodium ethane-1-hydroxy-1,1-diphosphonate (EHDP^{TM}): renal handling of phosphorus and the renal response to parathyroid hormone, J. Lab. Clin. Med. 81: 258-266 (1973).

4. R. Rizzoli, H. Fleisch, and J.-P. Bonjour, Role of 1,25-dihydroxyvitamin D_3 on intestinal phosphate absorption in rats with a normal vitamin D supply, J. Clin. Invest. 60: 639-647 (1977).

5. M.W. Walling, Intestinal calcium and phosphate transport: differential responses in vitamin D_3 and D_3 metabolites, Am. J. Physiol. 233: E488-E494 (1977).

6. T.H. Steele, J.E. Engle, Y. Tanaka, R.S. Lorenc, K.L. Dudgeon, and H.F. DeLuca, Phosphatemic action of 1,25-dihydroxyvitamin D_3, Am. J. Physiol. 229: 489-495 (1975).

7. J.-P. Bonjour, C. Preston, and H. Fleisch, Effect of 1,25-dihydroxyvitamin D_3 on the renal handling of Pi in thyroparathyroidectomized rats, J.Clin. Invest. 60: 1419-1428 (1977).

8. J.-P. Bonjour, and H. Fleisch, Calcium supply and renal handling of phosphate, Min.Electrol.Metab. 3: 261-267 (1980).

9. M. Davies, C.M. Taylor, L.F. Hill, and S.W. Stanbury, 1,25-Dihydroxycholecalciferol in hypoparathyroidism, Lancet i, 55-59 (1977).

10. J.F. Rosen, A.R. Fleischman, L. Finberg, J. Eisman, and H.F. DeLuca, 1,25-dihydroxycholecalciferol: its use in the long-term management of idiopathic hypoparathyroidism in children, J. Clin. Endocrinol. 45: 457-468 (1977).

11. J. Lemann jr,, W.J. Maierhofer, N.D. Adams, and R.W. Gray, Increased serum 1,25(OH)$_2$D$_3$ concentrations fails to affect serum or urine phosphate in humans, in: Regulation of phosphate and mineral, S.G. Massry, J.M. Letteri and E. Ritz (eds.) Plenum, New York and London (1982).

12. J.-P. Bonjour, U. Tröhler, R. Mühlbauer, C. Preston and H. Fleisch, Is there a bone-kidney link in the homeostasis of inorganic phosphate (Pi)? in: Phosphate Metabolism (Vol. 81 in Advances in Experimental Medicine and Biology). Proc. 2nd International Workshop on Phosphate, Heidelberg, 1976. S.G. Massry and E. Ritz, eds. Plenum Press, New York - London, (1977), pp. 319-322.

13. J.-P. Bonjour, J. Caverzasio, R. Mühlbauer, H. Fleisch, and U. Trechsel, Acute and chronic effects of vitamin D metabolites on the renal handling of phosphate, in: Vitamin D, Basic Research and its Clinical Application, A.W. Norman, K. Schaefer, D. v. Herrath, H.-G. Grigoleit, J.W. Coburn, H.F. DeLuca, E.B. Mawer and T. Suda, eds. W. de Gruyter, Berlin (1979), pp. 307-314.

EARLY RENAL ADAPTATION TO DIETARY PHOSPHORUS RESTRICTION

Barton S. Levine, Kiyoshi Kurokawa, and Jack W. Coburn

Nephrology Division, Research and Medical Services, VA Wadsworth Medical Center and Department of Medicine UCLA School of Medicine, Los Angeles, California 90073

INTRODUCTION

An important consequence of dietary phosphorus (P) restriction is the ability of the kidney to virtually clear the urine of phosphate (Pi) (1). This adaptation can occur in the normal, thyroparathyroidectomized (1), and vitamin D-deficient state (2). The adaptation has been demonstrated in isolated perfused proximal tubules (3) as well as in vesicles formed by tubule brush border membranes (BBM) of proximal tubules (4, 5), and has been demonstrated as early as two days in renal BBM of the pig (6). The underlying mechanism for this renal adaptation is unknown. Several reports have suggested that an increased alkaline phosphatase (AlPase) in the BBM is responsible for increased Pi reabsorption during P-depletion (4, 5). Other studies suggest that the adaptation may occur without concomitant changes in AlPase and there is no causal relationship between the two phenomena (7, 8, 9). The present study was designed to assess how rapid renal adaptation by BBM vesicles (BBMV) to dietary P-restriction develops and whether significant changes in BBM AlPase activity occur prior to changes in BBMV Pi transport. The results demonstrate that Pi uptake by the BBMV increases within 4 hours after dietary P restriction preceding any detectable increase in the AlPase.

MATERIALS AND METHODS

Male Sprague-Dawley rats, weighing between 150-175 grams were used. For 3 days prior to the day of study, rats were fed a diet of normal P (+P) content (0.6% P) between 8 a.m. and noon only. At 8 a.m. on the morning of the experiment the rats were divided into 3 groups; group 1 rats were given a low P (-P) diet (0.03% P), group 2 rats were given the +P diet, and no food was given to group 3 rats (fasted). The animals were allowed free access to distilled water throughout the experiment. After 4 hours, the amount of food eaten was determined and the animals anesthetized with pentobarbital, 40 mg/kg, and arterial blood samples were obtained from the abdominal aorta. The kidneys were rapidly excised and the BBMV was obtained as described below. In additional experiments, rats were given either the -P or +P diet for 1, 3 or 14 days. The +P rats in the 3 and 14 day experiments were pair-fed with their -P counterparts. Phosphate was measured in serum and urine using an Autoanalyzer (Technicon). Serum and urine creatinine levels were measured by a Beckman Creatinine Analyzer (Beckman Instruments, Inc., Fullerton, CA). Blood pH and pCO_2 were measured on blood gas analyzer IL-213 (Instrumentation Lab, Lexington, MA) and plasma bicarbonate was calculated utilizing the standard Henderson-Hasselbach equation.

The BBMV were prepared using the method of Beck and Sacktor (10) with modifications. The renal cortex was minced and then homogenized in 320 mM sorbitol, pH 7.5 (1 gm/8 ml), using a Polytron Homogenizer at 27,000 rpm for 20 sec and 15 strokes/specimen. $CaCl_2$ was then added at a final concentration of 10 mM) to the pooled homogenate, which was stirred for 15 min, and centrifuged at 1,500 x g for 5 min. The resultant supernate was then centrifuged at 35,000 x g for 20 min; the pellet was resuspended in 320 mM sorbitol and recentrifuged at 35,000 x g for 20 min. The final pellet was then resuspended in 320 mM sorbitol to give a protein concentration of approximately 2 mg/ml. All the above steps were performed at 0-4°C.

Transport studies were done using standard millipore filtration techniques (11). Briefly, 50 ul of the vesicle suspension were added to 100 ul of uptake solution, pH 7.5 at 22°C. The final incubation medium contained 100 mM NaCl, 0.1 mM $K_2H^{32}PO_4$ (1 uCi/tube) and 120 mM sorbitol. For glucose transport, K_2HPO_4 was replaced with 0.1 mM U-^{14}C-D-glucose (1 uCi/tube). The reaction was stopped by adding 800 ul of ice-cold 320 mM sorbitol and rapidly filtering through a 0.45 um millipore filter. After washing with 4 ml of ice-cold 320 mM sorbitol, the filter was placed in BioFluor scintillation liquid (New England Nuclear, Boston, MA) and counted for radioactivity by a liquid scintillation counter. Values obtained at time zero by adding vesicles to the stop solution were used to indicate non-specific binding to the filter rather than transport and were subtracted from experimental values. Statistical analyses were done using paired or unpaired t-tests as appropriate (12).

Activities of various marker enzymes were assayed to identify and establish the purity of BBM preparations. To measure AlPase activity, samples were diluted with 320 mM sorbitol to a protein concentration that assurred zero order kinetics. The samples were then placed in assay buffer and preincubated at 37°C for 15 min. The reaction was started by the addition of the substrate, P-nitrophenol phosphate. The final reaction medium (pH 9.5) consists of 10 mM $MgCl_2$, 0.5 mM $CaCl_2$, 0.5 mM $ZnCl_2$, and 100 mM Tris maleate at a volume of 1.0 ml. The reaction was carried out for 10 min at 37°C and was quenched with 2.0 ml iced 1.0N NaOH. Absorbance was measured spectrophotometrically using P-nitrophenol as a standard. For each group of experiments, AlPase measurements were carried out with the same reaction medium but at pH 7.5. Values at pH 7.5 were 85-90% lower than at pH 9.5 , but for at any given experiment the relative difference between the groups were unchanged from that at pH 9.5. Protein, maltase, Na-K-ATPase, succinic dehydrogenease and NADPH cytochrome C-reductase were measured as previously described (13).

RESULTS

In rats studied 4 hours after a change in diet, food intake in the +P and -P groups were similar; 6.6±0.5 gm/4 hours in +P and 6.3±0.7 in -P. **Table 1** shows serum Pi and creatinine and arterial blood gasses for the three groups. Serum Pi was lower in -P and unchanged in the fasted group when compared to +P while there was no significant differences in pH, pCO_2 or serum HCO_3 among the 3 groups. **Figure 1** shows the uptake of Pi and glucose by BBMV in the 3 groups. Phosphate uptake was greater at 15 sec and 1.5 min in -P compared to +P and fasting while Pi uptake was similar in +P and fasting; glucose uptake was similar in all three groups. Thus, Pi uptake was increased within 4 hours on -P diet.

Pi-uptake by BBMV was also measured 24 hours after changing diet P. The BBMV were incubated for 15 sec and the Pi concentration in the incubation media was varied from 0.01 to 5 mM in the presence of a 100 mM sodium gradient. Initial uptake values were higher in BBMV of -P rats at each concentration of Pi used. Saturation of Pi uptake tended to occur at a Pi concentration close to 1 mM, similar to previous reports (6). After subtracting uptake values obtained when KCl instead of NaCl was used in the incubation media, an Eadie-Hofstee plot was constructed as shown in **Figure 2.** The Km values derived from this plot were 0.13 mM in +P and 0.15 in -P. By contrast, the Vmax increased from 0.95 nmol/mg protein/15 sec in +P to 1.66 in -P.

Table 1. Blood Chemistries in Rats Fed Normal or Low Dietary Phosphorus

Dietary P	Phosphate	Creatinine	pH	pCO_2	HCO_3
%	mg/dl		Units	mmHg	mM
0.6 (14)[a]	8.05±0.32	0.60±0.09	7.37±.02	40.1±1.4	22.9±1.2
0.03 (14)	5.42±0.34[b]	0.67±0.08	7.37±.01	39.3±0.9	22.1±0.5
Fasted (14)	7.80±0.32	0.69±0.14	7.39±.01	37.5±0.8	22.3±0.7

Data are mean ± SEM
a: values in parentheses represent number of observations.
b: significantly different (p less than 0.01) than appropriate 0.6% dietary P group.

The time course of the change in specific activity and enrichments for AlPase and maltase in -P expressed as a percent of +P are shown in **Figure 3**. Data are shown for both the renal cortical homogenate and BBM. The AlPase and maltase activities were similar between groups at 4 and 24 hours. AlPase values were increased both in the renal cortical homogenates and BBM fraction in -P animals at 3 and 14 days. Maltase activity, on the other hand, did not increase. The fraction of AlPase present in BBM was 22-24% of that in the total homogenate with no difference between the diet groups. Results for the other enzymes measured showed that Na-K ATPase was enriched by 2.1±0.3 while enrichment ratios for succinic dehydrogenase, NADPH cytochrome C-reductase, and DNA were 0.4±0.06, 0.7±0.12 and 0.3±0.04, respectively. These ratios indicate a high proportion of BBM with little contamination by basolateral membranes, mitochondria, endoplasmic reticulum or nuclear material.

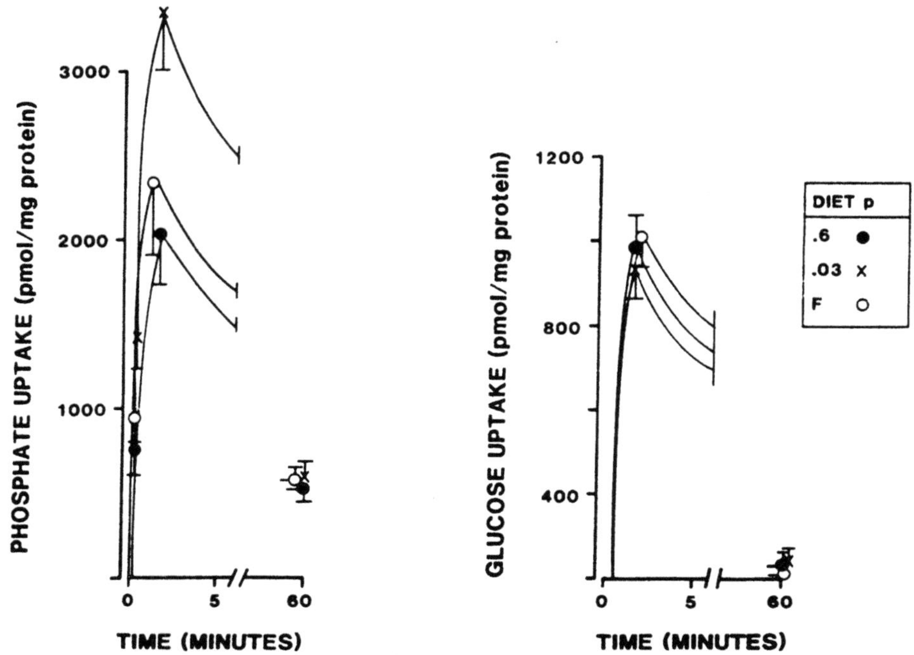

Figure 1. Uptake of Pi and glucose by BBMV prepared from rats fed on a normal (0.6% P) or low (0.03% P) P diet for 4 hours or not fed (fasted; F). Each point represents mean $\pm$ SEM; N=3 rats per group per experiment. Values of Pi uptake of 0.03% P diet at 15 sec and 1.5 min are significantly different (p less than 0.01) from values of normal P diet.

DISCUSSION

The present study demonstrates that Pi uptake by renal BBMV was increased within 4 hours of P-deprivation prior to any detectable change in AlPase activity. This effect is specific for Pi, as glucose uptake was unchanged.

Kinetic studies by Barrett et al (6) demonstrated that Vmax for Na^+-dependent Pi transport increases, while Km remains unchanged, evidence for an increase in membrane carrier or an increase in flux for Pi or both rather than increased carrier affinity. The studies by Barrett et al (6) demonstrated that the increase in Pi-uptake is not due to a change in Na permeability per se which alters the rate of dissipation of the Na^+ gradient. The fact that Na-dependent glucose uptake was unaffected by

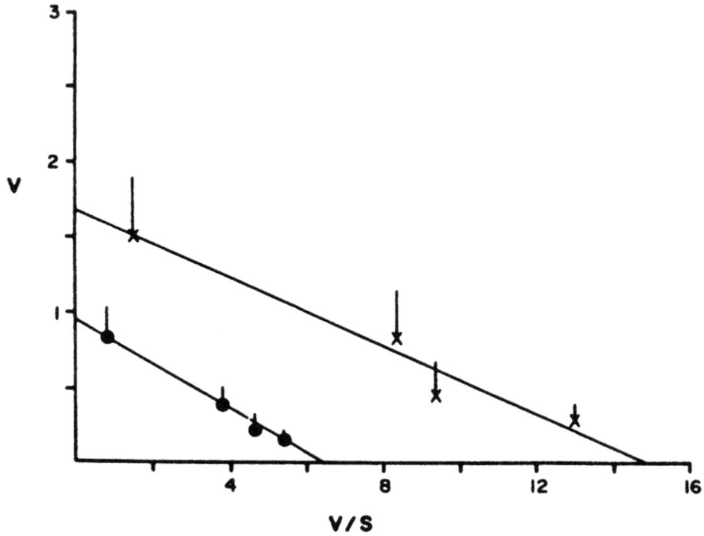

Figure 2. Eadie-Hofstee plot of initial Pi uptake by BBMV from rats fed normal (0.6%) or low (0.03%) P diet for one day. Transport was measured under the same conditions described in Figure 2 except the concentration of Pi varied from 0.01 to 5.0 mM and the incubation time was 15 seconds.

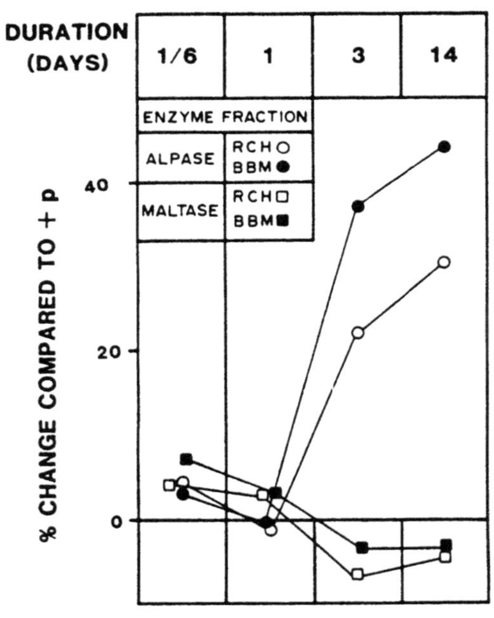

Figure 3. The percent change in alkaline phosphatase (AlPase) and maltase activities in rats fed a 0.03% P diet compared to rats fed a 0.6% P diet. Values for both the renal cortical homogenate (RCH) and brush border membrane (BBM) function are obtained at 4 hours, 1, 3, and 14 days after being placed on a low phosphate diet.

dietary P restriction suggests that the rate of dissipation of the Na gradient did not play a significant role. However, it will be necessary to directly measure Na uptake by BBM to prove this conclusively.

Kempson and Dousa (4) found increased AlPase activity in BBM after 14 days of P-depletion. In addition, adminstration of actinomycin D to rats fed on a P-diet prevented both the rise in AlPase activities and the decrease in urinary Pi excretion (5). These data suggested that AlPase may play a role in the renal adaptation to P-depletion. However, the present study demonstrates that changes in AlPase activity do not occur at a time when the Pi uptake by the BBMV has markedly increased i.e., Vmax already increased 74% by 24 hours, prior to any detectable changes in AlPase levels. These data suggest that a change in AlPase activity does not play a significant role in the early stages of renal adaptation to P-deprivation. The subsequent increase in AlPase activity demonstrated by others (4) as well as the present study could arise as a result of, rather than be the cause for, increased Pi transport. In vitro studies, using inhibitors of AlPase (9) and other studies in vitamin D-deficient rats (7) and in congenital hypophosphatemic mice (8) do not support a major role for AlPase in the adaptation to P-depletion. The rapid onset of the adaptive process shown in the present study may indicate that at least in the early adaptive period, the change in Vmax could represent an increased availability of carrier already present rather than an increased synthesis of new carriers. Further studies are needed, however, to clarify this point.

The early increase in Pi-uptake by the BBMV observed in the present study suggests that a decrease in urinary Pi during the initial period of P-deprivation occurs not only due to a decrese in serum Pi and hence filtered load, but also involves changes in activity of the proximal tubular cells. Whether the change in serum Pi or filtered load of Pi is the signal for tubular adaptation has yet to be determined. Studies by Brazy et al (3) have demonstrated an increase in Pi-flux in the isolated perfused proximal tubule of the rabbit 14 days after dietary P restriction. However, increasing the filtered load of Pi by uninephrectomy did not induce changes in Pi-transport by the isolated tubule contrary to the effect of increasing the filtered load of Pi by dietary means. Preliminary studies in our laboratory suggest that a fall in serum Pi precedes any change in BBM transport. However, it is not known whether the change in serum Pi is a prerequisite for the BBM adaptation.

Finally, the present study demonstrates that early BBM adaptation to P-deprivation requires the ingestion of a diet free of P. Thus, BBM prepared from rats fasted overnight failed to show a significant increase in Pi uptake. Similar to studies by Trohler et al (4), we were unable to demonstrate the presence of a metabolic acidosis in the fasted rats. Studies by Beck et al (15) in rats starved for 3 days suggested that metabolic acidosis may prevent the adaptation to Pi-depletion. Our studies suggest that the lack of dietary ingestion per se rather than metabolic acidosis plays a role in the lack of adaptation, at least at the BBM level.

Acknowledgements: The present study was supported by the Veterans Administration and in part by USPHS grant AM-21351. B.S.L. is a Research Associate of the Veterans Admiunistration.

REFERENCES

1. U. Trohler, J. -P. Bonjour, and H. Fleisch. Inorganic phosphate homeostasis: Renal adaptation to the dietary intake in intact and thyroparathyroidectomized rats. J. Clin. Invest. 57:264 (1976).

2. N. Brautbar, M. W. Walling, and J. W. Coburn. Interaction between vitamin D deficiency and phosphorus depletion in the rat. J. Clin. Invest. 63:335 (1979).

3. P. C. Brazy, J. W. McKeown, R. H. Harris, and V. W. Dennis. Comparative effects of dietary phosphate, unilateral nephectomy, parathyroid hormone on phosphate transport by the rabbit proximal tubule. Kidney Int. 17:788 (1980).

4. S. A. Kempson, and T. P. Dousa. Phosphate transport across renal cortical brush border membrane vesicles from rats stabilized on a normal, high or low phosphate diet. Life Sciences 24:881 (1979).

5. S. V. Shah, S. A. Kempson, T. E. Northrup, and T. P. Dousa. Renal adaptation to low phosphate diet in rats: blockade by actinomycin D. J. Clin. Invest. 64:955 (1979).

6. P. W. Barrett, J. M. Gertner, and H. Rasmussen. Effect of dietary phosphate on transport of pig microvillus vesicles. Am. J. Physiol. 8:F353 (1980).

7. M. W. Walling, B. S. Levine, N. Brautbar, D. B. N. Lee, and J. W. Coburn. Renal cortical alkaline phosphatase activity and renal phosphate retention during phosphate depletion in vitamin D deficient rats. Kidney Int. 14:643 (1978).

8. H. S. Tenenhouse, and C. R. L. Scriver. Alkaline phosphatase activity does not mediate phosphate transport in the renal-cortical brush border membrane. Biochem. J. 190:473 (1980).

9. C. Storelli, and H. Murer. On the correlation between alkaline phosphate and phospahte transport in rat renal brush border membrane vesicles. Pflugers Archiv. 384:149 (1980).

10. J. C. Beck, and B. Sacktor. The sodium electrochemical potential mediated uphill transport of D-glucose in renal brush border membrane vesicles. J. Biol. Chem. 253:5531 (1978).

11. P. S. Aronson, and B. Sacktor. The Na+ gradient-dependent transport of D-glucose in renal brush border membrane. J. Biol. Chem. 250:6032 (1975).

12. G. W. Snedecor, and W. G. Cochran. in: Statistical methods, Iowa State University Press, Iowa (1967).

13. B.S. Levine, K. Ho, J.A. Kraut, J.W. Coburn, and K. Kurokawa. Effect of metabollc acidosis on phosphate transport by the renal brush border membrane. Biochim. Biophys. Acta 727: 7, 1983.

14. U. Trohler, J.-P. Bonjour, and H. Fleisch. Plasma level and renal handling of Pi. Effect of overnight fasting with and without Pi supply, Am. J. Physiol. 240:F509 (1981).

15. N. Beck, S. K. Webster, and H. J. Reineck. Effect of fasting on tubular phosphorus reabsorption, Am. J. Physiol. 237:F241 (1979).

PHOSPHATURIA OF AGING: STUDIES ON MECHANISMS

D.B.N. Lee, N. Yanagawa, O. Jo, B.P. Yu and N. Beck

Department of Medicine, Sepulveda VAMC, University of California at Los Angeles, and Departments of Physiology and Medicine, University of Texas Health Sciences Center, San Antonio, Texas, USA

INTRODUCTION

Corvilain and Abramow (1) reported a lower serum inorganic phosphorus level associated with a reduction in maximum tubular reabsorption of phosphate (TmP) in adults when compared to children in active growth. Insogna and associates (2) also noted a reduction in serum phosphorus level and renal TmP in the elderly when compared to younger adult subjects. In addition, these investigators observed increases in immunoassayable parathyroid hormone (PTH) level in the blood and cyclic AMP (cAMP) excretion in the urine of the elderly subjects. Based on the observations that intestinal calcium absorption is reduced in elderly subjects (3,4) these authors suggested that the increased PTH was secondary to the suboptimal enteral calcium absorption and that this hyperparathyroidism in turn led to "renal phosphate wasting" and hypophosphatemia in the elderly. Berlyne and coworkers (5) confirmed the observation of an increase in PTH secretion and a decrease in TmP, as well as a reduction in glomerular filtration rate, in the elderly. They postulated that the hyperparathyroidism may, in addition, caused an increase in calcium mobilization from the skeleton and thus contributed towards the development of senile osteoporosis.

The observation that endorgan response to polypeptide hormones is reduced in several tissue systems in the elderly (6), raises the question whether the phosphaturia seen in these subjects could simply be attributed to the observed increase in PTH. Moreover, it has been shown that both PTH secretion and its catabolism are markedly influenced by aging (2,3,7), suggesting a need for caution in interpreting the biologic significance of changes in immunoassayble PTH in the elderly. Of additional interest is the observation of Fujita and associates (7) that the baseline PTH levels in young (1M) and old (18M) rats were not different. Furthermore, the response to hypocalcemic stimulation was, in fact, attenuated in the older rats. These findings taken together suggest the possibility that the decrease in renal phosphate (P) reabsorptive capacity associated with aginig may not be totally explicable on the basis of the observed increase in immunoassayable PTH.

The present study is designed to examine the interrelationship between PTH and renal P handling and to measure the P uptake by renal brush border membrane vesicles in senile, 28-29 month-old rats. The results are compared with those obtained from younger, 12-15 month-old rats.

METHODS

Senile, 28-29 month-old and younger 12-15 month-old, male Fischer 344 rats were obtained from Charles River Laboratories (Boston) through the National Institute on Aging. Studies were carried out 10 days after the rats were received from the supplier. During this period, the animals were fed equal amounts of Purina Rat Chow (15-20g/day). Thyroparathyroidectomy (TPTX) was carried out under Nembutal anesthesia at around 0800 h. An initial 0.8 ml blood was obtained from a femoral vein and the animal was maintained on a 120 mM NaCl solution containing 15mg/ml inulin and 4 ul/ml Nembutal, infused intravenously at a rate of 0.1 ml/min. 2.5 h after the initiation of infusion a 20-min urine sample was obtained, following which either one or five units of PTH (Beckman Biosynthetic PTH, N1-N34) was given intravenously as a single bolus. Three 20-min urine collections were than obtained and the experiment terminated after a final blood sample was obtained from the aorta.

The preparation of renal brush border membrane vesicles and the measurement of P uptake and alkaline phosphatase in these resealed vesicles were carried out using standard, published methods (8-12). Renal cortical cAMP concentration and urinary cAMP excretion were measured by methods previously published (13).

RESULTS

In rats fed equal amounts of dietary phosphorus we have observed an increase in urinary P excretion in the older rats. In order to examine the role of endogenous PTH on this observed difference in renal handling of P, the effect of acute TPTX on P excretion was studied. The fractional excretion of phosphate (FEP) in TPTX rats (figure 1, "0" unit PTH) remained high in senile rats (open dots) when compared to younger rats (solid dots). Increasing

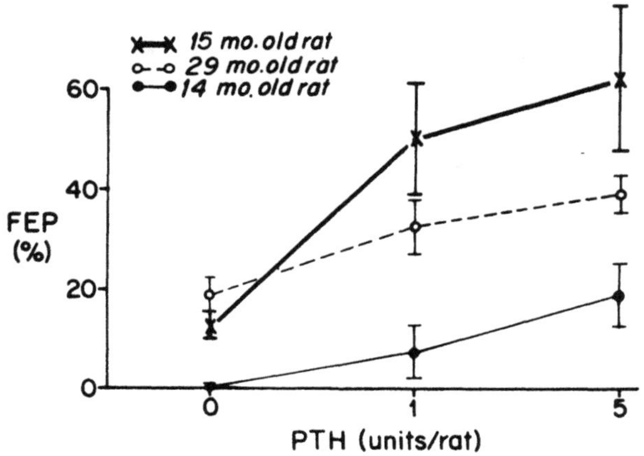

Figure 1.

doses of exogenous PTH caused proportionate increases in FEP in both age groups. Based on percent increase in FEP per unit PTH adminstered the senile rats did not appear to demonstrate an enhanced "phosphaturic" response to PTH. In order to examine the possibility that the initial high FEP in the senile rats may have caused a "blunting" of the subsequent phosphaturic response to PTH, an additional study was carried out in a group of younger, 15 month-old rats (figure 1, crosses and continuous line). In these rats, intravenous P was given following TPTX so that the pre-PTH FEP was not different from that observed in the senile rats. When PTH was given to these rats, the increase in FEP was in fact higher than those observed in senile rats. These data indicate that in the absence of endogenous PTH, senile rats continues to excrete a greater proportion of filtered P than the younger rats. In addition, the kidneys of the aged rats did not exhibit any increase in phosphaturic response to exogenously administered PTH.

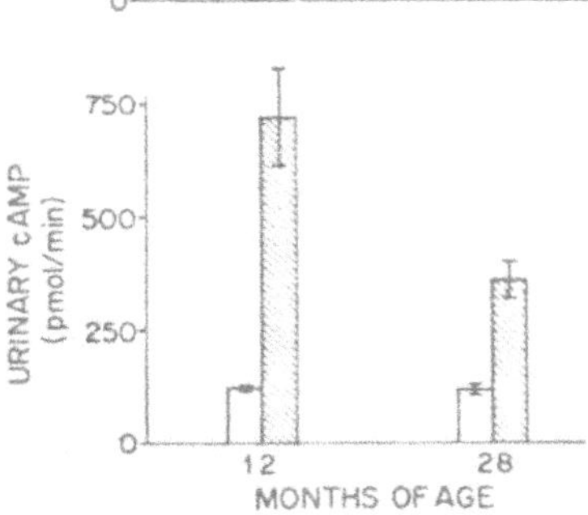

Figure 2.

Figure 2 summarizes the effect of 5 units of PTH on renal cortical cAMP concentration and urinary cAMP excretion. The basal renal cortical cAMP concentration (upper panel, open bars) was not different between 12M and 28M rats. PTH treatment (hatched bars) caused a marked increase in renal corticrl cAMP in the 12M old rats (N=10, P<0.01), while in the 28M rats the response was clearly attenuated (N=10, P>0.05). Similar remarks apply to the data on urinary cAMP excretion, with the exception that PTH also increased this parameter in the 28M rats, but when compared to that observed in the 12M rats the response was clearly attenuated.

Table I.

Age	Vmax	Km	Alk. P'ase
12M	1582.4 ± 395.5	150.5 ± 31.7	28.1 ± 4.0
28M	784.3 ± 242.9	87.8 ± 15.8	24.4 ± 3.4
P	<0.01	<0.01	n.s.

Phosphate uptake by brush border vesicles was clearly reduced in 28M rats (820.6 +/- 74.5 pmole/mg protein/2 min) when compared to that measured in the 12M rats (1247.7 +/- 151.1, P<0.01). Table I summarizes the data from kinetic studies and demonstrated a reduction in both Vmax (pmole/mg protein/6 sec) and Km (nM) in the older rats. Alkaline phosphatase concentration (umole paranitrophenol/mg protein/30 min) was not different between the two groups.

DISCUSSIONS

Our finding of a reduced renal reabsorption for P in senile rats echos similar observations in elderly human subjects (1,2,5). In man the increase in renal P excretion has been attributed to hyperparathyroidsm. Our study however demonstrates that an alteration in endogenous PTH activities alone cannot account for the reduced renal P reabsorption in the senile rats, because the FEP in these rats after TPTX remained higher than that found in similarly treated younger rats. Both groups were fed equal amount of dietary phosphorus.

We also examined the possibility that the "phosphaturia"

associated with aging may be the result of enhanced renal response to the action of PTH. We first examined the renal phosphaturic response to known doses of exogenous PTH in TPTX rats. The results indicated that the increase in FEP was not measurably different between the 15 and 29 month-old rats. In fact when the pre-PTH FEP in the younger rats was first elevated (by P infusion) to the level found in the older rats, subsequent administration of equal doses of PTH caused a lower, rather than higher, phosphaturic response in the aged rats. We also compared the renal response to PTH in terms of cAMP generation in the two age groups after TPTX. The basal values of either renal cortical cAMP generation or urinary cAPM excretion were not different between the two age groups. Furthermore, the increase in both parameters after PTH administration were clearly decreased, rather than increased, in the 29 month-old rats. These results support the thesis that the renal response to PTH, in terms of both cAMP generation and phosphaturia, is not enhanced in the aged rats. Since the observed difference in renal P reabsorption between the aged and the younger rats cannot be attributed to either a dysfunction of the parathyroid glands or an enhanced renal sensitivity to PTH, we examined P transport mechanism at steps distal the PTH-cAMP axis. For this purpose, we measured P uptake across the brush border membrane vesicles. The results demonstrated a clear decrease in P uptake by the vesicles prepared from the senile rats. Kinetic analysis revealed a reduction in Vmax as well as Km in the old rats when compared to the younger rats. Alkaline phosphatase activity was not different in the two age groups, confirming the common observation of a lack of correlation between the activity of this enzyme and P uptake.

SUMMARY

In rats fed equal amounts of dietary phosphorus we have observed an increase in urinary P excretion in the older rats. The increase in renal P excretion in these old rats is PTH-independent, since the observed phosphaturia was not reversed by TPTX, and the renal response (phosphaturia and cAMP generation) to exogenous PTH was not exaggerated in the senile rats when compared to the younger rats. P uptake across renal brush border membrane vesicles, however, was significantly reduced in preparations derived from the aged rats when compared to that derived from younger rats. The detail mechanism for the reduced renal P reabsorption in senile rats remained to be elucidated.

REFERECNCES.

1. J. Corvilain and M. Abramow: Growth and renal control of plasma phosphate. J Clin Endocrinol Metab 34:452-459, 1972.
2. K. L. Insogna, A. M. Lewis, B. A. Lipinski, C. Bryant and D. T. Baran: Effect of age on serum immunoreactive parathyroid hormone

and its bilogical effects. J Clin Endocrinol Metab 53:1072-1075, 1981.
3. J. C. Gallagher, B. L. Riggs, C. M. Jerpbak and C.D. Arnaud: The effect of age on serum immunoreactive parathyroid hormone in normal and osteoporotic woman. J Lab Clin Med 95:373-384, 1981.
4. J. R. Bullamore, R. Wilkinson, J.C. Gallagher, B.E.C. Nordin and D. H. Marshall: Effects of age on calcium absorption. Lancet II:535-537, 1970.2-4.
5. G.M. Berlyne, J. Ben-Ari, A. Kushelevsky, A. Idelman, D. Galinsky, M. Hirsch, R. Schainkin, R. Yagil and M. Zlotnik: The etiology of senile osteoporosis: secondary hyperparathyroidism due to renal failure. Quart J Med 175:505-521, 1975.
6. S.W. O'Connor, P.J. Scarpace and I.B. Abrass: Age-associated decrease of adenylate cyclase activity in rat myocardium. Mechanism of Aging and Development 16:91-95, 1981.
7. T. Fujita, M. Ohata, K. Ota, T. Tsuda, A Uezu, K Okano and M. Yoshikawa: Aging and parathyroid hormone secretion. J Gerontology 31:523-529, 1976.
8. W. Berner, R. Kinne and H, Murer: Phosphate transport into brush-border membrane vesicles isolated from rat small intestine. Biochem J 160:467-474, 1976.
9. C. Evers, H. Murer and R. Kinne: Effect of parathyrin on the transport properties of isolated brush-border vesicles. Biochem J 172:46-56, 1978.
10. W. Haase, A. Schafer, H. Murer and R. Kinne: Studies on the orientation of brush-border membrane vesicles. Biochem J 172:57-62, 1978.
11. K.A. Hruska, S.C. Mills, S. Khalifa and M.R. Hammerman: Phosphorylation of renal brush-border membrane vesicles. Effect of calcium uptake and membrane content of polyphosphoinositides. J Biological Chem 258:2501-2507, 1983.
12. H.S. Tenenhouse, C.R. Scriver and E.J. Vizel: Alkaline phosphatase activity does not mediate phosphate transport in renal-cortical brush-border membrane. Biochem J 190:473-476, 1980.
13. N. Beck, B.P. Yu: Effect of aging on urinary concentrating mechanism and vasopressin-dependent cAMP in rats. Am J Physiol 243:F121-F125, 1982.

ACKNOWLEGMENTS

This work was supported by NIH-AG 03425, Veterans Administration Research Support and Nelly W. Citron Reseach Fund.

CALCIUM AND MAGNESIUM TRANSPORT

THE ASSESSMENT OF RENAL CALCIUM REABSORPTION

O.L.M. Bijvoet and H.I.J. Harinck

Clinical Investigation Unit of the Dept.
of Endocrinology, University Hospital
Leiden, The Netherlands

Renal clearances studies rest upon comparisons of concentrations in the plasma (P; mass/vol) with simultaneously measured urinary excretion rates (UV; mass/time). Their value depends on adequacy of the assumption, that the function that relates excretion rate to plasma concentration, contains a minimum of variables and, that those variables are relevant as to the behaviour of the kidney.

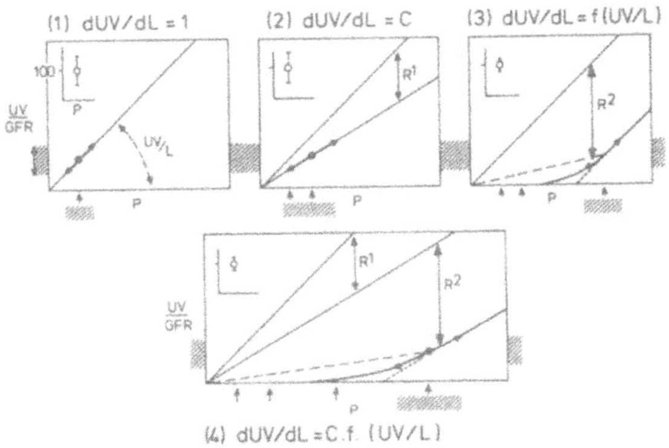

Fig. 1. Four models of renal electrolyte transport. Details are explained in text.

The simplest case is inulin clearance. The function is

$$UV = f.P$$

Simultaneous measurement of UV and P yields the value of f, which is equal to glomerular filtration rate (GFR). This function, written in the form

$$\frac{UV}{GFR} = P$$

is represented in fig. 1 in the left hand graph. UV/GFR (mass/vol) can be thought of as the amount excreted per unit volume of GFR. For inulin, and in humans the same holds for creatinine, the relation between UV/GFR and P can be represented by a 45° line. Clearance studies are often used to determine fractional excretion, i.e. the fraction (f) of filtrate retained in the urine.

$$\frac{UV}{GFR} = f.P$$

It so happens that when this is done, for instance for sodium, and when measurements are made of creatinine concentrations in the same samples, f can be derived by merely comparing concentrations in urine (U_{Na};U_{Creat}) and plasma (P_{Na}; P_{creat}):

$$f = \frac{U_{Na}.P_{creat}}{U_{creat}.P_{Na}}$$

The relation between UV/GFR and P, when f has a constant value smaller than unity, is given in the second graph of fig. 1. In persons who are in a steady state, excretion rate has a constant value which is equal to the sum of net intestinal absorption and/or metabolic production, and UV, taken together with GFR determines UV/GFR. Fractional excretion being the complement of fractional reabsorption, fractional reabsorption ensures a higher serum concentration at the same value of UV/GFR relative to the model in the first graph of the figure. The variability of P (shown in left upper corner) in this as well as in the first model, is proportional to the variability of UV. According to the second model fractional excretion (the efficiency of excretion) is fixed, regardless the actual values of UV/GFR or serum concentration. This model is referred to when one assesses fractional reabsorption (called TR, for instance TRP for fractional reabsorption of phosphate), and it is often used because concept and calculations are simple. However the results are difficult to interpret because generally this function is not adequate as a description of renal function, since TR is not a constant.

The third model, given in fig. 1 is more realistic and does apply to renal handling of, for instance glucose (1), amino-acids (2), magnesium (3) and phosphate (4) and for the last substance its properties have been worked out in some detail (4). It reflects the observation that the amount of phosphate reabsorbed per unit volume of glomerular filtrate (T/GFR; mass/vol) attains a constant and maximal value (TmP/GFR) when plasma phosphate concentrations are artificially raised by intravenous infusion. At these high values of P, TmP/GFR can be calculated by simpel subtraction:

$$TmP/GFR = P - UV/GFR$$

It is easily seen in the figure that TmP/GFR is equal to the value of P at which the line, representing this function, cuts the abscissa. At more normal plasma concentrations however, this function is found to "deviate" in a curvilinear fashion. This curvilinear part of the function is called "splay". Unfortunately phosphate reabsorption is normally "within splay" so that it is rather inadequate to consider splay as a deviation. More true would be the statement that the normal relation between UV/GFR and P is a curvilineair one, which attains a limit at high values of P. It has been found that the degree of curvature of phosphate splay (this appears to hold also for other substances) is proportional to the value of TmP/GFR (fig. 2), and attains its limit, regard-

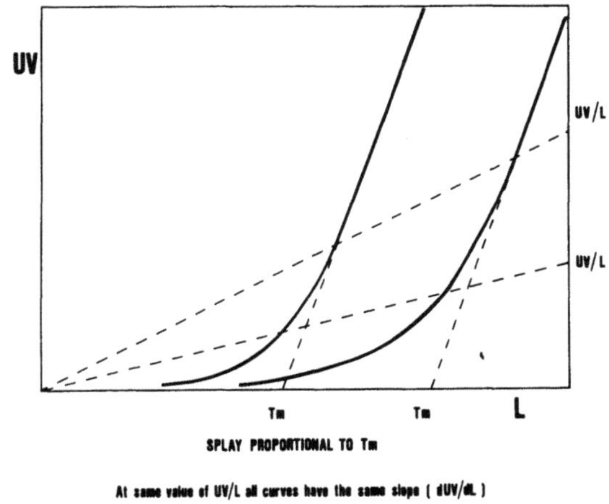

Fig. 2. Illustrating consequences of proportionality between degree of splay and value of Tm. At a given value of UV/L the slope of splay (dUV/dL) is constant and independent of the actual value of Tm.

less of the actual value of TmP/GFR when fractional excretion exceeds the value of 0.20 (5).
Note: that fractional excretion, or excreted fraction of filtered load, is defined here as (UV/GFR)/P. Since this becomes cumbersome, we will, when fractions are used, abbreviate this to UV/L, where L represents filtered load. Of course L = P.GFR.

The physiological meaningfulness of splay becomes clear when one considers that the tangent to this function, dUV/dL, representing the efficiency at which an *increment* of filtered load is excreted, attains a higher value to the extent that P, plasma concentration increases relative to the "intercept" TmP/GFR. TmP/GFR is therefore called threshold concentration (4). Below this, phosphate excretion is less efficient than above.

This type of regulation results, at a given phosphate production and GFR (i.a. at a given value of UV/GFR), in a plasma phosphate the value of which depends upon the phosphate threshold and the variation of which is relatively insensitive to variations in production (see left upper corner).

Repeated measurements in many conditions have made it possible to give an empirical description of splay, allowing construction of a nomogram (6,7). Using this nomogram the value of the phosphate threshold can be derived from a simultaneous measurement of plasma and urine phosphate and creatinine concentrations. Phosphate threshold is usually considered to be proportional to net total transport capacity of transporting "enzymes" in tubules. The cause and nature of splay is still subject to speculation (4).

The fourth model in fig. 1 has been proposed by Mioni et al (8) in an attempt to understand the renal handling of calcium. It describes the normal relation between UV/GFR and P without, and during infusion with calcium. Again, during infusion, the relation between UV/GFR and P approaches linearity, but the slope of this line is less than unity even when taking into account that only 56% of plasma calcium is ultrafiltrable (9). This has been explained by recalling that part of ultrafiltered calcium is reabsorbed along the proximal tubule together with sodium and that a second, sodium independent, parathyroid hormone (PTH) sensitive reabsorption system exists in the late distal tubule (10). The model states that a constant proportion (60%) of filtered calcium is reabsorbed together with sodium in the proximal tubule and that distal reabsorption obeys the Tm/GFR model. There are two difficulties that hinder the application of this model to analysis of clinical data: the first is that splay has as yet eluded empirical description because values in normal man are normally at the upper end of splay (11). The second is that micropuncture data indicate that proximal calcium reabsorption exceeds 60% and is more in the order of 85%. A value of 85% is incompatible with this model (12,13).

In the analysis of renal calcium handling which is now reported we arrive at the proposition that a curvilinear relation between UV/GFR and P is normal for electrolyte excretion. It is the consequence of a stochastic distribution of bidirectional fluxes along the length of renal tubules and, ultimately results in a simple power function containing only two constants:

$$\frac{dUV}{dL} = \left(\frac{P}{Th_m}\right)^{(c-1)}$$

One constant (Th_m) is directly proportional to the net total transport capacity of the renal tubules and has, like the classic threshold, the dimension of a concentration. The other constant (c), is specific to the transported substance and defines the affi-

nity of the transporting system to the substance. The function attains a natural limit when any further increment of filtered load is entirely excreted. (When $dUV/dL = 1$ and $P = Th_m$).
In the case of calcium, the relation between plasma concentration and excretion can be defined by a combination of two such functions which are of sufficiently different nature to be distinguished as separate. Since the function is simple yet accurate, it allows uniform interpretation of clearance studies.

The analysis is based on repeated measurements of calcium clearance in 80 patients suffering from osteitis deformance, before and during oral treatment with APD ((3-amino-1-hydroxypropilidene)-1,1-bisphosphonate) 600 mg per day. Treatment resulted in simultaneous lowering of urine and serum calcium (14,15). Use was further made of published material decribing clearance studies in healthy persons (17) and in patients with hypo- or hyperparathyreoidism (18) to whom calcium was administered by oral or intravenous route.

(a) (b)

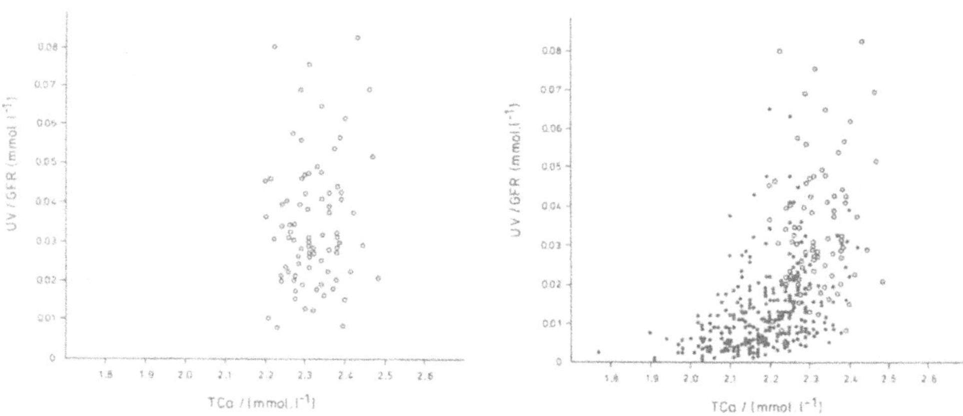

Fig. 3a/b. Comparison of fasting calcium excretion per unit volume of GFR (UV/GFR) with serum calcium concentration (T_{Ca}) in 80 patients with Pagets disease (a) before and (b) before and during treatment with APD.

The fasting urinary excretion of calcium per 1 of GFR is compared with simultaneous total plasma calcium for 80 untreated patients with Paget's disease in fig. 3a. Despite considerable variation in UV/GFR plasma calcium is maintained within narrow normal limits. In fig. 3b clearance values, obtained in the same patients during treatment with APD, have been added. There is an indication of curvilinearity, but the data seems not easily accessible to analysis, one of the probable reasons for this may be variation, between individuals, of calcium threshold.

One may recall the experience, schematically depicted in fig. 2, that the degree of "splay" is proportional to threshold (4). This implies, that the slope of (tangent to) splay, measured as dUV/dL, has a constant value at a given fractional excretion (UV/L), regardless of the actual value of the threshold. It was therefore decided to calculate for the individual patients rendered in fig. 3b the change in UV/GFR (Δ(UV/GFR)) and in serum calcium (ΔCa) between subsequent days, as well as the average of UV/GFR and serum calcium for these subsequent observations. From this a graph was constructed relating (ΔUV/ΔL) to UV/L.

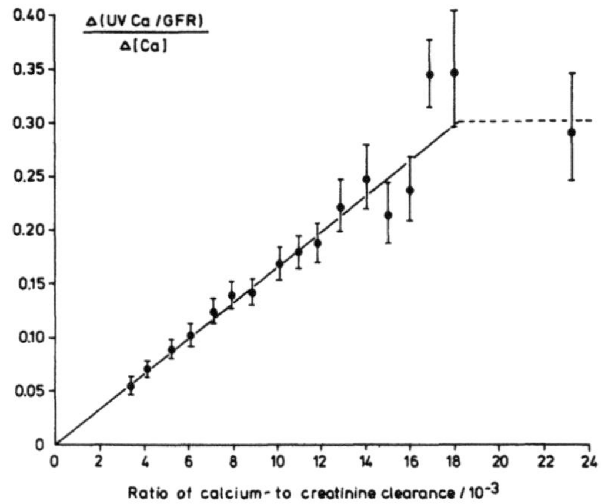

Fig. 4. Relation between Δ(UV/GFR)/ΔCa = ΔUV/ΔL and UV/L during APD treatment of 80 patients with Paget's disease.

Since the error in ΔL is much greater than the error in ΔUV, geometric averages rather than arithmetic averages were used for ΔUV/ΔL and the averages were calculated for subsequent overlapping intervals of 2.10^{-3} in UV/L. Each average contains around 25 measurements.

The result of this procedure is striking in that the regression of ΔUV/ΔL on UV/L appears to be linear, up to ΔUV/ΔL = 0.3, and does pass through the origin. The value ΔUV/ΔL = 0.3 occurs where, in fig. 1,[4] the curve describing the relation between UV/GFR and P ends and changes into a straight line with a slope of 0.3. The meaning of this result is apparent:

$$\frac{dUV}{dL} = c. \frac{UV}{L}$$

At any given value of fractional excretion, the fractional excretion of an increment in filtered load is proportional to the prevalent fractional excretion.

Assuming, for the time being, that the model given in fig.1,[4] is adequate, then the actual filtered load arriving at the distal tubule would be only 30% of serum calcium, but the increment of filtered load, ΔL would also be only 30% of the increment of serum calcium. Therefore the value of c which applies to the "Splay" in distal reabsorption is independent of the degree of ultrafiltrability and/or degree of fractional reabsorption in the proximal tubule. The actual value of c obtained in this study was 17.

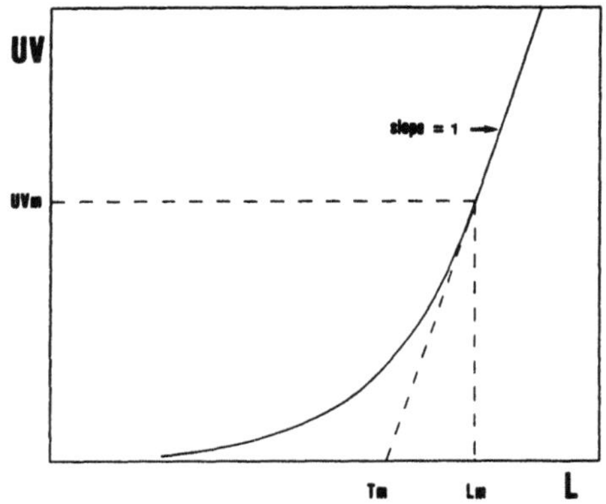

$$\frac{dUV}{dL} = c\frac{UV}{L} \rightarrow c = \frac{Lm}{UVm}$$

$$\frac{UV}{UVm} = \left(\frac{L}{Lm}\right)^{c} \rightarrow \frac{UV}{L} = \frac{1}{c}\left(\frac{L}{Lm}\right)^{(c-1)}$$

$$Tm = \left(1 - \frac{1}{c}\right) Lm$$

Fig. 5. Analysis of splay. Details are explained in text.

In order to simplify further analysis, we will immediately move on to the hypothesis, that the function we have found has general validity, and will also apply to splay in reabsorption of other electrolytes. dUV/dL = c(UV/L) is a differential equation and before applying it to analysis of the excretion of electrolytes it should be integrated. The consequences of this procedure and all relevant equations so obtained are rendered in fig. 5. The integration constant, Lm, refers to the filtered load at which splay ends (then dUV/dL = 1 and cannot increase any more). UVm should be read as the corresponding value of UV. When we would express excretion rate in terms of excretions per unit of GFR, UV/GFR, and in accordance with this, filtered load in units of GFR, as P, the entity Lm/GFR is the plasma concentration at which splay ends. In the past this concentration has been termed "maximal threshold", Th_m, in contrast to the normal threshold (Tm/GFR). The latter is equal to the plasma concentration at which the linear part of the function relating UV/GFR to P would cut the x-axis, when it is extrapolated downwards. From the formula:

$$\frac{dUV}{dL} = c.\frac{UV}{L}$$

follows, that when splay ends, dUV/dL = 1, UV = UV_m and L = L_m, then

$$c = \frac{Lm}{Uvm} \quad \text{and} \quad 1/c = \frac{UVm}{Lm}$$

Therefore 1/c corresponds to the value of fractional excretion when splay ends.

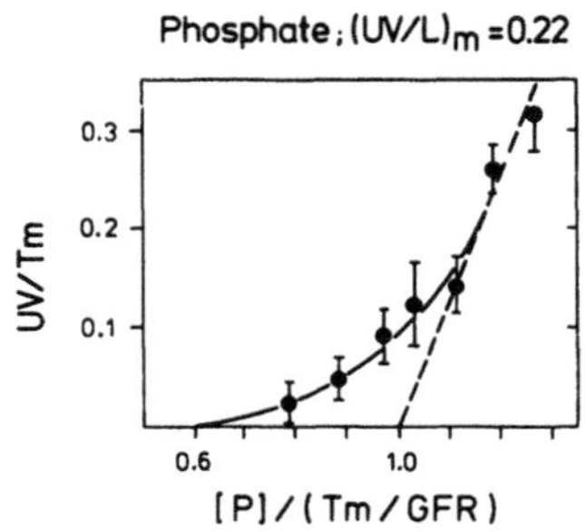

Fig. 6. Comparison of splay in phosphate excretion as measured empirically (closed circles) and splay as predicted by the model explained in the text (continuous line) using a value of 0.22 for the value of fractional excretion when splay ends $(UV/L)_m$.

We have mentioned in the previous section that for phosphate UVm/Lm equals 0.20. Using a slightly higher value of 0.22 for UVm/Lm and hence of 4.55 for c, the fit of the derived function with splay as empirically determined (4) is quite satisfactory (fig. 6).

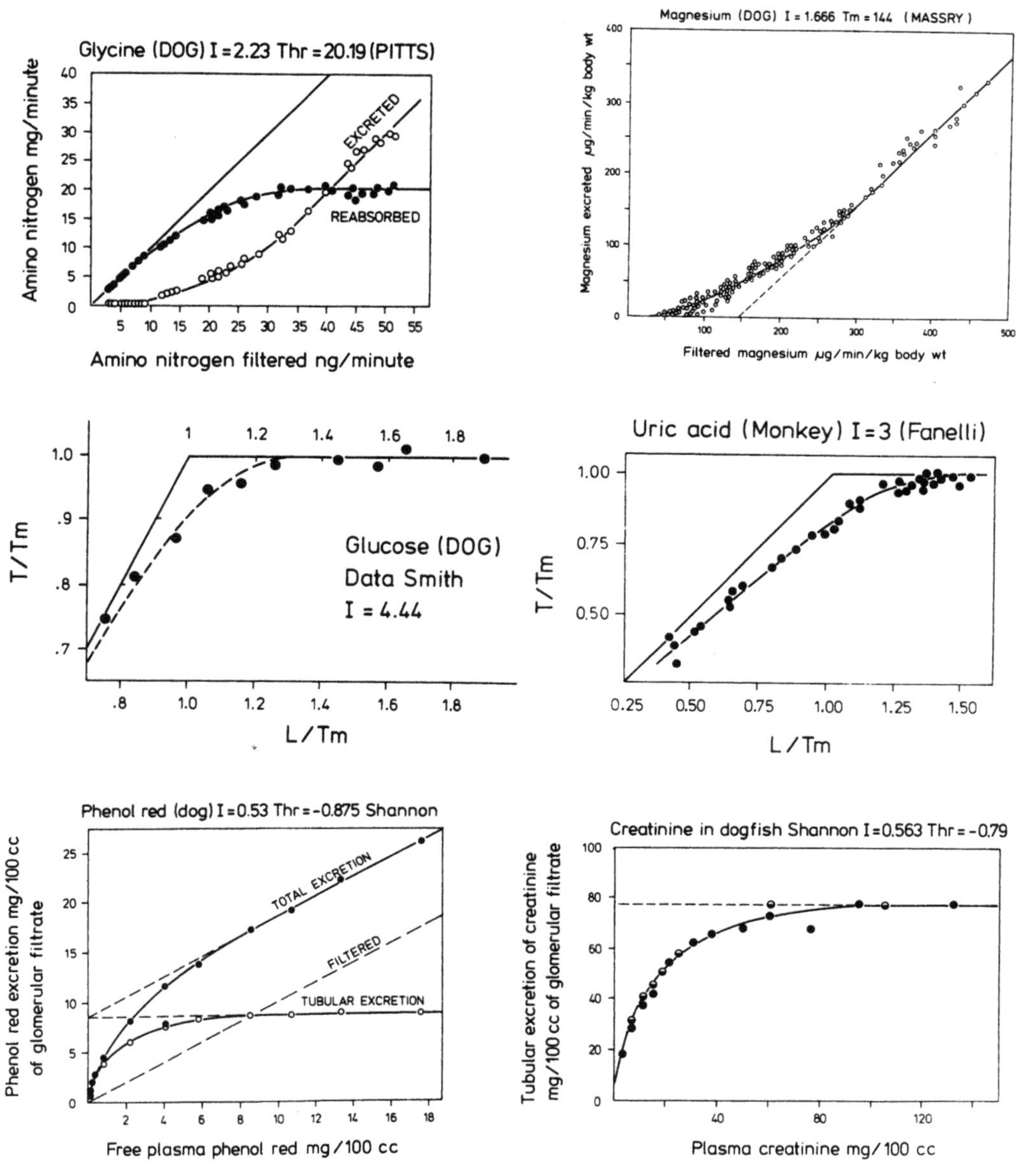

Fig. 7. Comparison of empirical measurements of splay with splay predicted by the model explained in the text. The symbol I corresponds to the symbol c used in the text. The figures refer to renal handling of glycine (2), magnesium (3), glucose (1), uric acid (18), phenol red (19) and creatinine (20). The format in which respective authors have presented their data is retained. The curves represent splay as calculated.

In fig. 7 such an analysis has been applied to all electrolytes and non-electrolytes for which, in traditional textbook literature (1-3, 18-20) sufficient data were available. In this figure the actual manner in which authors have presented their results is retained. This means that results have, in some instances, been given in terms of tubular reabsorption and sometimes factorized for T_m. It is seen that the form is not only satisfactory as a description of reabsorptive processes, but equally for secretion if $c<1$.

In fig. 5 the equation

$$\frac{dUV}{dL} = c \ \frac{UV}{L}$$

has been integrated to:

$$\frac{UV}{L} = 1/c\left(\frac{L}{Lm}\right)^{(c-1)}$$

Combining these equations, and calling $Lm/GFR = Th_m$ we obtain

$$\frac{dUV}{dL} = \left(\frac{P}{Th_m}\right)^{(c-1)}$$

The implications contained in this formula are easy to understand. The formula states that the efficiency of excretion of an *increment* in filtered load (dUV/dL) depends of the value of P relative to a reference concentration (Th_m) and increases as P increases relative to Th_m. The degree to which this happend depends upon the actual value of c. The value of the maximum threshold (Th_m) is determined by the capacity of the transporting system and is modulated by hormones. The constant c can be seen as an affinity constant, which is specific for the affinity between transporting enzyme and a given substrate. The greater this affinity, c, the smaller the splay.

It was mentioned in the introduction that the Mioni (8) model for renal calcium handling was unsatisfactory in that it underestimates sodium-linked proximal renal tubular reabsorption of calcium. In stead of assuming a constant fractional reabsorption for this process we propose that a curvilinear model with low affinity and high capacity can describe proximal calcium reabsorption. Total calcium reabsorption would then be explicable in terms of two processes, one sodium linked, high capacity low affinity process and one, PTH modulated, low capacity high affinity process.

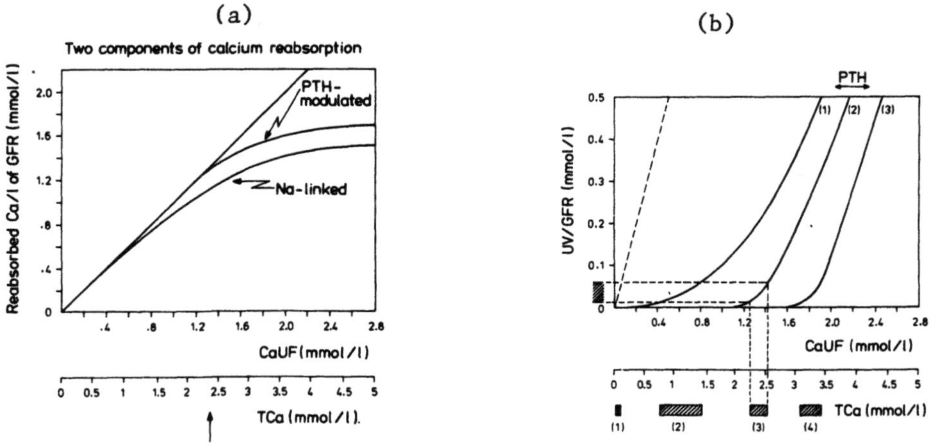

Fig. 8a. Renal tubular reabsorption of calcium as a function of total (TCa) or ultrafiltrable (CaUF) calcium in serum and represented as being composed from two separate processes, a proximal tubular sodium-linked, high capacity and low affinity process and a PTH-modulated, low capacity, high affinity process in the distal tubule.

8b. The same analysis in terms of excreted calcium per unit volume of GFR. (1) is the result of proximal reabsorption (2) the relationship subsequent to additional distal reabsorption and (3) the relationship when distal reabsorption is maximally stimulated. Shaded area: normal value of UV/GFR and of total calcium under the different circumstances.

Details of the following analysis will be published elsewhere (21). Suffice to say here that in the case of calcium, splay would be a combination of splay in sodium-linked calcium reabsorption and splay in the activity of PTH modulated reabsorption operating on the product of the first process. If we denote that product by the symbol X and characterize the first splay by c_1, the second by c_2 and the resulting splay by c, it is easy to show that $c = c_1 . c_2$, because from:

$$\frac{dUV}{dL} = c.\frac{UV}{L} \qquad \text{follows:} \quad \frac{dUV}{UV} = c.\frac{dL}{L}$$

We may write:

$$\frac{dUV}{UV} = c_2.\frac{dX}{X} \quad \text{and} \quad \frac{dX}{X} = c_1.\frac{dL}{L} \quad \text{hence} \quad \frac{dUV}{UV} = c_1.c_2.\frac{dL}{L}$$

From this follows:

$$\frac{dUV}{UV} = c_1.c_2.\frac{dL}{L} \quad \text{and} \quad \frac{dUV}{dL} = c_1.c_2.\frac{UV}{L}$$

Since we have already characterized the "combined" splay by:

$$\frac{dUV}{dL} = c. \frac{UV}{L}$$

it follows that $c = c_1.c_2$.

The data of Peacock and Nordin pertaining to healthy persons during intravenous or oral calcium load (16,17) were used to derive the value of c_1 for proximal calcium reabsorption in the following way. Assuming that distal reabsorption is saturated during calcium load, and deriving averages for UV/GFR and P at three different points of their saturation curve, one can algebraically solve for c_1,Lm_1 and Lm_2. The numerical results are given in table 1.

Table 1. Constants defining normal values for capacity and affinity of Na-linked, and of PTH-modulated calcium reabsorption.

	c	Th_m(mmol/1 in Ultrafiltr.Ca)
Na-linked	2.5	2.51
PTH-modulated	6.8	0.211
Total	17	-

Figs. 8a and 8b give the graphical results of the analysis in terms of total and of ultrafiltrable calcium. It is now evident that a value for proximal tubular calcium reabsorption is obtained which, at a normal total serum calcium, is realistic. Furthermore using data in familial benign hypercalcemia (22) and in primary hyperparathyroidism (17) one can make an estimate of a maximum possible value for distal tubular reabsorption of calcium. The normal range and the estimated limits for hyper- and hypoparathyroidism are given in fig. 9a and b.

(a) (b)

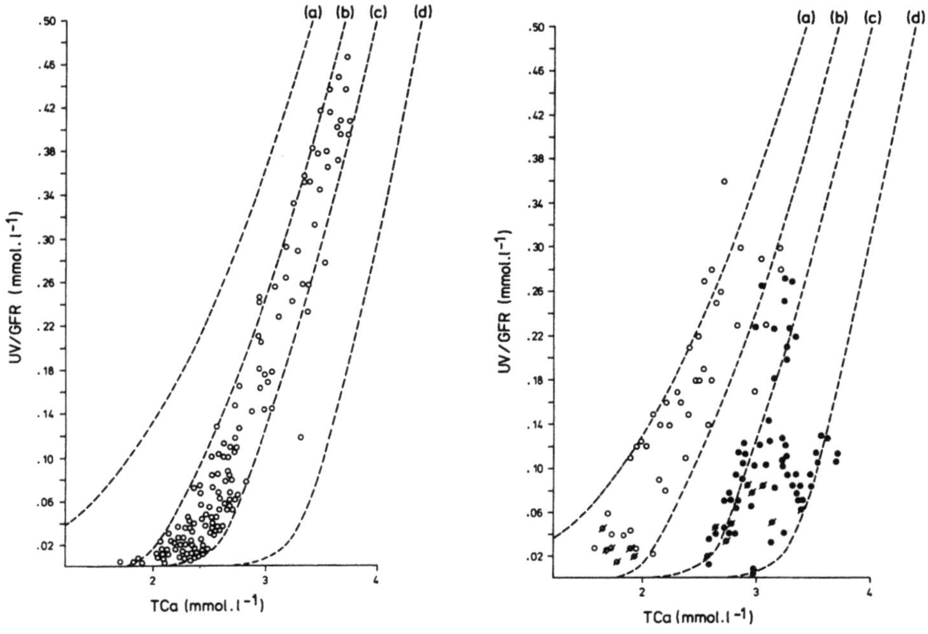

Fig. 9a/b. Relation between calcium excreted per unit volume of GFR (UV/GFR) and total serum calcium. The interrupted lines (a) and (d) denote absence and maximal stimulation of PTH-modulated calcium transport. The lines (b) and (c) delineate normal relationship. Left hand figure: open circles represent data in healthy persons without and during calcium load. Right hand: open circles patients suffering from hypoparathyroidism, closed circles, patients suffering from primary hyperparathyroidism, before and during calcium load. (data from ref. 16 and 17).

The main purpose of this paper was to demonstrate the possibility of formulating a general description of mineral excretion and to use this for the analysis of renal tubular calcium transport. This analysis has been carried further to include effects of volume depletion on calcium excretion as well as to derive a method for simple clinical assessment of renal tubular handling of calcium. Both will be described elsewhere (21). At the present however it may suffice to present in fig. 10 a summary of primary abnormalities of calcium homeostases within the framework of the preceding analysis.

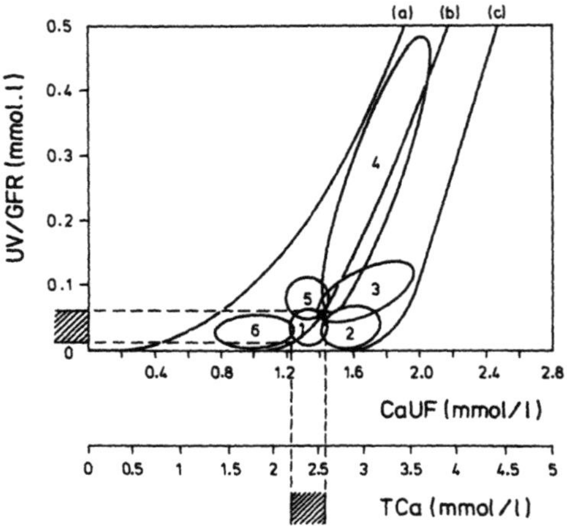

Fig. 10. Summary of the results of a number of disturbances of calcium metabolism on the relation between UV/GFR and serum calcium. The lines represent the relationship for minimal (a) normal (b) and maximal (c) stimulation of distal renal tubular reabsorption of calcium. The figure is further explained in the text.

In this figure familiar benign hypercalcaemia (2) is defined as hypercalcaemia entirely due congenital fixation of PTH-dependent renal tubular calcium reabsorption at a high value. In contrast (4) depicts hypercalcaemia due to excessive calcium production in hypercalcaemia of malignancy. Primary hyperparathyroidism (3) is a mixed form combining increased calcium reabsorption with excessive calcium production from gut and bone and is contrasted with hypoparathyroidism (6). Finally normocalcaemic hypercalciuria (5) is defined as increased production compensated by decreased reabsorption - or its converse.

REFERENCES

1. Smith, P.K., Ollayos, R.W., Winkler, A.W. Tubular reabsorption of phosphate in the dog. J.Clin.Invest. 22:143 (1943).
2. Pitts, R.F. A renal reabsorptive mechanism in the dog common to glycine and creatinine. Amer.J.Physiol. 140:156(1943).
3. Massry, S.G., Coburn, J.W., Kleeman, C.R. Renal handling of magnesium in the dog. Amer.J.Physiol. 216:1460(1969).
4. Bijvoet, O.L.M. Relation of plasma phosphate concentration to renal tubular reabsorption of phosphate. Clin.Sci. 37:23 (1969).

5. Bijvoet, O.L.M. Measurement of renal handling of phosphate. In: Renal handling of Phosphate, edited by S.G. Massry and H.Fleisch; Plenum Medical Book Cy. New York, 1980, pp. 1-37.
6. Bijvoet, O.L.M., Morgan, D.B. The tubular reabsorption of phosphate in man. In: Phosphate et Métabolisme Phosphocalcique, edited by D.J. Hiocco; L'Expansion Scientifique Francaise, Paris, 1971, pp. 153-80.
7. Walton, R.J., Bijvoet, O.L.M. Nomogram for the derivation of renal threshold phosphate concentration. Lancet 2:309(1975).
8. Mioni, G., d'Angelo, A., Ossi, E., Bertaglia, E., Marconi, G., Maschio, G. The renal handling of calcium in normal Subjects and in renal disease. Rev.Eur.Etud.Clin.Biol. 16:881 (1971).
9. Marshall, R.W. Calcium fraction in Plasma. In: Calcium, Phosphate and Magnesium Metabolism. Edited by B.E.C. Nordin, Churchill, London, 1976, pp. 162-178.
10. Bijvoet, O.L.M. Kidney function in Calcium and Phosphate Metabolism. In: Metabolic Bone Disease I, Edited by L.V. Avioli and S.M. Krane. Academic Press Inc., New York, 1977, pp. 49-140.
11. Marshall, D.H. Calcium and Phosphate Kinetics. In: Calcium, Phosphate and Magnesium Metabolism. Edited by B.E.C. Nordin, Churchill, London, 1976, pp. 257-297.
12. Le Grimmellec, C., Roinel, N., Morel, F. Simultaneous Mg, Ca, P, K, Na and Cl analysis in rat tubular fluid. III, During acute Ca plasma loading. Pflügers Arch. 346:171(1974).
13. Edwards, B.R., Sutton, R.A.L., Dirks, J.H. Effect of calcium infusion on renal tubular reabsorption in the dog. Amer.J. Physiol. 227:13(1974).
14. Frijlink, W.B., Bijvoet, O.L.M., Te Velde, J., Heynen, G. Treatment of Paget's disease with (3-amino-1-hydroxypropylidene)-1,1-bisphosphonate (APD). Lancet i:799(1979).
15. Adami, S., Frijlink, W.B., Bijvoet, O.L.M., O'Riordan, J.L.H., Clemens, T.L., Papapoulos, S.E. Regulation of Calcium Absorption by 1,25 Dihydroxy-Vitamin D-Studies of the Effects of a Bisphosphonate Treatment. Calcif.Tiss. Int. 34:317(1982).
16. Marshall, D.H., Peacock, M., Nordin, B.E.C. Plasma calcium homeostasis. In: Rein et Calcium, edited by D. Hioco, Rueil-Malmaison: Sandoz Editions (1973) pp. 15-25.
17. Peacock, M., Robertson, W.G., Nordin, B.E.C. Relation between serum and urinary calcium with particular reference to parathyroid hormone. Lancet i:384(1969).
18. Fanelli, G.M., Jr., Hohn, D.L., Stafford, S. Functional characteristics of renal urate transport in the Cebus Monkey. Amer.J.Physiol. 218:627(1970).
19. Shannon, J.A. The excretion of phenol red by the dog. Amer.J.Physiol. 113:602(1935).

20. Shannon, J.A. On the mechanism of the renal tubular excretion of creatinine in the dog fish, squalus acanthias. J.Cell. and Comp.Physiol. 16:285(1940).
21. Bijvoet, O.L.M., Harinck, H.I.J. in preparation.
22. Menko, F.H., Bijvoet, O.L.M., Fronen, J.L.H.H., Sandler, L.M., Adami, S., O'Riordan, J.L.H., Schopman, P. and Heynen, G. Familial benign hypercalcemia. Study of a large family. Quarterly J. of Medicine, in press. (1983)

CIS-PLATIN INDUCED HYPERMAGNESIURIA AND HYPERCALCIURIA IN RATS

V. Mavichak, N.L.M. Wong, J.H. Dirks and R.A.L. Sutton

Department of Medicine
University of British Columbia
Vancouver, B.C., Canada V6T 1W5

INTRODUCTION

Cisplatin (cis-diammine dichloroplatinum), an effective chemotherapeutic agent that is being increasingly used against solid tumors, frequently causes renal impairment and electrolyte disturbances in man, particularly hypomagnesemia and renal magnesium wasting (1,2,3,4). In one report, 76% of patients became hypomagnesemic during cisplatin therapy and of these 50% had remained persistently hypomagnesemic for as long as 3 years following discontinuation of cisplatin treatment (4). The pathogenesis and mechanism(s) of hypomagnesemia and inappropriate renal magnesium wasting induced by cisplatin is still unknown.

We have produced an animal model of renal magnesium wasting with cisplatin in the rat and have also examined renal handling of calcium in these animals.

METHODS

Two groups of male Wistar rats weighing 200-225 grams were studied.

Group A animals (N=44) were fed a normal diet (Purina Lab Chow, USA: Magnesium content = 0.21 gm%, and calcium content = 1.2 gm%).

Group B animals N=44) were fed a low magnesium and calcium diet (ICN, USA: Magnesium content = 0.03 gm%, calcium content = 0.41 gm%).

Each group was divided into 3 subgroups, as follows:

Subgroup I (control, n=12) received 0.9% NaCl solution (vehicle for cisplatin injection) 5 ml/Kg I.P. weekly for 3 weeks.

Subgroup II (n=16) received cisplatin (Bristol Laboratories, Canada) 2.5 mg/Kg I.P. weekly for 3 weeks.

Subgroup III (n=16) received cisplatin 5 mg/kg I.P. weekly for 3 weeks.

All animals were in metabolic cages, and they had free access to food and distilled water. Twenty-four hour urines were collected and analyzed for creatinine and electrolytes. Blood samples were drawn from tail veins every week for 6 weeks.

RESULTS

The effect of cisplatin on whole kidney function and on renal handling of magnesium and calcium were examined at the end of the 6th week of the experiment (3 weeks after completion of cisplatin injections).

Table I shows the effect of cisplatin on glomerular filtration rate (GFR). There was no significant difference in GFR between the normal diet group or the Low Mg/Low Ca diet group in subgroup I (control animals) or in subgroup II (low-dose cisplatin 2.5 mg/kg weekly x 3 weeks). However, there was a significant reduction of GFR in subgroup III (high-dose cisplatin, 5 mg/kg weekly x 3 weeks) compared with control rats in the normal diet group (GFR = 1.25 ± 0.10 vs 1.47 ± 0.08 ml/min, respectively, $p<0.01$). There was also a small but not significant decrease in GFR in subgroup III animals compared to controls in the Low Mg/Low Ca diet groups.

Table 1. GFR (creatinine clearance, ml/min)

	NORMAL DIET	LOW Mg, LOW Ca DIET
I Control (N=12)	1.47 ± 0.08	1.59 ± 0.11
II Cis (N=16) (2.5 mg/kg weekly x 3)	1.49 ± 0.05	1.44 ± 0.02
III Cis (N=16)	1.25 ± 0.10 *§	1.39 ± 0.09

* $p<0.01$ compared to I
§ $p<0.01$ compared to II

Table II shows the plasma Mg concentration and the fractional excretion of filtered Mg in both normal diet and Low Mg/Low Ca diet animals. In the normal diet group, after 3 weeks of cisplatin injections, plasma Mg levels were slightly but not significantly lower in animals that received low and high-dose cisplatin than in controls (P Mg = 0.92±0.01 mM, and 0.91±0.02 mM respectively compared 0.95±0.04 mM in control animals. However, fractional excretion of Mg (FE Mg) was significantly higher in cisplatin treated animals. Fractional urinary magnesium excretion correlated with the dose of cisplatin administration [FE Mg = 10.0±0.7% in control, 18.2±1.4% in subgroup II, and 24.0±2.1% in subgroup III). In the Low Mg/Low Ca diet group, P Mg was significantly lower in subgroup II than in controls (P Mg = 0.74±0.02 mM vs 0.81±0.02 mM, $p<0.01$). This was also accompanied by a higher FE Mg (0.13±0.09% in controls vs 2.94±0.88% in subgroup II, $p<0.01$), which indicated inappropriate renal magnesium wasting in the presence of a reduced plasma Mg.

Table 2. MAGNESIUM DATA

	NORMAL DIET		LOW Mg, LOW Ca DIET	
	Plasma Mg (mM)	FE Mg (%)	Plasma Mg (mM)	FE Mg (%)
I Control (N=12)	0.95±0.04	10.0±0.7	0.81±0.02	0.13±0.09
II Cis (N=16) (2.5 mg/kg weekly x 3)	0.92±0.01	18.2±1.4 *	0.74±0.02 *	2.94±0.88 *
III Cis (N=16) (5 mg/kg weekly x 3)	0.91±0.02	24.0±2.1 *§	0.79±0.02	5.13±0.88 *§

FE = fractional urinary excretion of filtered load.
* $p<0.01$ compared to I
§ $p<0.01$ compared to II.

Table III shows Plasma Ca and FECa in both groups. Cisplatin treated rats had significantly higher FECa than control rats. FE Ca in these rats also correlated with the dose of cisplatin administered.

Table 3. CALCIUM DATA

		NORMAL DIET		LOW Mg, LOW Ca DIET	
		Plasma Ca (mM)	FE Ca (%)	Plasma Ca (mM)	FE Ca (%)
I	Control (N=12)	2.62±0.01	0.58±0.06	2.65±0.02	0.47±0.17
II	Cis (N=16) (2.5 mg/kg weekly x 3)	2.62±0.02	1.70±0.34 *	2.66±0.02	1.04±0.14 *
III	Cis (N=16) (5 mg/kg weekly x 3)	2.62±0.03	4.02±0.6 *§	2.66±0.03	1.91±0.29 *§

* $p<0.01$ compared to I
§ $p<0.01$ compared to II

Figure I and II show that whole kidney absolute Mg and Ca reabsorption was consistently lower in cisplatin-treated rats than in controls at any level of filtered load of Mg and Ca respectively.

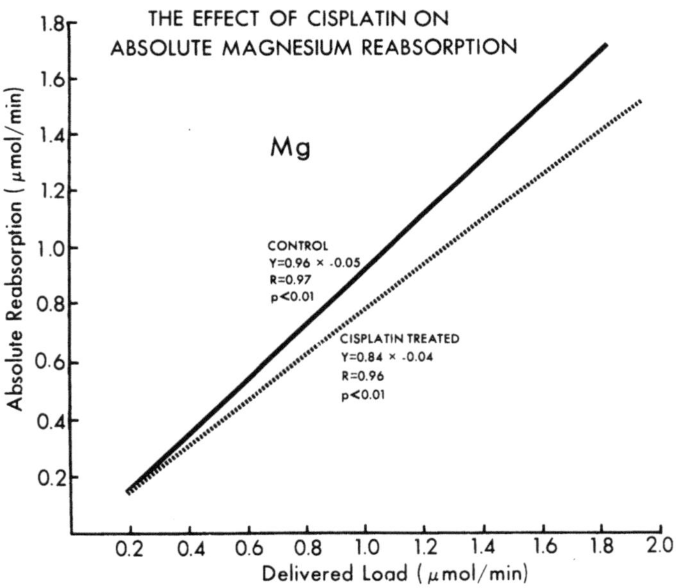

FIGURE 1

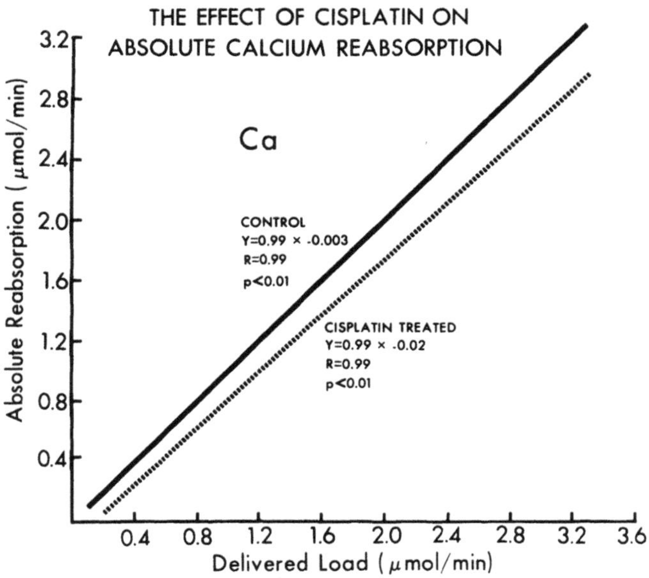

FIGURE 2

DISCUSSION

The nephrotoxicity associated with cisplatin chemotherapy is manifested not only as a decrease in glomerular filtration rate but also, in many patients, as a specific defect in renal tubular Mg conservation. The latter problem may persist for years following completion of cisplatin chemotherapy (4). Although, most of these patients are asymptomatic, the long term effects of chronic hypomagnesemia in man are unknown. Little is known about the pathogenesis of cisplatin induced hypomagnesemia and renal magnesium wasting, or about the long term effect of cisplatin on kidney. Our present studies have demonstrated that:

1) Cisplatin can induce hypomagnesemia in the rat, which is associated with inappropriate renal magnesium wasting and hypercalciuria.
2) The degree of renal magnesium wasting and hypercalciuria correlate with the dose of cisplatin administered.
3) Cisplatin-treated rats are able to maintain their plasma magnesium concentration and compensate for abnormal renal magnesium losses while they are on a high magnesium diet (Mg = 0.21 gm%). However, these animals become hypomagnesemic and are unable to conserve magnesium normally when placed on low magnesium diet (Mg = 0.03 gm%).

Under normal conditions, the kidney represents the primary regulator of magnesium balance in the body. Present evidence suggests that the renal excretion of magnesium occurs by glomerular filtration and tubular reabsorptive process. The major portion of filtered magnesium (65%) is reabsorbed in the loop of Henle, mainly in the thick ascending limb (5,6), and this segment is the primary site at which magnesium transport is modulated by factors such as diuretics, osmotic agents, and states of magnesium deficiency and excess. However, whether or not the hypermagnesiuric and hypercalciuric effects of cisplatin are the consequence of tubular transport defects in the ascending limb of Henle's loop in rats, needs further study. Furthermore, the role of extra- renal factors which regulate renal magnesium and calcium transport such as PTH, aldosterone, Vitamin D, etc. also requires study.

In summary, this animal model will facilitate the study of the pathogenesis and mechanism(s) of cisplatin-induced renal magnesium wasting. It should be also useful for the study of the relationship between renal magnesium and calcium handling.

ACKNOWLEDGEMENTS

These studies were supported by the Medical Research Council of Canada (MT-1915, MA-5279). Cis-platin used in these studies was supplied by Bristol Laboratories of Canada.

REFERENCES

1. N.E. Madias, J.T. Harrington. Platinum nephrotoxicity, a review. American Journal of Medicine, Volume 65, p. 307 (1978).
2. R.L. Schilsky, T. Anderson. Hypomagnesemia and renal magnesium wasting in patients receiving cisplatin. Annals of Internal Medicine, 90: 929-931 (1979).
3. J.D. Blachley, J.B. Hill. Renal and electrolyte disturbances associated with cisplatin. Ann. Intern. Med. 95: 628-632 (1981).
4. R.L. Schilsky, A. Barlock, R.F. Ozols. Persistent hypomagnesemia following cisplatin chemotherapy for testicular cancer. Cancer Treatment Reports Vol. 66; No. 9, p. 1767 (1982).
5. S. Carney, N.L.M. Wong, G.A. Quamme, J.H. Dirks. Effect of magnesium deficiency on renal magnesium and calcium transport in the rat. J. Clin. Invest. 65: 180, 1980.
6. G.A. Quamme, J.H. Dirks. Magnesium transport in the nephron: (editorial reviews). Am. J. Phys. 239 (Renal Fluid Electrolyte Physiology 8): F393, 1980.

BRUSH BORDER VESICLE TRANSPORT EFFECTS OF 1,25-DIHYDROXY VITAMIN D_3

Jules B. Puschett, J. Egel and J. Pfanstiel

Renal-Electrolyte Division
Department of Medicine
University of Pittsburgh
Pittsburgh, PA 15261, USA

Evidence has accumulated from investigations performed in this laboratory and in others that the renal tubular effect of 1,25-dihydroxy vitamin D_3 (1,25 D_3), the active form of the vitamin, is to increase phosphate reabsorption by the kidney (1-3). We recently reported that the infusion of 2.5 ng of 1,25 D_3 per hour along with 0.2 U of PTH/hr. for six hours resulted in an antiphosphaturia in thyroparathyroidectomized (TPTX), vitamin D-deficient (-D) rats (3). This dose of the metabolite has been considered to be in the physiological range, and was not effective unless given with the non-phosphaturic "permissive" dose of PTH. The development of the brush border vesicle (BBV) transport technique (4) provided us with an opportunity to study the locus of this antiphosphaturic action of the metabolite. Furthermore, glucose metabolism has been reported to be linked to phosphate (Pi) transport events; Rasmussen and his coworkers have reported (5) that parathyroid hormone (PTH), a substance which diminishes phosphate uptake by brush border vesicles (4), increases gluconeogenesis (GNG). Accordingly, we examined the effect of the antiphosphaturic agent 1,25 D_3, on BBV Pi uptake and on GNG.

Studies were performed in weanling vitamin D-depleted rats maintained on a -D diet containing 0.4% calcium and phosphorus for 2-4 wks. The animals were subjected to TPTX, a bladder catheter was placed, and they were infused with a replacement solution overnight. Control urine collections were taken, following which the rats received either 2.5 ng of 1,25 D_3 plus 0.2 U PTH/hr. for 6 hours, or the vehicles only (propylene glycol and saline). The animals were sacrificed and the kidneys were processed at once for BBV Pi transport studies or for measurements of GNG.

The preliminary results showed an antiphosphaturia in the rats given both the metabolite and the hormone (experimental rats) with a fall in absolute Pi excretion of approximately 30% from control levels, whereas there were no alterations in Pi excretion in the control rats. Furthermore, there were no changes in inulin excretion in either group of rats. Brush border membrane vesicles prepared from kidneys harvested from the experimental rats showed a reduction in Pi uptake compared to those from control rats at all of the early time periods (0.15, 0.5 and 1.0 min). In addition, GNG in experimental animals was reduced by almost 30% from the levels of control rats.

We conclude from these observations that the BBV Pi transport technique confirms earlier whole kidney observations that 1,25 D_3 promotes Pi reabsorption when given with permissive doses of PTH. This effect therefore seems to occur, at least in part, at the level of the proximal tubule. Furthermore, the combination of the metabolite and the hormone lowers renal cortical glucose production, an effect opposite to that of a pharmacological dose of PTH (5).

REFERENCES

1. Puschett JB, Kuhrman MS: Renal tubular effects of 1,25-dihydroxy vitamin D_3: Interactions with vasopressin and parathyroid hormone in the vitamin D-depleted rat. J Lab Clin Med 92:895, 1978.
2. Popovtzer MM, Robinette JB, DeLuca HF and Holick MF: The acute effect of 25-hydroxycholecalciferol on renal handling of phosphorus. J Clin Invest 53:913, 1974.
3. Puschett JB, Georgaki H: Acute effect of a "physiological" dose of 1,25-dihydroxy vitamin D_3 on renal phosphate transport. Endocr Res Comm 9:135, 1982.
4. Puschett JB, Kempson SA and Kowalski JC: Inhibition of renal brush border phosphate transport and stimulation of renal gluconeogenesis by cyclic AMP and parathyroid hormone. (In press).
5. Rasmussen H, Nagata N: Renal gluconeogenesis: Effects of parathyroid hormone and dibutyryl 3′,5′-AMP. Biochim Biophys Acta 215:17, 1970.

ACTIVE CALCIUM TRANSPORT IN FROG SKIN: STIMULATION BY CYCLIC AMP

Ellie Kelepouris, Mortimer Civan, and
Zalman S. Agus

Departments of Medicine and Physiology
University of Pennsylvania School of Medicine
Philadelphia, Pennsylvania

Cytosolic calcium activity is regulated at extremely low levels (10^{-7}M). This is accomplished in part by maintenance of a balance between calcium entry and exit via Ca-Mg-ATPase activity and Na/Ca exchange as defined in red cells and excitable tissue.[1] The distal nephron, in addition to maintaining cytosolic calcium activity must simultaneously regulate transepithelial calcium transport under the influence of parathyroid hormone and cyclic AMP.[2] Little is known at present about cellular mechanisms which regulate this transport and the relationship of this process to cytosolic calcium regulation. In this report, we present preliminary data demonstrating CAMP sensitive active transepithelial calcium transport in frog skin.

METHODS

Studies were performed utilizing standard electrophysiologic techniques and bidirectional Ca^{45} flux measurements in paired, continuously short-circuited, abdominal hemiskins from female Rana pipiens frogs mounted in double Ussing chambers. Studies were performed with symmetrical solutions in standard bicarbonate buffered amphibian Ringers containing 0.9 mM calcium. The data are presented as mean values of calcium flux for the average of two consecutive 30 minute collections before and after an experimental maneuver. The outer or apical surface is referred to as mucosa and the inner or basolateral surface as serosa. Studies were performed to evaluate the effect of serosal 8-P-chloro CAMP (10^{-4}M) on bidirectional and net flux and the effect of amiloride and replacement of mucosal sodium with choline on these effects.

RESULTS

Effects of Cyclic AMP

In 4 paired skins, cyclic AMP increased mucosal to serosal calcium flux from 0.65 ± 0.18 $nmol/hr/cm^2$ to 1.30 ± 0.18. Serosal to mucosal flux increased more markedly from 0.32 ± 0.11 to -2.95 ± 0.58. Thus frog skin exhibits net calcium absorption in the untreated state. Cyclic AMP stimulates both unidirectional fluxes but results in net secretion.

Effects of Amiloride

In 3 paired skins, unidirectional fluxes were measured before and after addition of mucosal amiloride (10^{-4}M), and after addition of serosal 8-p-chloro CAMP to the amiloride treated skins. Net Ca^{45} flux was 0.21 ± 0.14 during control, 0.30 ± 0.1 after amiloride and -0.9 ± 0.2 after cyclic AMP addition. Thus amiloride did not alter the effect of CAMP to induce net secretion.

Effects of Choline

In 4 paired skins, the effects of 8-p-chloro CAMP on serosal to mucosal flux were evaluated with one hemiskin bathed in standard sodium containing Ringers solution and the other paired hemiskin bathed in Ringers solution in which mucosal sodium was replaced with choline. Secretory flux increased significantly in both pairs; from 0.40 ± 0.01 to 1.5 ± 0.3 ($p<0.05$) in controls and from 0.17 ± 0.1 to 1.4 ± 0.3 ($p<0.05$) in the choline group. Thus sodium transport and/or Na/Ca exchange are not necessary for the stimulation of calcium secretion by cyclic AMP.

DISCUSSION

These studies establish the presence of net transepithelial calcium transport in frog skin. Net transport occurs in the absence of transepithelial electrochemical gradients, is independent of sodium transport, and is stimulated by cyclic AMP. As frog skin is easily accessible and amenable to study with a variety of micro and macrotechniques, this tissue may represent a useful model epithelium for the study of hormonally regulated transepithelial calcium transport.

Cyclic AMP stimulates net active secretion by increasing the serosal to mucosal flux out of proportion to the mucosal to serosal flux. As sodium/calcium exchange does not appear to play a significant role in the stimulation of secretion, this effect of CAMP is presumably due to a direct activation of mucosal Ca-Mg-ATPase or a selective increase in the permeability to calcium. A single effect to enhance calcium entry at the serosal side or stimulate calcium exit at the mucosal side however cannot explain the increase in mucosal to serosal flux which was also observed following cyclic AMP addition. The data are therefore compatible with either of several hypotheses. First, cyclic AMP could primarily stimulate exit mechanisms at both membranes, Ca-Mg-ATPase at the mucosal side and either Ca-Mg-ATPase or Na/Ca exchange at the serosal side. In this instance, there would have to be a preferential increase in ATPase activity at the mucosal side. Alternatively, the primary effect of cyclic AMP could be to increase membrane permeability to calcium with the serosal effect predominating. Exit at the mucosal side via Ca-Mg-ATPase and at the serosal side via either Na/Ca exchange would be increased secondarily due to the increase in cytosolic calcium concentration consequent to the increased permeability.

REFERENCES

1. A. P. Borle, Control, modulation and regulation of cell calcium. Rev. Phys. Biochem. Pharm. 90:13 (1981).
2. Z. S. Agus, A. Wasserstein, and S. Goldfarb, PTH, calcitonin, cyclic nucleotides and the kidney. Ann. Rev. Physiol. 43: 583 (1981).

ATP AS A FACTOR IN THE RESPONSE OF THE cAMP SYSTEM TO PTH IN PROXIMAL AND DISTAL CONVOLUTED TUBULES

Thomas P. Dousa, Gary M. Kiebzak, Ahad N. K. Yusufi, Eiji Kusano, and Julie Braun-Werness

Nephrology Research Unit, Division of Nephrology and Internal Medicine, Department of Physiology and Biophysics, Mayo Clinic, Rochester, MN U.S.A.

INTRODUCTION

Since the discovery of cyclic 3',5'-AMP (cAMP) as an intracellular mediator in hormone-responsive tissues by E. W. Sutherland (1), it was well recognized that ATP serves as a substrate for the key enzyme of cAMP metabolism--adenylate cyclase (AdC). Later it was also found that ATP may modulate cAMP catabolism by inhibiting cAMP-phosphodiesterase (cAMP-PDIE) (2). However, in recent years little attention was paid to cellular levels of ATP as a potential determinant of hormone-sensitive cAMP metabolism.

Recently an enormous diversity of cAMP-mediated hormonal responses in mammalian nephron became well recognized (3). In a concise way, cAMP-mediated cellular responses of specific tubular segments to a given hormone are often tacitly equated with the presence and responsiveness of hormone-sensitive AdC. Several recent observations brought to our attention that cellular factors other than activity of AdC, as assayed <u>in vitro</u> in the broken-cell system, may determine quantitatively and qualitatively, the hormone-elicited changes in cAMP content of tubular cells.

As an example, ADH fails to increase cAMP levels in medullary collecting tubules from mice with hereditary diabetes insipidus, in spite of the presence of an active AdC which is well sensitive to ADH stimulation in a standard assay <u>in vitro</u> (4). The pathologically high activity of cAMP-PDIE and the high rate of cAMP catabolism most likely accounts for the lack of cAMP increase in response to ADH in this tubular segment (4). In rat collecting tubules, PGE_2 has no detectable effect on ADH-sensitive AdC assayed in disrupted tubules; yet, PGE_2 markedly inhibits the stimulatory effect of ADH on cAMP levels in tubules with intact cells (5).

In our recent studies on the PTH-sensitive cAMP system of mouse cortical tubules, we observed that cellular ATP levels may be a factor which determines the response of the cAMP system to PTH.

RESULTS AND DISCUSSION

Studies were conducted on functionally normal mice. Microdissection of tubules, assays of AdC, cAMP-PDIE, and measurements of cAMP accumulation in samples of undisrupted tubules were conducted by techniques described in our laboratory, as well as by others (4,6,7). ATP levels were determined in samples of intact tubules with use of firefly luciferase microbioluminescence assay (8), adapted for this purpose recently by Doctor Yusufi in our laboratory (9). In this study we examined specifically the response of the cAMP system to PTH in proximal convoluted tubules (PCT) and in distal convoluted tubules (DCT) microdissected from mouse cortex.

In complete agreement with the results of Brunette, et al. (10), we found that both PCT and DCT dissected from mouse kidney cortex contain AdC highly responsive to PTH, as assayed in disrupted ("permeabilized") tubules (3,7,10). Although the absolute specific activity was considerably lower in PCT than in DCT, in both segments the AdC responded to 10 U PTH/ml by many-fold increase in activity (in PCT increase $\cong \Delta\% + 1500$; in DCT increase $\cong \Delta\% + 2800$); i.e. the relative stimulation of AdC by PTH was similar in PCT and in DCT.

In sharp contrast, both segments greatly differed in their response to PTH stimulation in terms of cAMP accumulation in intact tubules. In DCT incubated with high doses of PTH the cAMP level increased greatly ($\Delta + 1225\%$), but in PCT dissected from the same kidneys the same dose of PTH barely changed the level of cAMP ($\Delta + 50\%$). Having in mind our observations on mice with nephrogenic diabetes insipidus (4), we considered whether PCT may be endowed with a high activity of cAMP-PDIE. However, when compared under the same conditions (substrate cAMP level was 10^{-6} M cAMP) the activity of cAMP-PDIE was in fact lower ($\Delta -46\%$) in PCT than in DCT (9).

Next, we measured ATP levels in tubular samples, and we found that ATP levels in PCT were about 100 times lower than ATP levels in DCT. Taken into account tubular protein content in PCT and DCT which we measured in separate experiments, and the ratio of renal tissue wet weight to cellular protein, we estimated that ATP concentrations in DCT were about 0.3 mM, while ATP concentrations in PCT were about 0.003 mM. We tried to enhance ATP levels in PCT by using complete tissue culture media instead of Krebs Ringer solution, by the addition of various substrates (namely α-ketoglutarate) and/or membrane stabilizers (hydrocortisone), as well as by exploring various times and temperatures of incubation. None of these maneuvers improved cAMP response to PTH in PCT.

To learn whether a difference in ATP levels between PCT and DCT can indeed account for different responsiveness of PCT and DCT in terms of cAMP accumulation, we maneuvered ATP levels in DCT with the use of a metabolic inhibitor, rotenone (11). The addition of rotenone, an inhibitor of mitochondrial respiration, lowered ATP levels in DCT to values (about 0.009 mM) which are virtually indistinguishable from those found in PCT. Indeed, we found that in DCT with ATP levels depleted by incubation with rotenone, PTH failed to increase cAMP levels, similarly as in PCT. In control experiments, we documented that rotenone did not interfere with PTH stimulation of AdC in disrupted DCT under assay conditions when substrate ATP is supplied exogenously into the incubation medium (7,10).

Our interpretation of the observations recounted above is that a very low level of ATP in PCT was the major cause for failure of PTH to increase cAMP levels, inspite of the presence of highly active PTH-sensitive AdC in this tubule segment (9). As reported by others (12), the K_m for ATP of renal cortical AdC (and AdC in general) was estimated to be in the range of 0.1 - 0.2 mM ATP (12). Comparing estimated cellular concentrations of ATP in PCT and DCT, the simplest explanation to be offered is that in PCT (or in ATP-depleted DCT), ATP levels as a substrate for AdC are far below the 1/2 substrate saturation level needed for enzymatic catalysis of cAMP generation by AdC.

Nevertheless, even under conditions of very low ATP levels in PCT some minimal cAMP formation does occur; we observed that the addition of 0.5 mM isomethyl-butyl xanthine, a cAMP-PDIE inhibitor (4), to PCT increased cAMP accumulation in the presence of PTH about ten times. It is of interest to consider that the rate of cAMP catabolism is likely very high even at low cAMP levels since "low K_m - high affinity" cAMP-PDIE is active at a low concentration range (10^{-7} - 10^{-6} M) of cAMP (2,6). It is thus likely that a small quanta of cAMP generated in PCT in the presence of very low ATP levels are promptly catabolized by cAMP-PDIE.

Our present results are of interest in considering the interpretation of studies done in the past and present on mixed cortical tubule preparations; it was assumed and/or documented that such suspension of cortical tubules consist predominantly of PCT segments (13). Although direct comparison was not made, cortical tubules isolated either as a suspension, or isolated by microdissection techniques, are usually exposed to similar preparative factors: kidney perfusion, incubation with collagenase and extensive washing in incubation media (7,13). If ATP levels, and consequently cAMP responses to PTH, in DCT and PCT portions of such mixed cortical suspensions would be similar to those found in our present study (9), the major component of the cortical tubular mixture that accounts for increased cAMP content after the addition of PTH is likely DCT rather than PCT. Therefore, even apparently negligible admixture of DCT (> 10%) in suspensions of cortical tubules could contribute substantially to PTH-stimulated cAMP levels.

ATP levels in PCT were found to be lower than in DCT also with the use of the method more closely approximating conditions *in vivo* (14); the differences were not quantitatively so prominent (14) as in our present studies. Therefore, rather dramatic differences between ATP levels in PCT and DCT seen in our experiments may be due to greater sensitivity of PCT compared to DCT, towards adverse chemical and physical factors which are inherent in current procedures employed for preparation of isolated tubules (7,13).

It is not a far-fetched speculation to consider that due to higher lability of ATP levels in PCT compared to DCT, the cAMP-mediated functional responses of PCT to PTH *in vivo* may be particularly vulnerable in renal ischemia, phosphate depletion, fructose overload (14), and other pathophysiologic conditions in which renal cortical ATP content decreases (9). Indeed, according to current knowledge, cAMP-mediated proximal tubular responses to PTH are rather inconstant and more subject to the metabolic state of the kidney than PTH actions on distal nephron (15).

ACKNOWLEDGEMENTS

We gratefully acknowledge the technical assistance of Mrs. R. Holets and Ms. M. Keller as well as the secretarial assistance of Mrs. Bonnie Becker. Doctor Kiebzak is the recipient of an NIH research fellowship (Renal Diseases Research Training NIH Grant AM-07013). Dr. Kusano is a postdoctoral fellow of the American Heart Association, Minnesota Affiliate, Inc. This research was supported by NIH grant AM-30759 and by the Mayo Foundation.

REFERENCES

1. E. W. Sutherland, On the biological role of cyclic AMP, *JAMA* 214:1281 (1970).

2. T. P. Dousa, Cyclic nucleotides in renal pathophysiology, in: "Hormonal Function and the Kidney," B. Brenner and J. Stein, ed., Churchill Livingstone, New York (1979).
3. F. Morel, Sites of hormone action in the mammalian nephron. Am. J. Physiol. 240:F159 (1981).
4. B. A. Jackson, R. M. Edwards, H. Valtin, and T. P. Dousa, Cellular action of vasopressin in medullary tubules of mice with hereditary nephrogenic diabetes insipidus, J. Clin. Invest. 66:110 (1980).
5. R. M. Edwards, B. A. Jackson, and T. P. Dousa, ADH-sensitive cAMP system in papillary collecting duct: Effect of osmolality and PGE_2, Am. J. Physiol. 240:F311 (1981).
6. T. P. Dousa, B. A. Jackson, and R. M. Edwards. Cellular action of vasopressin in medullary collecting tubules and in ascending limbs of Henle's loop, in: "Antidiuretic Hormone," S. Yoshida, L. Share, and K. Yagi, ed., Japan Scientific Societies Press, Tokyo (1980).
7. F. Morel, D. Chabardes, and M. Imbert-Teboul, Methodology for enzymatic studies of isolated tubular segments: Adenylate cyclase, in: "Methods in Pharmacology: Renal Pharmacology," M. Martinez-Maldonado, ed., Plenum Press, New York (1976).
8. J. J. LeMasters, and C. R. Hackenbrock, Firefly luciferase assay for ATP production by mitochondria, in: "Methods in Enzymology," M. A. DeLuca, ed., Academic Press, New York (1978).
9. G. M. Kiebzak, A. N. K. Yusufi, E. Kusano, J. Werness, and T. P. Dousa, Low ATP levels in the proximal convoluted tubule of the mouse nephron, Fed. Proc. 42:1259 (1983).
10. M. G. Brunette, D. Chabardes, M. Imbert-Teboul, A. Clique, M. Montegut, and F. Morel, Hormone-sensitive adenylate cyclase along the nephron of genetically hypophosphatemic mice, Kidney Int. 15:357 (1979).
11. S. R. Gullans, P. C. Brazy, S. P. Soltoff, V. W. Dennis, and L. J. Mandel, Metabolic inhibitors: Effects on metabolism and transport in the proximal tubule, Am. J. Physiol. 243:F133 (1982).
12. M. K. Drezner, and W. M. Burch, Altered activity of the nucleotide regulatory site in the parathyroid hormone-sensitive adenylate cyclase from the renal cortex of a patient with pseudohypoparathyroidism, J. Clin. Invest. 62:1222 (1978).
13. W. G. Guder, and A. Rupprecht, Hormonal regulation of gluconeogenesis in isolated rat kidney tubule fragments, in: "Use of Isolated Liver Cells and Kidney Tubules in Metabolic Studies," J. M. Tager, H. D. Soling, and J. R. Williamson, ed., North-Holland Publishing Company, Amsterdam, (1976).

14. H. B. Burch, S. Choi, C. N. Dence, T. R. Alvey, B. R. Cole, and O. H. Lowry, Metabolic effects of large fructose loads in different parts of the rat nephron, J. Biol. Chem. 255:8239 (1980).
15. C. Amiel, D. Chabardes, and C. Bailly. Effects of parathyroid hormone on the kidney: Sites and mechanisms of action, in: "Advances in Nephrology," J. Hamburger, J. Crosnier, J. Greenfield, and M. Maxwell, ed., Year Book Medical Publishers, Inc., Chicago, (1982).

DIFFERENT EFFECTS OF PARATHYROID HORMONE ON EPITHELIAL TRANSPORT

Sandra Sabatini, Roger Mola, James T McCreary, and
Neil A Kurtzman

Departments of Medicine & Physiology
University of Illinois College of Medicine
Chicago, Illinois

INTRODUCTION

Parathyroid hormone (PTH) has been shown to stimulate calcium (Ca) transport in many tissues including human red cells, cultured heart cells, isolated mitochondria, Hela cells, renal and Ehrlich ascites tumor cells (1-7). The effect of PTH on calcium transport appears to be independent of activation adenylate cyclase (8). Because of these findings, we proposed that PTH may act as a naturally occurring calcium ionophore (8).

We have previously shown that maneuvers which increase cytosolic calcium are associated with a decrease in sodium, water, and proton transport in isolated anuran membranes (9-12). We therefore postulated that, if PTH acted as a nonselective calcium ionophore, it should affect membrane transport and calcium transport similarly, regardless of the tissue studied and whether PTH receptors are present.

We compared the effect of PTH on transport in two membranes: the toad bladder and the turtle bladder. The toad responds to parathyroidectomy as do mammals (13). The turtle, however, does not alter plasma calcium either following parathyroidectomy or infusion of parathyroid extract. The primitive parathyroid tissue of this animal shows no mitochondria and very few granules. When citrate infusion is given to turtles to decrease plasma calcium, which should stimulate PTH release, the parathyroid cells from the turtle are totally unchanged (13); thus, it appears that the parathyroid gland in fresh-water turtles is a vestigial organ and plays no role in calcium metabolism.

MATERIALS AND METHODS

Urinary bladder from the freshwater turtle (Pseudemys scripta) and toads (Bufo marinus) were excised, divided into hemibladders, and mounted in plexiglass chambers as previously described (9,10). In the turtle and toad bladders, sodium transport was measured using the short-circuit current (SCC) for 60-90 minutes following the serosal addition of either 1 μgm/ml PTH (bovine, 1-84) or the calcium ionophore, A23187 (10^{-5}M) (9,10). Proton secretion was measured as the reverse short-circuit current (RSCC) in the turtle bladder, as previously described, for 60 minutes following the addition of 1 μgm/ml PTH or 10^{-5}M A23187 (9).

Turtle bladder (stripped mucosa) and toad bladder epithelial cells were isolated as previously described (9,10). Ca^{45} uptake was measured following a 60 minute preincubation with either 1 μgm/ml PTH or 10^{-5}M A23187.

The data for SCC or RSCC in the experimental periods are normalized and expressed as percent of control values. Ca^{45} uptake is expressed as nanomoles/mgm protein/5 minutes. Statistical analysis was performed using either paired or unpaired "t" test with significance chosen at the $p<0.05$ level.

RESULTS

Table I shows the effect of PTH and A23187 on SCC in both the toad bladder and the turtle bladder. In the toad bladder, SCC fell to 78.1±10.5% of control 60 minutes following PTH (n=8, $p<0.05$). Following A23187, SCC fell to 70.7±5.9% of control (n=6, $p<0.05$). In the turtle bladder, PTH had no effect on SCC; however, following the administration of A23187, sodium transport fell to 79.3±3.6% of control (n=6, $p<0.05$).

Table I. Effect of PTH (1 μgm/ml) and A23187 (10^{-5}M) on Sodium Transport in the Toad and Turtle Bladders ($\bar{x}$±SEM)

	SCC (% of control)		
	Control	PTH	A23187
Toad	99.0±2.5	78.1±10.5[a]	70.7±5.9[a]
Turtle	98.1±1.5	96.2±2.6	79.3±3.6[a]

[a]$p<0.05$ from Control.

As shown in Table II, Ca^{45} uptake by the toad bladder significantly increased following PTH; this concentration of PTH had no effect on calcium transport in the turtle bladder. The ionophore significantly increased Ca^{45} uptake in both the toad and turtle bladders.

Table II. The Effect of PTH and A23187 on Ca^{45} Uptake by Isolated Toad Bladder Epithelial Cells and Stripped Turtle Bladder Mucosa ($\bar{x}$±SEM)

Toad	nmols/mgm protein/5 min
Control (n=8)	4.9±0.3
PTH (n=8)	9.9±0.7[a]
A23187 (n=8)	8.2±1.5[a]
Turtle	
Control (n=8)	29.7±3.0
PTH (n=8)	27.4±4.9
A23187 (n=8)	36.1±3.2[a]

[a]$p<0.05$ from Control.

In the turtle bladder, the ionophore significantly inhibited proton secretion as measured with the RSCC (72.2±9.3% of control, n=8, $p<0.05$). PTH, in a concentration which significantly inhibited sodium transport in the toad bladder, had no effect on hydrogen ion secretion in the turtle bladder.

DISCUSSION

These studies demonstrate that both PTH and the calcium ionophore, A23187, inhibit sodium transport in the toad bladder. These effects are associated with an increase in Ca^{45} uptake in isolated toad bladder epithelial cells. PTH has no effect on either membrane transport or Ca^{45} uptake in the turtle bladder. The calcium ionophore, however, inhibits both sodium and hydrogen transport in this tissue in concert with an increase in Ca^{45} uptake.

PTH has been shown to stimulate calcium transport in many tissues, in addition to its well-known effect in activating adenylate cyclase. Indeed, the transport of calcium appears to be totally independent of the activation of adenylate cyclase. The ionophore A23187, a polyene antibiotic, is known to affect calcium transport in many cells as well (2-5,9,10). In some tissues the effect of the ionophore is independent of the activation of adenylate cyclase.

As shown in this study, however, PTH exerts an effect only in certain sensitive tissues; that is, those membranes from animals with parathyroid tissue and presumably receptors for PTH. The ionophore, by contrast, affects transport (i.e., inhibits it) in a nonselective manner. The present study supports the notion that membrane transport is inhibited in association with an increase in cytosolic calcium. The mechanisms whereby PTH and the ionophore exert their effects on membrane transport are likely different.

REFERENCES

1. Bogin E, Massry SG, Levi J, Djaldeti M, Bristol G, Smith J: Effect of parathyroid hormone on osmotic fragility of human erythrocytes. J Clin Invest 69:1017, 1982.
2. Meytes D, Bogin E, Ma A, Dukes PP, and Massry SG: Effect of parathyroid hormone on erythropoiesis. J. Clin. Invest. 67:1263, 1981.
3. Chausmer AB, Sherman BS, Wallach S: The effect of parathyroid hormone on hepatic cell transport of calcium. Endocrinology 90:663, 1972.
4. Tenebause A, Meier H, Rasmussen H: Parathyroid hormone and bone mobilization in vitro. J Biol Chem 241:1314, 1966.
5. Borle AB: Calcium metabolism in Hela cells and the effect of parathyroid hormone. J Cell Biol 36:567, 1968.
6. Borle AB: Calcium metabolism at the cellular level. Fed Proc 32:1955, 1973.
7. Borle AB: Parathyroid hormone and cell calcium. In Calcium, Parathyroid Hormone, and the Calcitonins, eds Talmage RV and Munson RL. Amsterdam, Excerpta Medical Foundation, 484, 1972.
8. Sabatini S, McCreary JT, Kurtzman NA: Parathyroid hormone - a naturally occurring Ca ionophore. Clin Res 30:788A, 1982.
9. Arruda JAL, Sabatini S: Effect of quinidine on Na, H+ and water transport by the turtle and toad bladders. J Membrane Biol 55:141, 1980.
10. Arruda JAL, Sabatini S: Cholinergic modulation of water transport in the toad bladder. Amer J Physiol 239:F154, 1980.
11. Arruda JAL, Sabatini S: Cholinergic inhibition of urinary acidification by the turtle bladder. Kidney Internat 17:622, 1980.

12. Sabatini S, Arruda JAL: Calcium and membrane transport. In The Role of Calcium in Biological Systems, eds Anghileri LJ and Truffet-Anghileri AM, vol 2. Boca Raton, CRC Press Inc, 2, 1982.
13. Clark NB: Experimental and histologic studies of the parathyroid glands of fresh-water turtles. Gen Compar Endocrinol 5:297, 1965.

ACKNOWLEDGEMENTS

This work was supported in part by Chicago Heart Association Grant 83-41 and National Institutes of Health Grant AM-20170.

James T. McCreary was a fellow of the National Kidney Foundation.

INTESTINAL ABSORPTION OF PHOSPHATE AND CALCIUM

VERAPAMIL IMPROVES DEFECTIVE INTESTINAL CALCIUM ABSORPTION IN UREMIA

M.S. Goligorsky, C. Chaimovitz, Sh. Shany, J. Rapoport and Y. Sharony

With the technical assistance of I. Suili and N. Yankovitz

Dept. of Nephrology, Soroka University Hospital
and Faculty of Health Sciences, Ben-Gurion Univ. of Negev
Beer-Sheba, Israel

INTRODUCTION

One of the recognized manifestations of renal insufficiency is a defect in intestinal absorption of calcium (1). There is substantial clinical and experimental evidence that this abnormality in intestinal absorption of calcium is secondary to uremia per se and to reduced ability of the diseased kidney to synthesize 1,25-(OH)$_2$vitamin D_3 (2-5). Interestingly, this impairment of intestinal transport of calcium has been described even in early stages of renal insufficiency when other parameters of renal function are relatively well preserved, and when plasma levels of 1,25 (OH)$_2$vitamin D_3 may be normal (5,6). Normal level of vitamin D in the face of reduced intestinal absorption of calcium suggests that renal 1α-hydroxylase activity is relatively suppressed in early uremia (7).

There is experimental evidence that cytosolic calcium concentration is one of the main factors regulating 1α-hydroxylase activity (8). Thus, extramitochondrial concentrations of calcium up to 10^{-5}M maintain 1α-hydroxylase activity of stimulated mitochondrial preparations (9)., whilst higher concentrations suppress 1α-hydroxylation (10). In this connection, renal parenchymal accumulation of calcium is a well-known feature of chronic renal failure (11,12). If this calcium accumulation involved the cytosolic compartment, it could play a role in 1α-hydroxylase suppression. The corollary of this assumption is that preventing cytosplasmic calcium accumulation in uremia might restore at least partially 1α-hydroxylase activity and, consequently, 1,25 (OH)$_2$vitamin D_3 synthesis. This hypothesis was tested by using the calcium influx blocker verapamil to prevent cytosolic calcium accumulation in uremic rats. rats.

MATERIALS AND METHODS

Studies were performed on male Charles River rats weighing 200-250 g. Four experimental groups, each consisting of 10 animals, were studied: Group A - rats were studied 3 weeks after renal failure was induced by single step 5/6 nephrectomy using a flank incision. Group B - rats with chronic renal failure induced as in group A, treated with verapamil 10 mcg/100 g body weight twice a day administered intramuscularly. Group C - Sham operated rats who underwent flank incision and kidney decapsulation. Group D - Sham operated rats (as in group C), who received verapamil 10 mcg/100 g body weight intramuscularly twice daily. All the animals were kept in individual metabolic cages for 3 weeks following 5/6 nephrectomy of sham operation. Rats of group A were fed standard chow and had free access to water. Rats of groups B and C were pair-fed with rats of group A during the 3-week period following operation.

Intestinal absorption of calcium was determined by the method of Omdahl et al (13). Briefly, a 10 cm segment of duodenal loop was isolated, and its lumen rinsed with 5 ml of phosphate-free bicarbonate solution. 0.5 ml of the solution containing 0.5 mcCi of ^{45}Ca with a final calcium chloride concentration of 1 mM/L was then injected into the loop. After 30 min the duodenal loop was excised and dry ashed in a dish at 600^{0}C for 24 hours. Radioactivity was estimated in a packard scintillation counter. Results were expressed as percentage of ^{45}Ca absorbed:

Percentage of ^{45}Ca absorbed $= (1 - {}^{45}Ca_{remaining} / {}^{45}Ca_{added})\,100$.

Following the above protocol, the kidneys were removed with special attention paid to removing the scarred capsule and to performing determinations on apparently non-necrotic cortical tissues. Light microscopy of hematoxylin-eosin and von Kossa-stained Kidney slices obtained after these procedures proved the absence of coarse tissue damage due to the surgical procedure.

After drying, renal cortical tissue was reweighed, and then hydrolyzed with 0.5 ml of concentrated hydrochloric acid for 60 min during which time complete tissue digestion occurred. The residue was then neutralized with sodium hydroxide solution to pH 7.9, and lanthanum chloride was added to each sample to a final concentration of 1%. Calcium concentration was determined by atomic absorption spectriphotometry (Varian 375).

25-hydroxy-vitamin D_3 was determined by competitive protein-binding assay (14). Briefly, plasma samples were subjected to the following procedures. 1. Sample extraction with chloroform-methanol (2:1.v/v). 2. Chromatography of lipid residues on Sephadex LH-20 Column. 3. Equilibration of collected fraction of 25-OH-vitamin D_3 and ^{3}H-labeled 25-OH-vitamin D_3 with the assay binding protein. 4. Absorption of "free" sterol by charcoal coated with dextran and 5. Counting of "bound" sterol .

1,25-dihydroxy-vitamin D_3 was measured by radioimmunoassay according to the technique of Clemens et al (15). Sheep antisera to 1,25 $(OH)_2$ vitamin D_3 were kindly supplied by Dr. J.L.H, O'Riordan. B riefly, plasma samples were extracted with ethanol and purified by chromatography on Sephadex LH 20 and then subjected to high pressure liquid chromatography (Gow Mac Instr Co., Model 080 - 20). Aliquots of the chromatographed plasma extracts were incubated with antiserum for 24 hours at 4^{0}C and then adsorbed on dextrancoated charcoal. Supernatants were transferred to a liquid scintillator and counted in a packard LSC at an efficiency of 35-40%.

Statistical analysis of data was carried out by Student's t test, and results expressed as mean$\pm$S.E.M.

RES ULTS

Verapamil administration to sham operated rats was not associated with any changes in the plasma concentrations of BUN, creatinine, calcium or inorganic phosphorus, as compared to the untreated sham operated group. 5/6 nephrectomy (group A) was followed by a rise in plasma creatinine to 1.2$\pm$0.3 (Mean$\pm$SE) , and BUN to 45$\pm$ 1 mg%, as compared to groups C and D ($p<0.01$) . Plasma calcium and inorganic phosphorus concentrations in group A rats were 10.2$\pm$0.2 and 8.8$\pm$0.4 mg/dl respectively. Administration of verapamil to 5/6 nephrectomized rats (group B) did not lead to any substantial change in the plasma concentration of BUN, creatinine, calcium or phosphorus, as compared to group A rats.

Fractional duodenal calcium absorption (FDA-Ca).

Figure 1 summarizes FDA-Ca in the experimental groups A-D, FDA-Ca was quite similar in groups C and D, 72$\pm$3% and 78$\pm$4% respectively. Untreated 5/6 nephrectomized rats exhibited a marked reduction in FDA-Ca, 25$\pm$4%, as compared to groups C and D ($p<0.01$) Verapamil administration to chronically uremic rats (group B) resulted in an almost 2-fold increase in FDA-Ca, 51$\pm$5%, compared to untrated 5/6 nephrectomized rats ($p<0.01$) . In order to exclude a possible effect of verapamil on the intestinal absorption of calcium via a mechanism independent of 1.25 $(OH)_2$ vitamin D_3 synthesis, FDA-Ca was determined in 8 rats 48 hours after bilateral nephrectomy. FDA-Ca in these rats was markedly depressed (8$\pm$2%) . However, when verapamil 10 mcg/100g body weight was given to another group of 8 bilaterally nephrectomized rats, FDA-Ca was even further reduced (3$\pm$1%) . These data strongly suggest that the presence of resudual renal parenchyma is necessary for the enhancement of FDA-Ca in uremic rats receiving verapamil.

Ca content of renal cortex.

In the untreated 5/6 nephrectomized rats (group A), renal calcium content was 1.29±0.234 mg/g dry weight, a value significantly higher than 0.566±0.106 mg/g dry weight seen in the sham operated group. ($p<0.01$). Following verapamil treatment of 5/6 nephrectomized rats, renal cortical calcium content (0.851±0.175 mg/g dry weight) was substantially decreased ($p<0.01$) as compared to the similar non-treated uremic animals.

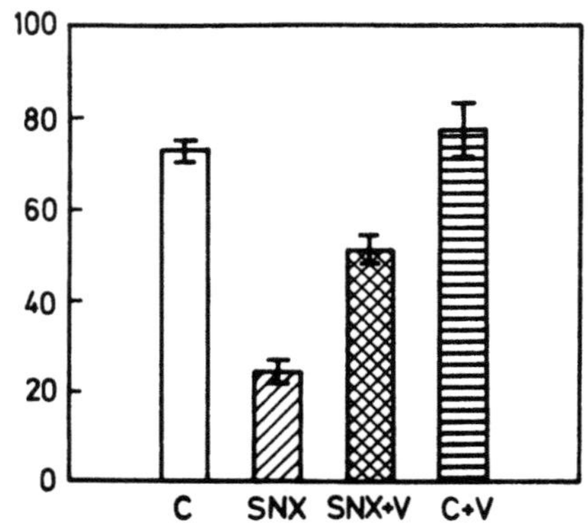

Fig. 1. Fractional duodenal absorption of ^{45}Ca in the four groups of experimental rats: C-sham operated, C+VE - verapamil treated sham operated rats, SNX - subtotally-nephrectomized, and SNX+VE - verapamil treated subtotally-nephrectomized rats.

Plasma concentration of vitamin D metabolites.

Figure 2 depicts the plasma concentration of 25 (OH) $_2$ vitamin D_3 and 1.25 (OH) $_2$ vitamin D_3 in rats of groups A, B and C. Plasma concentrations of 25 (OH) vitamin D_3 were not significantly different in these 3 experimental groups. Plasma concentration of 1.25 (OH) $_2$ vitamin D_3 in the untreated 5/6 nephrectomized rats - 29±8 pg/ml was not statistically different from the level of 32±5 pg/ml, in the sham operated animals. However, the administration of verapamil induced a marked increase in plasma 1.25 (OH) $_2$ vitamin D_3 to 50±9 pg/ml in 5/6 nephrectomized rats. This value was significantly higher ($p<0.05$) than values obtained in sham and in untreated 5/6 nephrectomized rats. Plasma concentration of 1.25 $(OH)_2$ vitamin D_3 in sham rats treated with verapamil (Group D) was similar to the non-treated sham rats (Group C).

DISCUSSION

The present study demonstrates that chronic verapamil administration to 5/6 nephrectomized rats leads to a marked improvement in the defective intestinal absorption of calcium. This effect was not related to changes in renal excretory function, since BUN and creatinine concentrations remained similar in VE-treated and untreated partially nephrectomized animals.

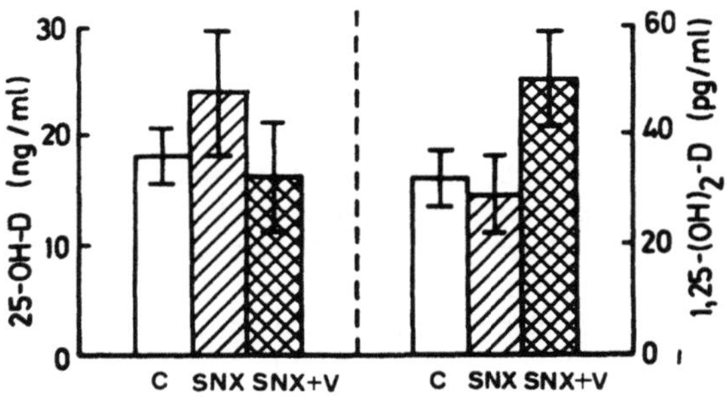

Fig. 2. Serum levels of 25-hydroxy-vitamin D (left panel), and 1.25-dihydroxy-vitaminD(right panel) in sham operated (C), 5/6 nephrectomized (SNX) and verapamil treated 5/6 nephrectomized (SNX+VE) rats.

It could be argued that the improved intestinal absorption of calcium following verapamil treatment may be due to a direct effect of this agent on intestinal transport of calcium. The administration of verapamil to bilaterally nephrectomized rats, however, did not improve the blunted ability of the duodenum to transport calcium. Thus, we found no evidence for a direct effect of verapamil in stimulating intestinal calcium transport in these animals. Hence, it can be concluded that verapamil-induced enhancement of FDA-Ca necessitated the presence of residual renal parenchyma.

In this connection, another major finding of the study was that verapamil administration caused an almost 2-fold increase in the serum 1,25 (OH) $_2$ vitamin D_3 concentration in partially nephrectomized animals. It should be noted that the normal plasma levels of 1,25 (OH) $_2$ vitamin D_3 found in non-treated uremic rats in the face of reduced intestinal calcium absorption are in agreement with similar findings in a previous study (6).

One of the factors controlling 1α-hydroxylase activity is the cytoplasmic calcium concentration of renal tubular cells; an increased concentration suppressed whilst a reduced concentration enhanced 1α-hydroxylase activity of mitochondrial preparations obtained from vitamin D-deficient animals (9,10). Similarly, in vivo studies in rats receiving high doses of diphosphonates demonstrated suppression of 1α-hydroxylase activity, a reduction in intestinal calcium transport and renal calcium accumulation (16-18). In order to demonstrate whether the enhanced serum 1,25 (OH) $_2$ vitamin D_3 levels found in the present study were related to renal calcium accumulation in the uremic rats, we measured the latter in partially nephrectomized animals with and without chronic verapamil administration. While non-treated uremic rats had elevated renal parenchymal calcium content, verapamil treated uremic rats revealed significantly lower renal calcium content similar to control values obtained in the sham group. These data suggest that the increased 1,25 (OH) $_2$ vitamin D_3 generation by the uremic kidney treated with verapamil and the normalization of renal calcium content might be related phenomena. It is well established that verapamil attenuats plasma membrane influx of calcium into the cytoplasma. In this context verapamil-induced correction of renal calcium accumulation in 5/6NX rats allows to assume that cellular calcium overload plays a pivotal role in the development of uremic nephrocalcinosis.

The present data cannot rule out the possibility that the augmented synthesis of 1,25 (OH) $_2$ vitamin D_3 may be mediated by an action on PTH on concentration of phosphate (9,19). Since plasma phosphate concentration in verapamil animals were similar to those seen in pair-fed, non-VE-treated rats, it is unlikely that there was significant alteration in phosphate homeostasis in verapamil treated animals.

Theoretically, the augmented intestinal calcium absorption and elevation in plasma level of 1,25 (OH) $_2$ vitamin D_3 could be due to a stimulatory effect of verapamil on PTH secretion. It was shown recently, however, that verapamil infusion directly into the parathyroid artery resulted in marked suppression of PTH secretion (20).

We have thus demonstrated that verapamil administration to chronically uremic rats reduces renal parenchymal calcium content, stimulates synthesis of 1,25 (OH) 2 vitamin D_3 and augments impaired intestinal calcium absorption. It is tempting to speculate that these phenomena are related. Hence, the primary effect of verapamil may be to decrease cytosolic calcium concentration of renal tubular cells, thereby enhancing 1α-hydroxylase activity, increasing production of 1,25 (OH) 2 vitamin D_3 and thus improving intestinal calcium absorption.

REFERENCES

1. Coburn, J. W.; Hartenbower, D.L.; Brickman, A.S.; Massry, S.G., and Kopple, J.D.: Intestinal absorption of calcium, magnesium and phosphorus in chronic renal insufficiency. In: Calcium metabolism in chronic renal failure and nephrolithiasis. Ed. by D.S. David. A Wiley medical publication, 1977, pp. 77-111.

2. Mawer, E. B.; Backhouse, J.; Taylor, C.M. Lumb, G.A., and Stanbury, S. W.: Failure of formation of 1,25 (OH) 2 vitamin D in chronic renal insufficiency. Lancet 1: 626-628 (1973).

3. Brumbaugh, P.F.; Haussler, D.H.; Bressler, R., and Haussler, M.R.: Radio-receptor assay for 1,25-dihydroxy-vitamin D_3. Science 183: 1089-1092 (1974).

4. Hartenbower, D.L.; Coburn, J. W.; Riddy, C.R. and Norman, A. W.: Calciferol metabolism and intestinal calcium transport in the chick with reduced renal function. J. Lab. Clin. Med. 83: 38-46 (1974).

5. Malluche, H.H.; Werner, E. and Ritz, E.: Intestinal absorption of calcium and whole-body calcium retention in incipient and advanced renal failure. Min. & Electr. Metab. 1: 263 - 270 (1978).

6. Slatopolsky, E.; Gray, R.; Adams, N.D.; Lewis, J.; Hruska, K.; Martin, K.; Klahr, S. and Deluca, H.F.: Low serum levels of 1,25 $(OH)_2D_3$ are not responsible for the development of secondary hyperparathyroidism in early renal failure. In: Proc. Amer. Soc. Nephrol. 11: 99A (1978).

7. Goldstein, D.A.; D.A.; Horowitz, R.E.; Petit, S.: Haldiman, B.; Massry, S.G.: The duodenal mucosa in patients with renal failure: Responce to 1,25 $(OH)_2D_3$. Kidney Int., 19: 324-331 (1981).

8. Fraser, D.: Regulation of the metabolism of vitamin D. Physiol. Rev. 60 (2): 551-613 (1980).

9. Bikle, D.D.; Murphy, E.W.; Rasmussen, H.: The ionic control of 1,25 (OH) $_2D_3$ synthesis in isolated chick renal mitochondria. The role of calcium as influenced by inorganic phosphate and hydrogen ion. J. Clin. Invest. 55: 299-304 (1975).

10. Horiuchi, N.; Suda, T.; Sasaki, S.; Ogata, E.; Ezawa, I.; Sano, Y. and Shimazawa, E.: The regulatory role of calcium in 25-OH-vitamin D_3 metabolism in chick kidney in vitro. Arch. Biochem. Biophys. 171: 540-548 (1975).

11. Ibels, L.S.; Alfrey, A.; and Huffer, W.E.: Calcification in end stage kidneys. Amer. J. Med. 71: 33-37 (1981).

12. Kuzela, D.C.; Huffer, W.E. and Conger, J.D.: Soft tissue calcification in chronic dialysis patients. Amer. J. Pathol. 86: 403-424 (1977).

13. Omdahl, J.; Holick, M.; Suda, T.; Tanaka, Y. and DeLuca, H.F.: Biological activity of 1,25-dihydroxycholecalciferol. Biochemistry 10: 2935-2940 (1971).

14. Edelstein, S.; Charman, M.; Lawson, D. and Kodicek, E.: 25-hydroxyvitamin D_3 determination by competitive binding protein assay. Clin. Sci. Mol. Med. 46: 231-240 (1974).

15. Clemens. T.L.; Hendy, G.M.; Papapoulas, S.E.; Fragher, L.J. and O'Riordan, J.L.H.: Measurement of 1,25-dihydroxycholecalciferol in man by radioimmunoassay. Clin. Endocrinol. 11: 225-234 (1979).

16. Gasser, A.B.; Morgan, D.B.; Fleisch, H.A. and Richelle, L.J.: The influence of two diphosphonates on calcium metabolism in the rat. Clin. Sci. 43: 31-45 (1972).

17. Baxter, L.A.; DeLuca, H.F.; Bonjour, J-P. and Fleisch, H.A.: Inhibition of vitamin D metabolism by ethane-1-hydroxy-1,1-diphosphonate. Arch. Biochem. Biophys. 164: 655-662 (1974).

18. Goulding, A. and Cameron, V.: Effects of diphosphonate on kidney calcium content and duodenal absorption of ^{45}Ca. Horm. Metab. Res. 10: 573-574 (1978).

19. Fraser, D.R. and Kodicek, E.: Regulation of 25-hydroxycholecalciferol-1-hydroxylase activity in kidney by parathyroid hormone. Nature (London) 241: 163-166 (1973).

20. Hove, K. and Sand, O.: Evidence for a role of calcium influx in

the stimulation-secretion coupling in parathyroid cells. In: Hormonal control of calcium metabolusm. Excerpta Medica 1981 p.346.

VITAMIN D ACTIVATES $(Na^{+}-K^{+})$ATPase: A POSSIBLE REGULATION OF PHOSPHATE AND CALCIUM UPTAKE BY CULTURED EMBRYONIC CHICK SMALL INTESTINE

Heide S. Cross and Meinrad Peterlik

Department of General and Experimental Pathology
University of Vienna, Austria

INTRODUCTION

The effect of vitamin D_3 and of its biologically most active metabolite, 1,25-dihydroxyvitamin D_3, on intestinal calcium and inorganic phosphate (P_i) absorptive mechanisms has been studied extensively in an organ culture system of embryonic chick small intestine (Corradino, 1973; Peterlik, 1978; Cross and Peterlik, 1982). Elevation of Ca and P_i uptake by vitamin D depends on prior gene activation by the sterol (cf. also Franceschi and DeLuca, 1981b). However, this vitamin D action is only partially expressed in undifferentiated absorptive cells, since they respond to the sterol solely by an increase in Ca but not in P_i uptake. Induction of the latter has been shown to require advanced target cell maturation (Cross and Peterlik, 1982).

Although lumen-to-blood transfer of Ca and P_i involves separate transepithelial routes (for review see Wasserman, 1981), a common linkage of these pathways may exist in the dependence of individual transfer steps on the transmembrane Na^{+} gradient which drives P_i entry across the brush-border membrane (Berner et al., 1976; Fuchs and Peterlik, 1980) as well as Ca exit via the basolateral Na^{+}/Ca^{++} exchanger (Hildmann et al., 1982). It is conceivable that vitamin D could stimulate transepithelial Ca and P_i transport in a coordinate fashion through an effect on transmembrane Na^{+} fluxes, thereby generating a steeper Na^{+} gradient. In fact, vitamin D has been shown to reduce Na^{+} permeability of brush-border vesicles derived from chick small intestine. The resultant elevation of the electrochemical Na^{+} potential could thus contribute to the vitamin D-related increase in Na^{+}-dependent solute transport (Peterlik,

Fuchs and Cross, 1981). Another possibility to step up the extra/intracellular Na^+ gradient would be stimulation of the basolateral (Na^+-K^+)ATPase by vitamin D. This was explored in the present study.

MATERIAL AND METHODS

Organ culture procedure

Embryonated eggs were incubated at 38.5°C and 80% relative humidity for 15-20 days. Proximal segments of the duodenum, jejunum and ileum were then excised, slit open and cultured mucosa side-up on stainless steel grids in serum-free McCoy's 5A mod. medium as described in detail elsewhere (Corradino, 1973). Culture time was 48 h, if not stated otherwise. Routinely, vitamin D_3 or 1,25-dihydroxyvitamin D_3 were dissolved in ethanol and added to the culture medium to achieve concentrations of 26 µM or 120 nM, respectively. Final ethanol concentration did not exceed 0.1%.

Ion transport measurements

For determination of radiotracer fluxes, 6-8 cultured guts were incubated together in 5.0 ml phosphate-free Krebs-Henseleit bicarbonate buffer at 37°C (pH 7.4), containing 0.5 µCi/ml of either $^{22}Na^+$, $^{42}K^+$ or $^{86}Rb^+$. Stable ion concentrations were 143 mM Na^+, 4.75 mM K^+ or 0.1 mM Rb^+. Incubation was terminated by rinsing the guts three times with ice-cold isotonic mannitol solution under continuous suction. Guts were then blotted, weighed and assayed for γ-radioactivity. Details of the method have been described previously (Corradino, 1973; Peterlik, 1978). When appropriate, ouabain was added to the incubation buffer at 1.0 mM.

Determination of (Na^+-K^+)ATPase

(Na^+-K^+)ATPase was assayed in mucosal scrapings of cultured guts according to Charney et al.(1974). Three independent determinations comprising a total of 18 segments were carried out for each group.

Presentation of data

Transport data were calculated on a mg tissue wet weight basis and converted, when appropriate, to "percent of vitamin D-free control" (means ± S.E.; n, 6-12). Difference from control group was considered significant when indicated by P values at least < 0.05

RESULTS AND DISCUSSION

(Na^+-K^+)ATPase activity determined by $^{86}Rb^+$ uptake

(Na^+-K^+)ATPase and, hence, sodium pump activity was measured by uptake of the K^+ tracer $^{86}Rb^+$. When cultured intestinal segments were incubated for 30 min in the presence and absence of ouabain, vitamin D_3 was found to increase ouabain-sensitive $^{86}Rb^+$ accumulation in duodenal, jejunal and ileal tissue by 36±4, 100±8 and 20±5 %, respectively, over controls. Since the jejunum was most sensitive to the sterol, this segment was exclusively used for subsequent experiments.

$^{86}Rb^+$ uptake is linear for up to 60 min in this tissue (Fig.1) and is stimulated by the presence of vitamin D_3 in the culture medium. Ouabain, when added to the incubation buffer, reduced $^{86}Rb^+$ uptake substantially and totally abolished the vitamin D increment. This suggests a distinct sensitivity of the Na^+ pump towards vitamin D. This appears to be in contrast to direct measurements of (Na^+-K^+)ATPase activity: In mucosal homogenates of jejunal segments cultured with and without vitamin D_3, no significant difference in

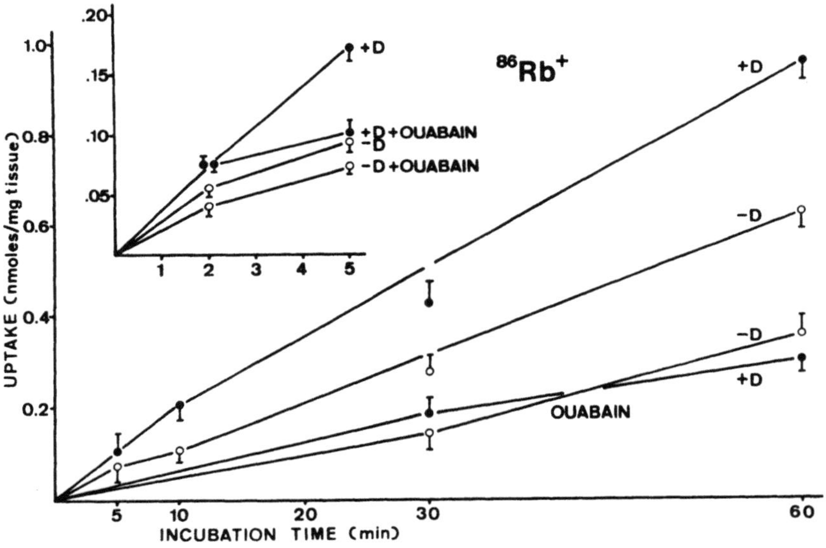

Fig. 1 Effect of vitamin D on $^{86}Rb^+$ uptake in embryonic jejunum (day 20). Ouabain present during total incubation time. Insert: Preincubation with or without ouabain for 20 min. ○-D, vitamin D-free controls; ● +D, 26 μM vitamin D_3.

hydrolytic enzyme activity could be detected (0.65±0.07 vs. 0.63±0.03 μmoles P_i liberated per mg protein in 1 h).

$^{86}Rb^+$ uptake by cultured jejunum in response to vitamin D_3 is first visible after 12 h culture, and rises then gradually until 48 h. This increment is brought about by vitamin D_3 and 1,25-dihydroxyvitamin D_3 alike. However, the sterols differ in their effectiveness to raise $^{86}Rb^+$ uptake: The least effective concentration of 1,25-dihydroxyvitamin D_3 tested was 12.5 nM. Maximum response (57±5% over controls) was elicited by 120 nM. Comparable effects were obtained by 0.26 to 26 μM vitamin D_3.

Since the degree of differentiation of enterocytes apparently determines the extent of vitamin D action (Cross and Peterlik, 1982) the influence of vitamin D on (Na^+-K^+)ATPase activity was measured in jejunal segments cultured at different stages of embryonic development. The highest vitamin D-related increment of ouabain-sensitive $^{86}Rb^+$ uptake was observed already in day 16 small intestines (Fig. 2). It declined until day 18-19, and then rose again shortly before hatching. In this, vitamin D stimulation of (Na^+-K^+)ATPase

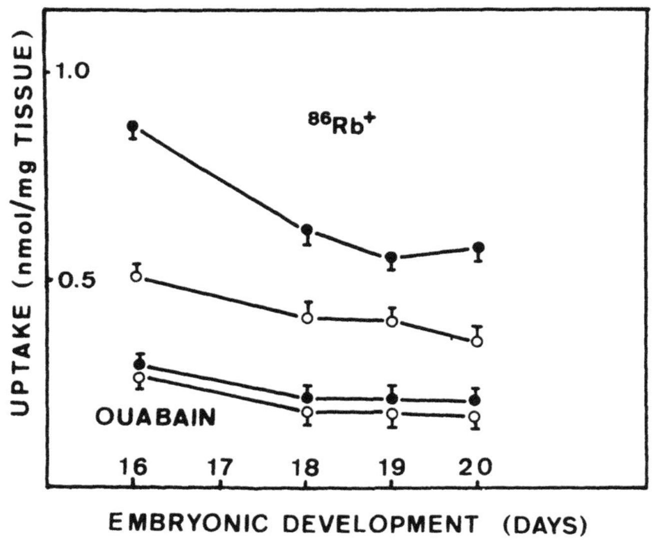

Fig. 2 Stimulation of ouabain-sensitive $^{86}Rb^+$ uptake by vitamin D in dependence of embryonic development. Preincubation 20 min with and without ouabain. Incubation time with radioisotope 30 min. ○ -D, vitamin D-free controls; ● +D, 26 μM vitamin D_3.

activity resembled very much the effect of the sterol on Ca uptake, though it is in contrast to Na^+-dependent P_i transport which is not affected by vitamin D until late in development on embryonic day 20 (Cross and Peterlik, 1982). This suggests that the vitamin D effect on Na^+-linked P_i transport is not solely mediated by its action on the sodium pump.

Stimulation of the sodium pump by vitamin D has some implications on the regulation of transepithelial transport of calcium. In addition to facilitation of the entry step, the steroid hormone could thereby provide an effective measure also for Ca exit. Activation of the (Na^+-K^+)ATPase leading to a steeper transmembrane Na^+ gradient might thus stimulate coupled Na^+/Ca^{++} exchange. Its existence in embryonic enterocytes can be inferred from the dependence of Ca accumulation on extracellular Na^+ (Corradino, 1978; Peterlik, 1978; Franceschi and DeLuca, 1981a). Since luminal Ca transfer is not affected by extracellular Na^+ (Corradino, 1978), the accentuation of Ca accumulation in the absence of buffer Na^+ could only be linked to an effective block of a Na^+-sensitive exit step. This would be most likely a Na^+/Ca^{++} antiport system, particularly since definite proof of its existence in the small intestine has been obtained in other species (Hildmann et al., 1982).

Activation of the (Na^+-K^+)ATPase by vitamin D bears on the possible role of the steroid as a trophic hormone (Birge and Alpers, 1973). Since elevated sodium pumping is regarded as one of the earliest signals for cell growth (Rozengurt and Mendoza, 1980), vitamin D may play an important role in proliferation of undifferentiated enterocytes.

Influence of vitamin D on luminal $^{22}Na^+$ uptake

A possible explanation for the failure to demonstrate a vitamin D-related change in hydrolytic activity of the (Na^+-K^+)ATPase, despite the increased $^{86}Rb^+$ uptake, may be that the sodium pump is activated not through a change of its intrinsic properties but rather by increased permeation of Na^+ into the cell. In this respect, Rozengurt and Mendoza (1980) have shown that serum and growth factors stimulate the translocation of Na^+ across cell membranes which, in turn, would enhance the pump by the increased availability of Na^+. Since a similar mechanism may be underlying the observed effect of vitamin D on the (Na^+-K^+)ATPase, we investigated a possible role of the hormone in Na^+ transport by embryonic chick intestine.

When tissue uptake of $^{22}Na^+$ was measured by 2.0 min incubation of cultured day 20 small intestine, an about equal increment due to vitamin D_3 or 1,25-dihydroxyvitamin D_3 (20-30% above basal values) was observed in all segments of the small intestine. This is obviously in contrast to the segment-specific increase in vitamin D-induced $^{86}Rb^+$ uptake.

Preincubation with 1.0 mM ouabain did by no means reduce the extent of the vitamin D effect on Na^+ uptake (Fig. 3). This excludes the possibility that the higher rate of Na^+ entry observed in guts cultured in the presence of vitamin D_3, was only a consequence of enhanced Na^+ pumping across the contralateral plasma membrane. In addition, it would be expected that ouabain, by blocking the Na^+ pump, would increase intracellular Na^+ and thereby affect Na^+ accumulation. The ineffectiveness of ouabain on basal Na^+ uptake (Fig. 3) therefore raises the question, whether Na^+ uptake as measured rather reflects Na^+ entry into the epithelium by a paracellu-

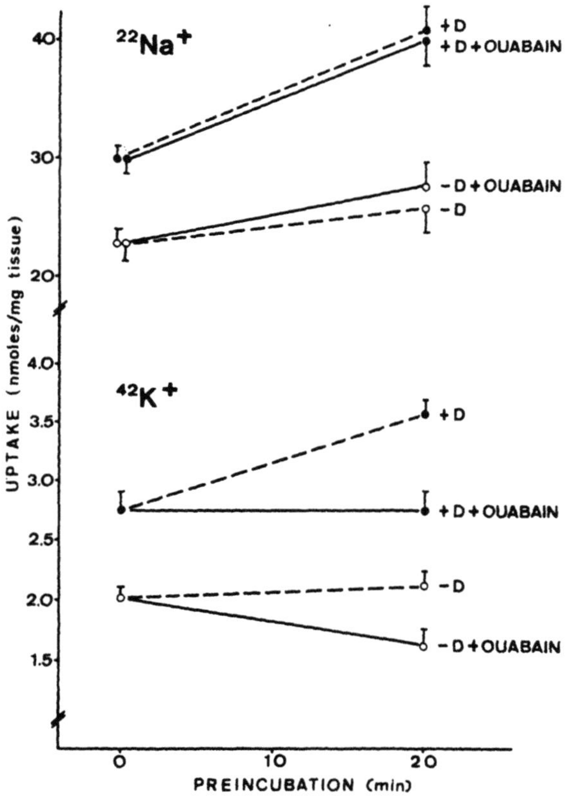

Fig. 3 Stimulation of $^{22}Na^+$ and $^{42}K^+$ uptake by vitamin D in embryonic jejunum (day 20). Preincubation with and without ouabain. Incubation time with radioisotopes 2 min. ○ -D, vitamin D-free controls; ● +D 26 μM vitamin D_3.

lar than a transcellular route. This has to be considered a likely possibility in view of the fact that in a "leaky" epithelium such as the small intestine transepithelial Na^+ transfer proceeds mainly via intercellular junctions (cf. Schultz, 1979).

In addition, any stimulatory effect of vitamin D on Na^+ entry into epithelial cells across the luminal plasma membrane would be difficult to reconcile with the finding, that vitamin D by reduction of potential-sensitive Na^+ flux as well as of Na^+/H^+ antiport inhibits any mode of Na^+ transfer in isolated intestinal brush-border membrane vesicles from four week-old chicks (Fuchs and Peterlik, manuscript in preparation).

Therefore, we assumed that the observed increase in $^{22}Na^+$ uptake was more likely to result from a change in Na^+ permeability of the junctional complex than of the apical enterocytic membrane. If this hypothesis was correct, the action of vitamin D should not be restricted specifically to Na^+ transfer but flux rates of other ions able to pass readily through intercellular junctions ought to be likewise affected. To test this hypothesis, we chose to determine $^{42}K^+$ uptake by cultured jejunum, primarily, because in "leaky" epithelia paracellular pathways show cation selectivity with K^+ permeability exceeding that of Na^+ (Schultz, 1979). Therefore, it seemed likely that, in comparison to Na^+, measurement of K^+ uptake under the conditions employed, would even more reflect paracellular flux into the intact epithelium.

Fig. 3 shows that K^+ enters more readily into the epithelium of guts cultured in the presence than in the absence of vitamin D_3. This effect of the steroid hormone persisted when incubations were carried out in the presence of ouabain, though basal K^+ flux was somewhat reduced. Apparently, the incubation time chosen is sufficient to allow a substantial amount of K^+ to enter the intercellular space, but is too short to allow major reuptake of K^+ through the basolateral Na^+/K^+ pump.

Similar results were obtained with $^{86}Rb^+$ (cf. Fig. 1, insert). Its junctional permeability in leaky epithelia is comparable to that of K^+ (cf. Schultz, 1979). When $^{86}Rb^+$ was allowed to enter the epithelium for 2.0 min, increased flux rates unaffected by ouabain were observed, when guts had been cultured with vitamin D_3 in the culture medium. After 5.0 min incubation, however, basal and vitamin D-related uptake was heavily diminished by ouabain.

CONCLUSIONS

Vitamin D stimulates (Na^+-K^+)ATPase activity in cultured embryonic small intestine and, consequently, through a higher rate of Na^+ pumping could give rise to steeper transmembrane Na^+

gradients. Conceptually, this effect may be related to the stimulatory action of vitamin D on transepithelial Ca transport since it would benefit Ca extrusion via Na^+/Ca^{++} antiport. Concurring variations during embryonic development of both vitamin D-induced Na^+ pump activity and of Ca uptake from the lumen support the notion that transcellular Ca transport might be coordinately regulated through vitamin D action on the entry as well as on the exit step. In contrast, vitamin D action on the (Na^+-K^+)ATPase could be dissociated from its effect on Na^+-dependent P_i transport showing a different developmental pattern. This excludes the possibility that vitamin D promotes Na^+ gradient-driven P_i transport solely by its action on the Na^+ gradient.

From a comparison of the vitamin D-related change in Na^+ pump activity (measured by $^{86}Rb^+$ uptake by intact epithelium) and the enzymatic activity of the (Na^+-K^+)ATPase in cell homogenates it is obvious that vitamin D does not alter intrinsic properties of the pump but raises its activity in intact cells by indirect means. Increased luminal influx of Na^+, which is considered likely to trigger basolateral Na^+ extrusion, was in fact observed in response to vitamin D. However, attempting to define the localization of this vitamin D-sensitive pathway within the epithelium, it appeared that Na^+ uptake as measured is predominantly on a paracellular route and, thus, had to be discounted as explanation for the stimulatory action of vitamin D on the (Na^+-K^+)ATPase. Although the exact mechanism by which this is accomplished remains unclear, these attempts at its elucidation have led to the discovery of another vitamin D effect: By inducing changes in ionic "shunt" permeability, which were observed also by measurements of ion fluxes in addition to Na^+ (viz. K^+, Rb^+), vitamin D may play a potentially important role as a hormonal regulator of epithelial ion transport in the small intestine.

ACKNOWLEDGMENTS

This work was supported by Grant No. 4422 of the Austrian National Research Foundation. 1,25-Dihydroxyvitamin D_3 was generously supplied by Dr. Milan Uskoković, Roche Inc., Nutley, N.J. The authors thank Peter Wyskovsky for skillful technical assistance.

REFERENCES

Berner, W., Kinne, R., and Murer, H.: Phosphate Transport into Brush-Border Membrane Vesicles Isolated from Rat Small Intestine. Biochem.J. 160:467-474 (1976).

Birge, S.J., and Alpers, D.H.: Stimulation of Intestinal Mucosal Proliferation by Vitamin D. Gastroenterol. 64:977-982 (1973).

Charney, A.N., Gots, R.E., and Gianella, R.A.: (Na^+-K^+)-Stimulated Adenosine Triphosphatase in Isolated Intestinal Villus Tip and Crypt Cells. Biochim.Biophys.Acta 367:265-270 (1974).
Corradino, R.A.: Embryonic chick intestine in organ culture: A unique system for the study of the intestinal calcium absorptive mechanism. J.Cell Biol. 58:64-78 (1973).
Corradino, R.A.: A Simple Technique for the Measurement of Unidirectional Calcium Influx at the Mucosal Surface of Organ-Cultured Embryonic Chick Duodenum. Analyt.Biochem. 91:60-69 (1978).
Cross, H.S., and Peterlik, M.: Differential Response of Enterocytes to Vitamin D during Embryonic Development: Induction of Intestinal Inorganic Phosphate, D-Glucose and Calcium Uptake. Horm.metabol.Res. 14:649-652 (1982).
Franceschi, R.T., and De Luca, H.F.: Characterization of 1,25-Dihydroxyvitamin D_3-dependent Calcium Uptake in Cultured Embryonic Chick Duodenum. J.Biol.Chem. 256:3840-3847 (1981a).
Franceschi, R.T., and De Luca, H.F.: The effect of inhibitors of protein and RNA synthesis on 1α,25-dihydroxyvitamin D_3-dependent calcium uptake in cultured embryonic chick duodenum. J.Biol.Chem. 256:3848-3852 (1981b).
Fuchs, R., and Peterlik, M.: Vitamin D-Induced Phosphate Transport in Intestinal Brush Border Membrane Vesicles. Biochem. Biophys.Res.Comm. 93:87-92 (1980).
Hildmann, B., Schmidt, A., and Murer, H.: Ca^{++}-Transport across Basal-Lateral Plasma Membranes from Rat Small Intestinal Epithelial Cells. J.Membrane Biol. 65:55-62 (1982).
Peterlik, M.: Phosphate transport by embryonic chick duodenum: Stimulation by vitamin D_3. Biochim.Biophys.Acta 514:164-171 (1978).
Peterlik, M., Fuchs, R., and Cross, H.S.: Stimulation of D-glucose transport. A novel effect of vitamin D on intestinal membrane transport. Biochim.Biophys.Acta 649:138-142 (1981).
Rozengurt, E., and Mendoza, S.: Monovalent Ion Fluxes and the Control of Cell Proliferation in Cultured Fibroblasts. Ann.N.Y. Acad.Sci. 339: 175-190 (1980).
Schultz, S.G.: Transport Across Small Intestine, in: "Membrane Transport in Biology" Vol. IVB, Giebisch, G., Tosteson, D.C., Ussing, H.H., eds., Springer Verlag New York (1979).
Wasserman, R.H.: Intestinal absorption of calcium and phosphorus. Fed.Proc. 40:68-72 (1981).

EFFECTS OF pH AND SODIUM ON PHOSPHATE TRANSPORT ACROSS BRUSH BORDER MEMBRANE VESICLES OF SMALL INTESTINE

Giustina Danisi, Heini Murer* and Ralph W. Straub

Dept of Pharmacology, University of Geneva, and
*Inst. of Physiology, University of Zürich
Switzerland

INTRODUCTION

It is known that, in isolated intact rat small intestine, the phosphate (P_i) transport from lumen to tissue increases when the pH of the luminal solution is reduced[1]. A similar observation has also been reported in brush border membrane vesicles (BBMV) from rat small intestine[2]. These results have suggested that the increase in mono- respective to divalent phosphate, which occurs when pH is reduced, was responsible for the higher uptake found at acidic pH, thus leading to the conclusion that primary P_i was transported across the brush border of small intestinal epithelium. Such a conclusion, however, is valid only if direct effects of pH on the phosphate transport system are excluded.

We have reinvestigated the effects of pH on phosphate transport by using BBMV from rabbit small intestine. We asked the following question : can the changes in P_i transport with pH be accounted by different amounts of mono- respective to divalent phosphate ? Or, alternatively, are they explained by direct effects of pH on the phosphate transport system ?

METHODS

BBMV from frozen rabbit duodenum were prepared by a Mg^2 -precipitation method and differential centrifugation as reported[3] with some modifications[4]. Purification of the brush border enzyme markers alkaline phosphatase and leucine aminopeptidase was 10-15 times over the initial homogenate and the recovery was 20-30 %. All animals were "group-fed" for four days and received an intravenous injection of 1.2 μg/kg b.w. of 1,25-dihydroxycholecalciferol 15 hours before sacrifice. Experiments were carried out with BBMV from rabbit duodenum because only this segment of rabbit small intestine appears to possess a Na-dependent P_i transport system at the brush border membrane level[5].

RESULTS AND DISCUSSION

When pH was 7.4 and in the absence of a pH gradient, the phosphate uptake into BBMV at 0.1 mM P_i was, in the presence of a Na gradient, higher than the uptake when Na was replaced by K. An overshoot 2-3 times the equilibrium values measured at 10-15 hours was observed. The equilibrium values in the presence of Na were similar to the levels measured in the presence of K. They were higher, however, than the D-glucose uptake equilibrium levels measured in parallel experiments under the same conditions for the P_i uptake above, thus suggesting that some binding of P_i occurs in these vesicles. This binding appeared to occur in the vesicles' interior because (i) it could not be displaced by the presence of 5 mM P_i in the "stop" solution and (ii) extrapolation of P_i uptake as a function of time to the origin resulted in intercepts not statistically different from zero[4]. In conclusion, BBMV prepared from frozen rabbit duodenum show a similar P_i transport system at the brush border membrane level as vesicles prepared from fresh tissue[6].

Fig. 1 shows how P_i uptake into vesicles prepared at a pH value of 7.4 changed when the extravesicular pH was varied from 5.7 to 8.1. The P_i uptake was studied under Na and K gradient conditions; the concentration of both cations was 100 mM and phosphate 0.1 mM. The P_i uptake in the presence of Na was only slightly affected by changes in pH from 5.7 to 6.9. With further increases in pH, however, there was a rapid decrease in P_i uptake which appeared to level off around a pH of 8. When Na was replaced by K, P_i uptake was markedly reduced compared to its level in the presence of Na in the whole range of pH investigated. It was highest, however, at pH 5.7 and decreased slowly when the pH was increased further. These results show that, when Na is present, the phosphate transport across the brush border of rabbit duodenum varies with pH as shown for the phosphate transport system found in rat small intestine[2]. In contrast to rat, however, in our preparation, Na-dependent P_i transport was present in the whole range of pH investigated. Na-dependent P_i transport was apparent at a pH value of 5.7, when 93 % of P_i is in the monovalent form, and also at a pH value of 8.1, when the divalent form of Pi accounts for 95 % of phosphate in solution. These results strongly suggest that both forms of phosphate are transported across the brush border membrane by a Na-dependent transport mechanism. In these experiments a pH gradient was present across the vesicles' membrane. Similar results however were obtained in the absence of pH gradients.

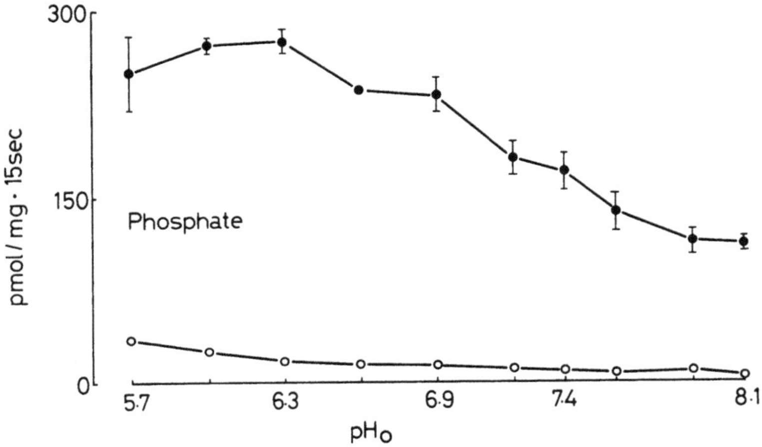

Fig. 1. Change of phosphate uptake with variations in extravesicular pH.

The variation of P_i uptake with pH was specific for the phosphate anion. D-glucose uptake, at the same substrate concentration as P_i, showed, in the presence of a Na gradient, an opposite dependence on pH. Uptake of D-glucose in the presence of K and the equilibrium values in the presence of Na or K were not affected by pH. These data suggest therefore that the results presented in Fig. 1 cannot be attributed to a general alteration of membrane permeability or to changes in the volume of the vesicles with pH.

The pH dependence of the P_i transport system was also investigated at a lower Na concentration, 25 mM. The results, carried out under Na gradient conditions and at a P_i concentration of 0.05 mM, are presented in Fig. 2, for two Na concentrations, 100 and 25 mM. When Na in the incubation media was 100 mM, similar changes of phosphate uptake with pH as in Fig. 1 were observed. Surprisingly, however, when Na was 25 mM, the change of phosphate uptake with pH was opposite to what was seen at the higher Na concentration. When Na in the media was low, the phosphate uptake above the pK_2 for phosphate, 6.8[7], was always higher than the uptake found below such a pH value. The data presented in Fig. 2 show that the pH dependence of phosphate transport depends strongly on the Na concentration in the medium. The pH dependence of phosphate transport at 100 mM and 25 mM further suggests that primary and secondary phosphate are both transported across the brush border membrane of small intestine.

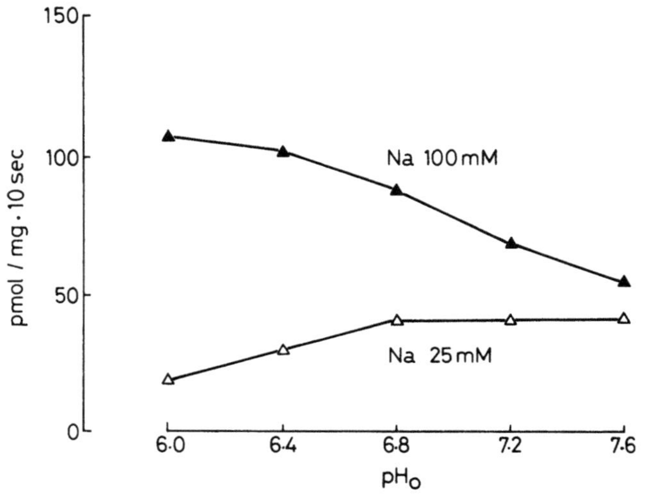

Fig. 2. pH dependence of phosphate transport at two external sodium concentrations.

The results shown in Fig. 1 and 2 suggested that the stimulation by Na of the Na-dependent phosphate transport system was a function of pH. Therefore the Na dependence of this transport was investigated at pH 6, 6.8 and 7.6, up to 300 mM Na, by stepwise replacement of Na by K. The first and last pH values were chosen in order to study the Na dependence of the P_i transport system when it interacted mainly with monovalent or divalent phosphate, respectively. The data are shown in Fig. 3. Phosphate uptake was a sigmoidal function of the external Na concentration at the three pH values investigated, thus suggesting that more than one

Na ion was transported with each phosphate. Estimation of Hill coefficients at each pH resulted in the following values : 2.1 ± 0.2 for pH 6, 2.2 ± 0.1 at pH 6.8 and 2.0 ± 0.3 for pH 7.6[4]. Therefore, two Na ions appear to be transported with each P_i in the pH range studied and there appeared to be no effect of pH on the number of Na ions which accompany phosphate. The apparent K_m of the phosphate transport system for Na, K_{Na}, changed with pH. Thus K_{Na} was lowest at pH 7.6, 19 ± 0.9 mM, but increased to 30 ± 3.7 mM at pH 6.8 and had a value of 90 ± 4.7 mM when pH was reduced to 6. Such results could be interpreted as a higher affinity of the P_i transporter for Na at higher pH values, a situation where the divalent P_i would be the transported species. The data presented in Fig. 3 also show that sodium stimulated the phosphate transport up to 300 mM at pH 6 while there was no further stimulation of the uptake by Na at pH 6.8 and 7.6 above approximately 50 and 75 mM, respectively. Thus it is likely that pH affected the affinity of the P_i transporter for Na independently of the presence of mono- or divalent phosphate.

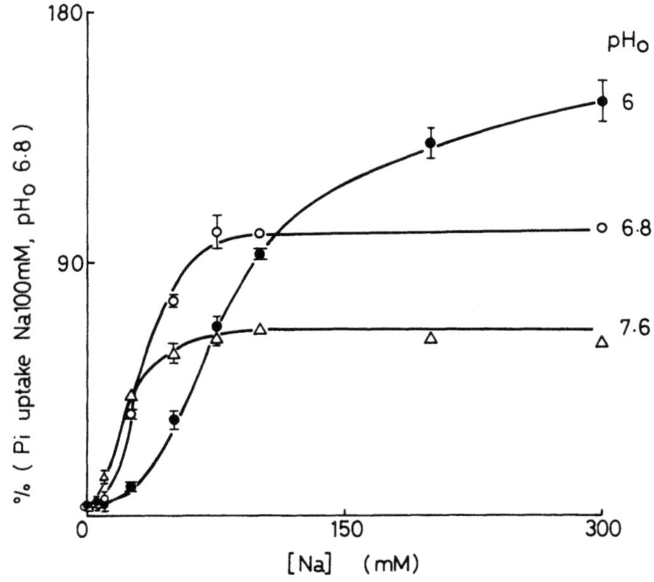

Fig. 3. Phosphate uptake into BBMV as a function of the medium sodium concentration.

In order to further clarify which form of P_i was the transported species, we investigated the change of phosphate uptake with the external P_i concentration at pH 6, 6.8 and 7.6. The rationale for these experiments was that if primary or secondary phosphate were transported across the brush border, the K_m, measured as a function of total phosphate, would vary inversely with the increase of the transported form when changing pH. When the P_i concentration was raised up to 1 mM in incubation media, the phosphate uptake showed a tendency to saturate at pH 6, 6.8 and 7.6[4]. Na-dependent P_i uptake was estimated by subtraction of the uptake in the presence of K from the total uptake measured when Na was present. K_m and V_{max} values of the P_i transporter were estimated by the Eadie-Hofstee linear transformation and are presented in Fig. 4 as a function of pH.

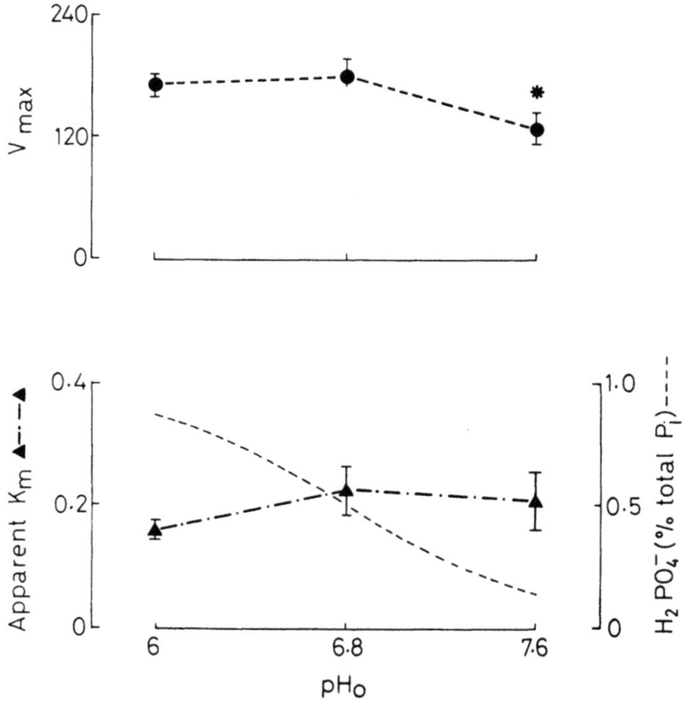

Fig. 4. Changes in K_m and V_{max} as a function of pH at 100 mM sodium.

The lower part of Fig. 4 shows that K_m at pH 6 and 7.6 was slightly decreased respective to its values at pH 6.8, but these changes were not statistically significant. The small changes in K_m which occurred between pH 6 and 7.6, did not correlate with the presence of monovalent phosphate in this pH range, shown as a dotted line in Fig. 4. Thus the changes of K_m with pH do not appear to depend on the ionic form of phosphate transported and may actually suggest that both forms of the substrate, primary and secondary phosphate, are transported by the phosphate transport system. The pH dependent changes in K_m might be related to an effect of pH on the substrate binding site. Furthermore, as shown in the upper part of Fig. 4, there is an additional effect of pH on the phosphate transport mechanism as shown by the significant reduction of V_{max} at pH 7.6 compared to the values observed at pH 6 and 6.8.

CONCLUSIONS

Our results on the change of phosphate uptake with pH are consistent with the transport of the monovalent and divalent forms of phosphate by a Na-dependent transport system across the brush border membrane of the small intestine. A similar conclusion has been reached in BBMV from rat kidney cortex[7]. In rabbit small intestine, the pH dependence of the phosphate uptake is strongly dependent on the sodium concentration in the medium. The pH dependence of the phosphate transport system across the brush border membrane appears to result mainly from direct effects of pH on the phosphate transport system, rather than from changes in the relative proportions of mono- and divalent phosphate with pH.

ACKNOWLEDGMENTS

Supported by 3.035.081 and 3.226.082 grants from the Swiss National Science Foundation. We are indebted to F. Hoffmann-La Roche & Co, Basel, Switzerland for the generous gift of 1,25-dihydroxycholecalciferol.

REFERENCES

1. M. W. Walling, Effects of 1α,25-dihydroxyvitamin D on active intestinal inorganic phosphate absorption, in : "Vitamin D, Biochemical, Chemical and Clinical Aspects Related to Calcium Metabolism," A. W. Norman, K. Schaefer, J. W. Coburn, H. F. DeLuca, D. Fraser, H. G. Grigoleit and D. V. Herrath, eds, Walter de Gruyter, New York, pp. 321-330 (1977).

2. W. Berner, R. Kinne and H. Murer, Phosphate transport into brush-border membrane vesicles isolated from rat small intestine, Biochem. J. 160:467-474 (1976).
3. J. Biber, B. Stieger, W. Haase and H. Murer, A high yield preparation for rat kidney brush border membranes. Different behaviour of lysosomal markers, Biochim. Biophys. Acta 647:169-176 (1981).
4. G. Danisi, H. Murer and R. W. Straub, The effect of pH on phosphate transport into intestinal brush border membrane vesicles. Am. J. Physiol., submitted.
5. G. Danisi and R. W. Straub, Unidirectional influx of phosphate across the mucosal membrane of rabbit small intestine, Pflügers Arch. 385:117-122 (1980).
6. B. Hildmann, C. Storelli, G. Danisi and H. Murer, Regulation of Na^+-P_i cotransport by 1,25-dihydroxyvitamin D_3 in rabbit duodenal brush-border membrane, Am. J. Physiol. 242:G533-G539 (1982).
7. G. Burckhardt, H. Stern and H. Murer, The influence of pH on phosphate transport into rat renal brush border membrane vesicles, Pflügers Arch. 390:191-197 (1981).

DIRECT IN VITRO EFFECTS OF 1,25(OH)2 VITAMIN D3 ON PHOSPHATE TRANSPORT IN ISOLATED ENTEROCYTES FROM NORMAL OR VITAMIN D DEFICIENT RATS

Gérard Karsenty, Bernard Lacour, André Ulmann, Evelyne Pierandreì and Tilman Drüeke

INSERM U.90 and Laboratoire de Physiologie Hôpital Necker, Paris, France

INTRODUCTION

1,25 dihydroxy vitamin D3 (1,25$(OH)_2$ D3), the main active metabolite of vitamin D3, stimulates intestinal phosphate (Pi) absorption (1). Pi transport across the enterocyte appears to involve at least three steps (2): 1) Pi entry across the luminal brush border membrane into the enterocyte, a secondary active or facilitated process requiring energy provided by the sodium (Na^+) gradient, 2) Pi transport from the mucosal to the serosal side of the cell, 3) Pi extrusion of the enterocyte into the extracellular space across the basolateral membrane. It has been proposed that 1,25$(OH)_2$ D3 could act by altering the rate of Na^+ dependent mucosal entry of Pi into the cell. However, the precise mechanism by which the hormone enhances intestinal Pi transport is still controversial.

The purpose of this study was to investigate whether the in vitro addition of 1,25$(OH)_2$ D3 to the incubation medium could alter the kinetics of Pi uptake by isolated enterocytes from vitamin D replete rats (D+) and vitamin D deficient rats (D-), and whether such an effect could occur independently of a de novo protein synthesis.

MATERIALS AND METHODS

Non fasted male Wistar AF rats weighing 100-180 g

were used. Before experiments, D(+) rats were fed at least during one week the standard diet of the laboratory. D(-) rats were maintained on a vitamin D deficient diet and were left in a dark room at least three weeks. Enterocytes were obtained from the duodeno-jejunum by a mechanical vibration procedure (3). No enzymatic digestion was performed. The working buffer always used was of the following composition (mM) : NaCl, 120 ; Tris, 20 ; $MgCl_2$, 1.0 ; $CaCl_2$, 1.0 ; glucose, 10 ; K_2HPO_4, 3.0. It contained also 1 mg/ml bovine serum albumin ; pH was 7.4 $\pm$ 0.1.

Pi uptake studies were performed as follows : the cell pellet obtained after mechanical vibration was divided into two parts. Each part was suspended in 10 ml of working buffer and maintained in constant agitation during a 20 min incubation period at 37°C. The test substance was added to one cell suspension and the vehicle to the other at the beginning of this time period. Then, 10 µCi of ^{33}P were added and aliquots of 500 µl each from both suspensions were obtained at the following time points : 15 sec, 1,2,3,4,5,6,7 and 8 min after ^{33}P addition. Each sample was immediately transferred into its respective vial containing 5.0 ml of ice-cold solution of the following composition (mM) : $MgCl_2$, 110 ; Tris, 1 ; pH was 7.4 $\pm$ 0.1. The cells were washed with this solution. Then, 1.0 ml of 10 % trichloroacetic acid solution was added to the last pellet. After centrifugation, a 500 µl aliquot of the supernatant was measured for its radioactivity. The other 500 µl were used to determine the protein content (4). The initial Pi influx velocity (iV_{Pi}) was estimated by linear regression between 15 sec and 8 min. Results were expressed as means $\pm$ S.E. Statistical analysis was carried out using Student's paired t test.

RESULTS

As shown in Fig. 1, the addition of $1{,}25(OH)_2$ D3 (1.0 pM) at the beginning of the incubation period induced a significant increase of iV_{Pi} after 20 min in D(+) enterocytes as well as in D(-) enterocytes. No significant enhancement of iV_{Pi} was observed after an exposure of the cells to the hormone of 15 min or less. The Na dependence of $1{,}25(OH)_2$ D3 effect was assessed by experiments where NaCl was removed from the working medium and replaced by choline chloride 120 mM. In the absence of Na^+ in the medium, $1{,}25(OH)_2$ D3 losts its ability to enhance initial Pi uptake in D(+) entero-

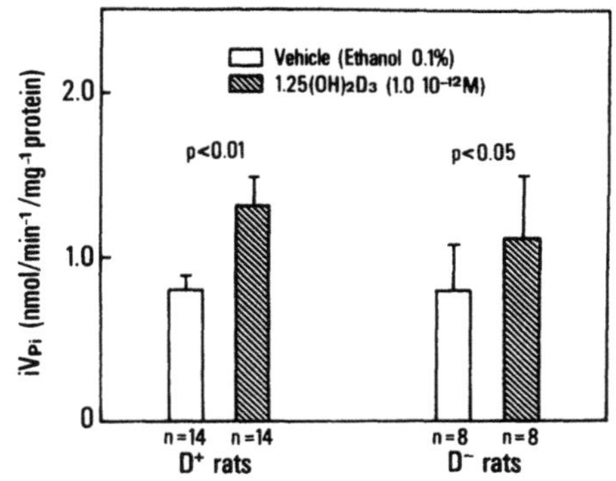

Fig. 1. Effect of 1,25$(OH)_2$ D3 (10^{-12}M) on enterocyte initial Pi uptake velocity (iV_{Pi}) in D replete and D deficient rats. Pi and Na concentrations in the medium were 3.0 and 120 mM respectively.

cytes : iV_{Pi} was 0.68 $\pm$ 0.31 $nmol.min^{-1}.mg^{-1}$prot. for cells incubated with vehicle and 0.84 $\pm$ 0.30 $nmol.min^{-1}$. mg^{-1}prot. for cells incubated in the presence of 1,25$(OH)_2$ D3 ($n = 6$, p = NS).

The possibility that the stimulatory effect of the hormone resulted from de novo protein synthesis was also studied. In D(+) rats, iV_{Pi} of enterocytes incubated with the hormone alone was not significantly different from that of enterocytes incubated with hormone and cycloheximide (5µg/ml). The latter is known to block de novo protein synthesis. iV_{Pi} was 1.25 $\pm$ 0.27 in the absence of cycloheximide and 1.26 $\pm$ 0.29 nmol. min^{-1}.mg $prot.^{-1}$ in the presence of cycloheximide. Furthermore, in other series of experiments performed in D(+) rats and in D(-) rats we have used a complex of 1,25$(OH)_2$ D3 linked to albumin at the C3 position corresponding to 10 pM of free hormone. Previous investigations in our laboratory have shown that this complex was able to bind to cytosol receptors of chick enterocytes. Moreover, the possibility of cleavage of the macromolecular derivative during the incubation was ruled out. In D(+) rats as well as in D(-) rats, the compound was able to significantly enhance iV_{Pi} after 20 min of incubation (Fig. 2).

The possibility that 1,25$(OH)_2$ D3 induced a change in the membrane fluidity was then studied. In D(+) rats the stimulatory effect of 1,25$(OH)_2$ D3 on iV_{Pi} was blunted when the cells were incubated in presence of the hormone and the methyl ester of transvaccinic acid (MTVA) 0.12 mM (Fig. 3a). This compound is known to decrease the fluidity of cell membranes (5). In D(-) rats, the methyl ester of cis vaccinic acid (MCVA) which is known to increase the fluidity of the enterocyte membrane (5) had the same stimulatory effects on iV_{Pi} as the hormone (Fig. 3b).

DISCUSSION

Previous investigations of intestinal Pi absorption have provided evidence for a secondary active transport of this ion. In most of the experimental models 1,25$(OH)_2$ D3 was found to enhance the Na dependent component of Pi absorption (2,6). The molecular mechanism of the hormonal action remains unclear. Peterlik and Wasserman (2) showed that this stimulatory effect of 1,25$(OH)_2$ D3 could be blocked through an inhibition of protein synthesis. Birge et al (7)

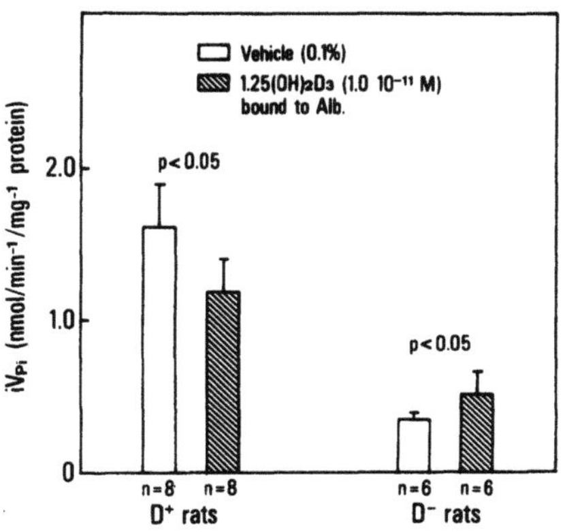

Fig. 2. Effect of 1,25$(OH)_2$ D3 (10^{-11}M) linked to albumin on enterocyte initial Pi uptake velocity (iV_{Pi}) in D replete and D deficient rats. Pi and Na concentrations in the medium were 3.0 and 120 mM respectively.

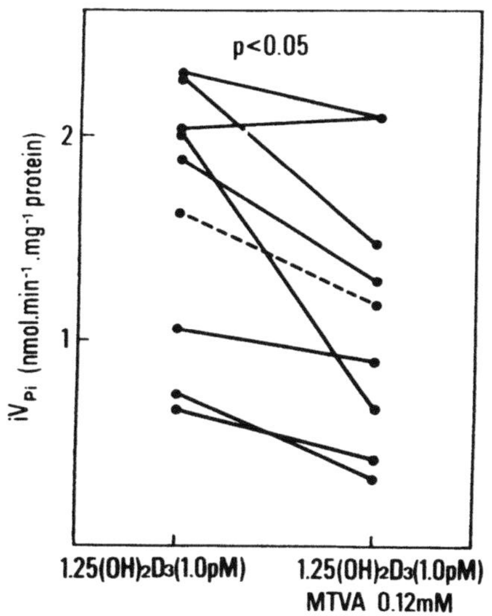

Fig. 3a. Enterocyte initial Pi uptake velocity (iV_{Pi}) in vitamin D replete rats, after incubation of cells with either 1,25$(OH)_2$ D3 alone or 1,25$(OH)_2$ D3 plus the methyl ester of transvaccinic acid (MTVA).

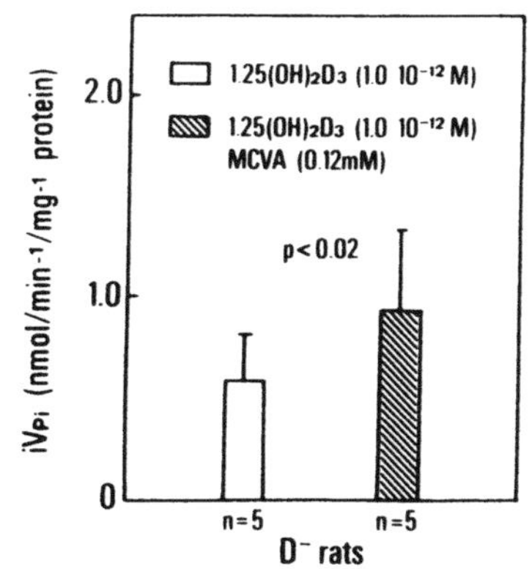

Fig. 3b. Enterocyte initial Pi uptake velocity (iV_{Pi}) in vitamin D deficient rats in the presence or absence of the methyl ester of cisvaccinic acid (MCVA). Pi and Na concentrations in the medium were 3.0 and 120mM respectively.

using chick ileum explants and Matsumoto et al (6) using brush border membrane vesicles have shown that $1,25(OH)_2$ D3 could exert a direct non genomic effect on Pi accumulation. However the in vivo administration of $1,25(OH)_2$ D3 in their studies did not allow to firmly exclude de novo protein synthesis.

In the present study we have used a model of mechanically isolated rat enterocytes. The hormone or other test substances were added only in vitro. We have demonstrated that $1,25(OH)_2$ D3 at a concentration of 1.0 pM increased iV_{Pi} as early as 20 min after starting incubation. This effect was observed only when Na^+ was present in the working medium. The effect did not seem to require de novo protein synthesis. As a matter of fact, cycloheximide, a potent inhibitor of protein synthesis failed to block the $1,25(OH)_2$ D3 mediated increase of iV_{Pi}. Furthermore , when $1,25(OH)_2$ D3 bound to albumin was used in order to prevent the hormone from entering the cell,we found a stimulation of iV_{Pi} in D(+) similar to that observed with free hormone.

This early effect of $1,25(OH)_2$ D3 may be due in part to a modification of the lipid composition of the cell membrane (5,8). In support of this hypothesis, we found MTVA which decreases the fluidity of the membrane, blunted the stimulatory effect of the hormone in D(+) rats. MCVA which increases the fluidity of the membrane mimicked the effect observed with the hormone in D(-) rats.

In conclusion, $1,25(OH)_2$ D3 appeared to exert in our model a rapid non genomic effect on enterocyte Pi uptake by stimulating iV_{Pi} similarly to its direct effect recently described in isolated kidney tubular epithelium (9).

REFERENCES

1. A. Murer, and B. Hillmann, Trancellular transport of calcium and inorganic phosphate in the small intestine. Am. J. Physiol. 240:409 (1981).
2. M. Peterlik, and R.H. Wasserman, Effect of vitamin D on transepithelial phosphate transport in chick intestine. Am. J. Physiol. 234:379 (1978).
3. B. Lacour, T. Drüeke, E. Pierandreï, B. Nabarra, and J.L. Funck-Brentano, Rat enterocyte Na^+ transport in vitro : action of parathyroid hormone and calcitonin. Biochim. Biophys. Acta 848:151 (1981).

4. O.H. Lowry, J.J. Rosebrough, A.L. Farr, and R.J. Randall, Protein measurement with the folin phenol reagent. J. Biol. Chem. 193:265 (1951).
5. O. Fontaine, T. Matsumoto, D.B.P. Goodman, and V.H. Rasmussen, Liponomic control of Ca^{2+} transport relationship to mechanism of action on 1,25 dihydroxyvitamin D3. Proc. Natl. Acad. Sci. USA 78:1751 (1981).
6. T. Matsumoto, O. Fontaine, and H. Rasmussen, Effect of 1,25 dihydroxyvitamin D3 on phosphate uptake into chick intestinal brush border membrane vesicles. Biochim. Biophys. Acta 599:13 (1980).
7. S.T. Birge, and R.A. Miller, The role of Pi in the action of vitamin D on the intestine. J. Clin. Invest. 60:980 (1977).
8. P.J.A. O'Doherty, 1,25 dihydroxyvitamin D3 increases the activity of the intestinal phosphatidyl choline deacylation reacylation cycle. Lipids 14:75 (1979).
9. C.T. Liang, J. Barnes, R. Balakir, L. Cheng, and B. Sacktor, In vitro stimulation of phosphate uptake in isolated chick renal cells by 1,25 dihydroxycholecalciferol. Proc. Natc. Acad. Sci. USA 79:3532 (1982).

1,25-DIHYDROXYVITAMIN D3 STIMULATES CALCIUM AND PHOSPHATE ABSORPTION BY DIFFERENT MECHANISMS: CONTRASTING REQUIREMENTS FOR SODIUM

David B. N. Lee, Marlin W. Walling*, Dalila B. Corry and Jack W. Coburn
Research and Medical Services, Sepulveda and Wadsworth VA Medical Centers. UCLA School of Medicine, Los Angeles, California

INTRODUCTION

Previous studies from our laboratory have demonstrated that 1,25-dihydroxyvitamin D3 (1,25D) stimulates separate calcium (Ca) and inorganic phosphate (P) absorptive mechanisms in rat intestine (1,2). The proportion of Ca to P "pumps" varies in different regions of the intestine. Thus, there is a preponderance of Ca pumps in the duodenum, a preponderance of P pumps in the jejunum and an equal distribution of Ca and P pumps in the ileum (3). Interestingly, the colon has only 1,25D-responsive Ca pumps (2). The active Ca absorptive mechanisms in duodenum, ileum and colon appear to share certain characteristics, all exhibiting a Km of approximately 1 mM (2,3). The expression of this 1,25D-induced Ca absorption in colon does not appear to require the presence of extracellular sodium ions (4). In the present study we examined the sodium (Na) requirement of 1,25D-stimulated P transport processes in rat jejunum.

METHODS

Vitamin D-deficient rats were raised according to the protocol previously described (1,2). Unless otherwise stated, 1,25D repletion was accomplished by intraperitoneal injection of 1.3 nmole of the metabolite in 0.2 ml of 1:1 n-propanediol:ethanol, 48 and 24 hours before experiment. Control rats were handled similarly but received only the vehicle without 1,25D. Transmural, P fluxes were studied *in vitro* using the

*The studies in the paper were carried out by Dr. Walling before his death on November 30, 1979.

modified Ussing technique described in detail in previous publications (1,2). Unidirectional absorptive or mucosal-to-serosal flux (Jms) and secretory or serosal-to-mucosal flux (Jsm) were measured under steady conditions and in the absence of transepithelial electrochemical gradients. Calculated net flux (Jnet=Jms-Jsm) represents active absorption. All fluxes are expressed in units of nmoles/cm2/hr. When indicated, buffer Na was bilaterally replaced by isosmotic substitution of choline chloride.

P influx across the brush border membrane of intact jejunal epithelium was measured using the same Ussing apparatus described for transmural flux studies, with the modification that the mucosal compartment could be rapidly drained (<2 seconds) and then flushed with ice-cold 0.3% mannitol (5 seconds). Jejunal epithelium was mounted as described for transmural flux measurements, and allowed to equilibrate for 45-60 minutes so that the ion transport should be at steady-state under short circuited conditions. Tracer amounts of 32-P-phosphate and 3-H-polyethylene glycol (3-H-PEG, MW=800-1000) were then added to the mucosal compartment and the mucosa was exposed for 1,2,4 and 8 minute intervals. Termination of exposure was defined as the time at which the mucosal compartment was drained and ice-cold mannitol rinse commensed. The exposed tissues were removed, blotted, digested overnight in 0.1N nitric acid and counted in a dual channel liquid scintillation counter. After correction for the trapped volume based on 3-H counts, P influx was calculated on the basis of the specific activity of the 32-P-phosphate.

All data are expressed as mean +/- SEM. Statistical comparisons of independent variables within treatment groups was made using one-way analysis of variance. When the analysis of variance indicated a difference between means, Dunnett's format for multiple t test comparisons was used to obtain probability estimate (5).

RESULTS

Active P absorption was present even in jejunum from vitamin D-deficient rats (Jnet=28.1 +/- 7.3, N=7). However, net P absorption increased markedly 24 hours after a single dose of 975 nmole of 1,25D (Jnet=101.8 +/- 5.7, N=7, P<0.001). The stimulatory action of 1,25D affected selectively Jms, with Jsm remaining unchanged.

Figure 1 summarizes the effect of reducing buffer (extracellular) Na concentration on short circuit current (Isc) and the 1,25D-stimulated, net phosphate absorption (Jnet) in jejunum. As one would anticipate, the progressive reduction in ambient Na concentrations was associated with a parallel reduction

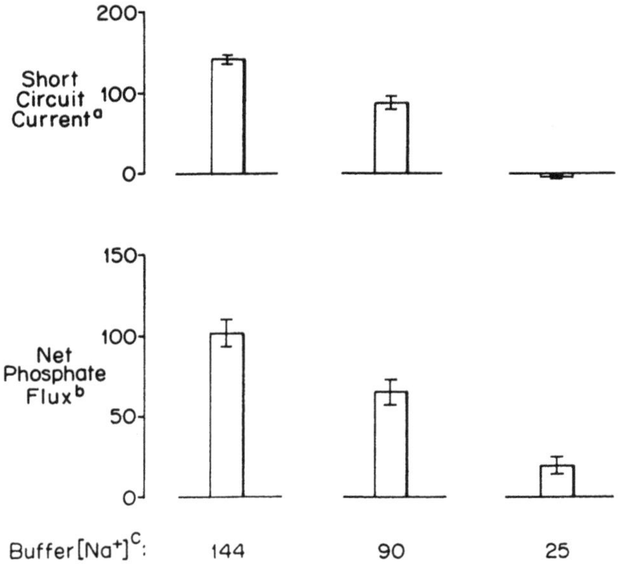

FIGURE 1

in Isc which is a reflection of active, transepithlial Na absorption. However, in contrast to the 1,25D-stimulated Ca transport in colon, which is not affected by complete substitution of buffer Na by choline (4), the 1,25D-stimulated P absorption decreased with decreases in ambient Na concentrations.

The interrelationship between Na and 1,25D-sensitive P transport was further analysed by measuring P influx across the brush border membrane of intact jejunal epithelium at different external sodium concentrations. The data (not shown) duplicated closely those obtained for transepithelial P transport studies, i.e. P influx and Isc decreased in parallel with stepwise reduction in buffer Na concentrations from 100 to 0 mM. However, a significant P influx remained in the total absence of external Na. We therefore carried out futher analysis of these two components of P influx, i.e. the sodium-dependent componet and the sodium-independent component, and examined if 1,25D affects either or both processes.

Figure 2, depicts P influx measured over a range of buffer P concentrations. The influx measured in the presence of Na was designated total influx, while the influx measured in the total absence of Na was designated Na-independent influx. The sodium-dependent influx was calculated by subtracting the Na-independent influx from the total influx and revealed a curve with nearly ideal carrier-kinetics. Thus the total P influx across

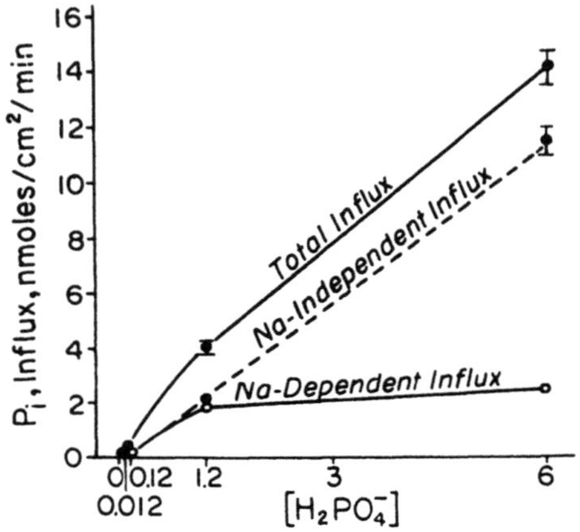

FIGURE 2

the brush border membrane consists of two components. A Na-indenpendent component demonstrating no tendency towards saturation and a Na-dependent component demonstrating saturable characteristics. Further analysis using jejunum from vitamin D-deficient rats and similar but 1,25D repleted rats revealed that the stimulatory effect of 1,25D on P influx was selectively mediated through the Na-dependent component.

DISCUSSIONS

Previous studies from our laboratory have demonstrated that 1,25D stimulates active absorption of both Ca and P in rat small intestine (1). The parallel induction of both transport mechanisms has led to the question whether 1,25D-stimulated Ca and P transport processes are coupled or separate (3). The question is answered, in large measure, by our studies in rat colon. In this intestinal segment, 1,25D selectively stimulates active Ca absorption with no discernible effect on P absorption at all (2). This Ca-only effect, provides compelling evidence for the existence of separate Ca and P transport processes in the intestine.

The present study provides further characterization of the differences between the 1,25D-responsive Ca "pumps" from the 1,25D-responsive P pumps. The former, as previously demonstrated in rat colon, is not influenced by the presence or absence of extracellular Na (4). On the other hand the 1,25D-induced intestinal P transport is clearly dependent on the extracellular Na concentrations. Brush border influx studies suggest that intestinal P transport consists of a Na-dependent and a Na-independet components and that 1,25D selectively stimulates the Na-dependent component of P transport.

Danisi and Straub (6), and Danisi, Bonjour and Straub (7), have reported unidirectional P influx across the mucosal membrane of rabbit small intestine and demonstrated that only the duodenum has a Na-dependent, carrier mediated phosphate transport mechanism and that 1,25D stimulates this process by modulating the number of carrier sites available at the mucosal membrane for Na-dependent P entry. No Na-dependent, carrier mediated P influx mechanism was demonstrated in the jejunum and the ileum of rabbit. Our finding of 1,25D-responsive, Na-dependent influx in rat jejunum therefore emphasizes the importance of species difference in these studies.

REFERENCES

1. Walling MW: Intestinal Ca and phosphate transport: differntial responses to vitamin D3 metabolites. Am J Physiol 233(b):E488-494, 1977.
2. Lee DBN, Walling MW, Silis V, Gafter U and Coburn JW: Calcium and inorganic phosphate tranport in rat colon: dissociated response to 1,25-dihydroxyvitamin D3. J Clin Invest 65:1326-1331, 1980.
3. Walling MW and Lee DBN: Theories on the mechanism of action of 1,25(OH)2D3 on active intestinal calcium and inorganic phosphate absorption: are the calcium and phosphate transport processes coupled, uncoupled or both? In : Norman AW, Schaefer K, Herrath DV, Grigoleit HG, Coburn JW, DeLuca HF, Mawer EB and Suda T (Eds), "Vitamin D: Basic Research and Its Clinical Applications", Walter de Gruyter, Berlin/New York, 1979, pp 687-692.
4. Lee DBN: Unanticipated stimulatory action of glucocorticoids on epithelial calcium absorption. Effect of dexamethasone on rat distal colon. J Clin Invest 71:322-328, 1983.
5. Dunnett CW: A multiple comparison procedure for comparing several treatments with a control. Am Statis Assoc J 50:1096-1121, 1955.
6. Danisi G and Staub RW: Unidirectional influx of phosphate across the mucosal membrane of rabbit small intestine. Pflugers Arch 385:117-122, 1980.
7. Danisi G, Bonjour J-Ph, Staub RW: Regulation of Na-dependent phosphate influx across the mucosal border of duodenum by 1,25-dihydroxycholecalciferol. Pflugers Arch 388:227-232, 1980.

ACKNOWLEDGMENTS This work was supported by U.S. Public Health Service Grant AM20-919, Veterans Administration Research Support and Nelly W. Citron Research Fund.

DISSOCIATION OF ABSORPTIONS OF CALCIUM AND PHOSPHATE IN DIFFERENT PATHOPHYSIOLOGICAL STATES IN MAN

Carlo Gennari, Marco Bernini, Paolo Nardi and Luciana Fusi

Institute of Medical Semeiotics
University of Siena, Italy

INTRODUCTION

Calcium (Ca) and inorganic phosphate (Pi) are absorbed by an active transport system, concentration and energy dependent, confined to the small intestine and depending on the presence of vitamin D.

In animals and man it has been shown that the active transport of Ca is more highly developed in the duodenum than in the jejunum or ileum[1-10]. On the contrary, Pi is rapidly trasported across all segments of the small intestine; in some species, including man, Pi absorption is greater in the jejunum than in the duodenum[11-15].

The administration of vitamin D increases both Ca and Pi absorption. Several workers have suggested that this constituted evidence for the two processes being linked. Vitamin D stimulates the intestinal Ca absorption both in animals and in man. There is a 12 hour lag between administration of vitamin D and any evidence of response; the time involved for the conversion of administered vitamin D into metabolically active forms by the liver and kidney and for the synthesis of Ca binding protein (CaBP) in the intestinal cell can account for part of this lag period[16]. Vitamin D enhances Pi absorption after a time lag of 16 hours, but a phosphate binder in the mucosal cell, equivalent to CaBP, has not been detected[17]; CaBP is evident at 12 hours, four hours earlier than the increased Pi absorption could be detected.

Pi absorption, measured in man by the intubation-perfusion

technique[18] or by in vitro gut segments technique[19] shows that it is similar to Ca absorption, consisting of two processes: the first, a saturable carrier mediated active transport; the second, a linear concentration-dependent diffusion process. The active Pi absorption is two times greater than Ca absorption, whereas the diffusion component is greater for Ca than for Pi, thus suggesting that the Ca and Pi transport systems are not identical.

A great many different methods of measuring Ca and Pi absorption in man exist, ranging from intubation with a triple lumen tube to balance procedures and procedures involving the oral administration of radioactive Ca or Pi or the simultaneous oral and intravenous administration of two Ca or Pi isotopes. From the recent comparison of the various methods the single tracer method has proven to give reasonable and sufficient estimates of absorption rates such to be useful for clinical purposes[20-22].

We have extensively employed the single tracer methods to measure the intestinal absorption of Ca and Pi in different pathophysiological states in man, including postmenopausal osteoporosis, nutritional or malabsorptive osteomalacia and chronic renal failure. In a certain number of patients, the digestive transport processes of both Ca and Pi have been simultaneously measured by a double tracer (radiocalcium and radiophosphate) method. In comparing values obtained from patients with those obtained in normal control subjects we frequently observed a dissociation between the two transport processes.

MATERIALS AND METHODS

The intestinal absorptions of Ca and Pi were measured by the single tracer methods (^{47}Ca or ^{32}P) or by the double tracer method (^{45}Ca and ^{32}P) in 250 individuals. Ca absorption and Pi absorption were simultaneously estimated following a combined oral dose of ^{45}Ca and ^{32}P in a carrier of 20 mg Ca (as calcium chloride) and 50 mg Pi (as disodium hydrogen phosphate) according to the method of Peacock et al.[23], based on plasma sampling during 4 hours after tracer administration. The activity of each single isotope has been distinguished by liquid scintillation counting of samples, since β-emissions of ^{32}P and ^{45}Ca differ substantially in energy content. Plasma radioactivity, expressed as a percentage of the dose per liter, has been corrected for extracellular fluid volume by multiplying by 15% of body weight. The circulating fraction (fx) of the absorbed dose for each isotope was calculated by using the simplified two compartment model of Marshall and Nordin[24]. Concerning

^{32}P absorption , the blood levels of radioactive Pi were related to the renal clearance of ^{32}P determined from the urine samples collected from the same sample period, since renal handling of Pi may significantly influence the circulating levels of Pi[14,15].

The intestinal absorption of Ca has been studied by the single tracer method (^{47}Ca) in 100 normal subjects (46 females and 54 males, age range 17-87 years). The intestinal absorption of Pi has been studied by the single tracer method (^{32}P) in 62 normal subjects (31 females and 31 males, age range 17-83 years). All normal subjects were selected on the basis of normal hepatic and renal function and presenting with normal values for the biochemical parameters of Ca and Pi metabolism and for bone mineral content as assessed by dual photon absorptiometry. The dietary intake of Ca was 600-1000 mg/day and 800-1000 mg/day for Pi.

Seventy-three osteoporotic females presenting with at least one vertebral crush fracture as indicated by X-ray were studied: the single ^{47}Ca tracer method has been employed in 37 patients, the single ^{32}P tracer method in 6 patients and the simultaneous double tracer (^{45}Ca and ^{32}P) method in 30 patients. The simultaneous double tracer method has been employed to study 21 cases of nutritional or malabsorptive osteomalacia, proved by iliac crest bone biopsy, and 23 patients with chronic renal failure (CRF). Thirty-three further patients with CRF were tested by the single methods for Ca (16 cases) or Pi (17 cases).

The double tracer method was repeated in some cases after a 10 day treatment period with the active metabolites of vitamin D: 25-hydroxycholecalciferol (25-OHD) in 4 normal subjects at 5 mcg/day, in 8 CRF patients at 5 mcg/day and in 7 CRF patients at 50 mcg/day; 1,25-dihydroxycholecalciferol (1,25$(OH)_2D$) in 5 normal subjects at 1 mcg/day and in 10 CRF patients at 5 mcg/day.

RESULTS

By utilizing the oral Ca and Pi radioisotopic tests permitted us to establish the levels of normality for the absorbed fraction of the two ions. These values, reported in Table 1, and obtained in selected normal adults, between the ages of 17 to 50 years indicate that the absorbed fraction of Ca and Pi are slightly higher in male than in female. This difference is not statistically significant. The control data collected from all normal subjects of both sexes between the ages of 17 to 87 years demonstrated that the absorbed fractions significantly decreased with increasing age: in 100 individuals the correlation between ^{47}Ca fx and age was r=-0.49

(p<0.001); in 62 individuals the correlation between ^{32}P fx and age was r=-0.45 (p<0.001).

Table 1. Circulating fraction of the absorbed dose (fx) of ^{47}Ca and ^{32}P in normal subjects (M±SD)

n	sex	age	^{47}Ca fx	
25	M	17-50	0.245±0.048	
24	F	19-50	0.226±0.026	
n	sex	age	^{32}P fx	Cp^{32}
16	M	17-50	0.230±0.040	10.78±3.95
16	F	24-50	0.206±0.037	10.21±3.17

The decline in intestinal transport of ^{47}Ca with age in postmenopausal osteoporotic women was more marked when compared to the decline in Ca absorption in age matched non osteoporotic women (Figure 1). No correlation was found between the intestinal absorption of ^{32}P and age in postmenopausal osteoporotic women (Figure 2).

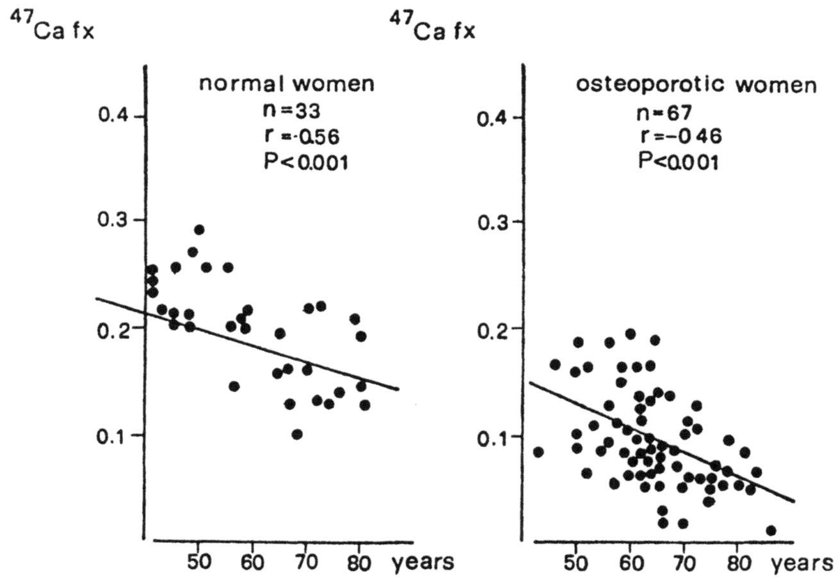

Fig. 1. Correlation between the intestinal absorption of radiocalcium and age in postmenopausal osteoporotic women and age matched non osteoporotic women.

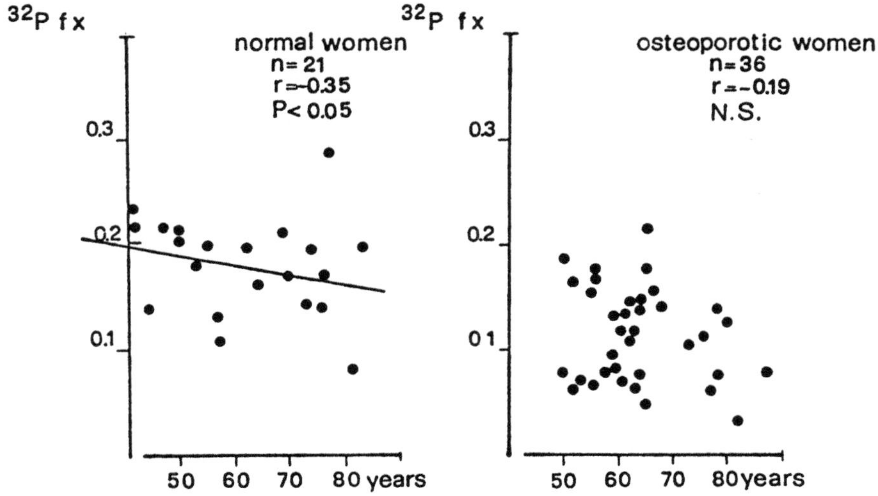

Fig. 2. Correlation between the intestinal absorption of radiophosphate and age in postmenopausal osteoporotic women and age-matched non osteoporotic women.

The comparison between the values obtained by the simultaneous double tracer method in 30 postmenopausal osteoporotic women and in 21 women with osteomalacia demonstrate that in both conditions a state of intestinal malabsorption of Ca and Pi exists; Ca malabsorption is notably marked in osteoporosis whereas Pi malabsorption is more so in osteomalacia (Table 2). These data indicate a dissociation between the two intestinal absorption processes.

Table 2. Intestinal absorption of Ca and Pi in postmenopausal osteoporosis and in nutritional or malabsorptive osteomalacia

	n	^{45}Ca fx	^{32}P fx
Osteoporosis	30	0.106±0.048	0.124±0.049
Osteomalacia	21	0.143±0.043	0.079±0.029
Normal values	100	0.219±0.046	
Normal values	62		0.194±0.049

Values given as mean±standard deviation.

We observed in patients with CRF an impairment in the intestinal absorption of Ca and Pi. The malabsorption of Ca and Pi significantly correlated with the glomerular filtration rate as as-

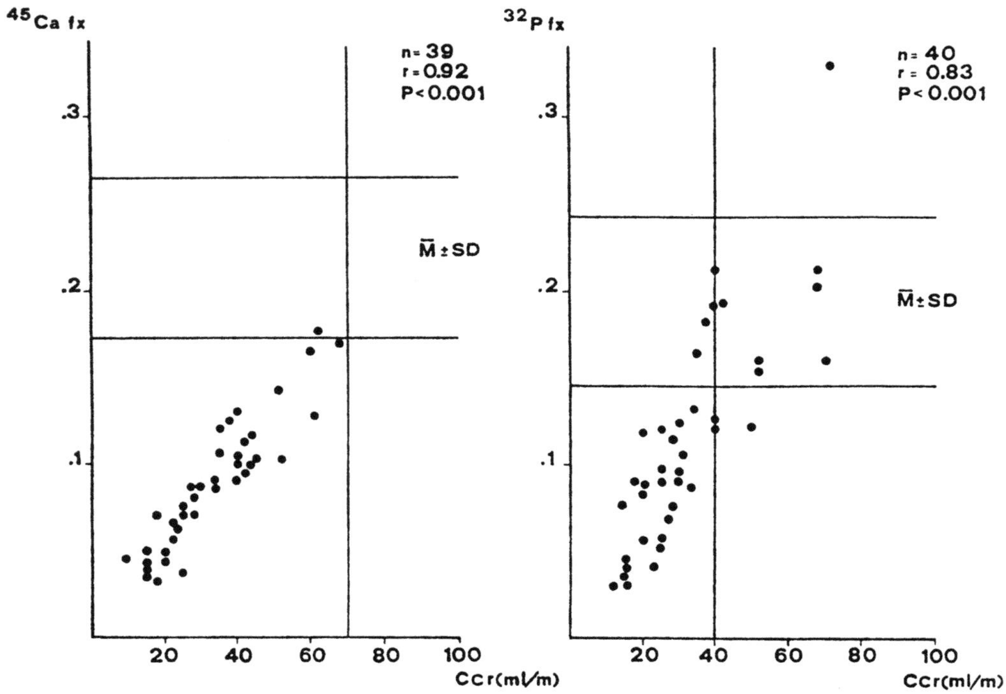

Fig. 3. Correlation between the intestinal absorption of ^{45}Ca and ^{32}P and the renal clearance of creatinine in CRF patients.

sessed by endogenous creatinine renal clearance (Figure 3). In this case, an earlier deterioration of Ca absorption was apparent when compared to Pi absorption with declining renal function.

It is well known that vitamin D and active metabolites stimulate the intestinal absorption of both Ca and Pi. In normal subjects the intestinal absorption of ^{45}Ca and ^{32}P significantly increased after 10 days of treatment with paraphysiologic doses of 25OHD or 1,25(OH)$_2$D (Table 3 and 4). In CRF patients the treatment with paraphysiologic doses of 25OHD was ineffective in modifying the Ca and Pi malabsorption, whereas pharmacologic doses of 25OHD resulted in an improvement in ^{45}Ca absorption with no changes in ^{32}P absorption (Table 3). Furthermore in patients with CRF on maintenance hemodialysis the treatment with pharmacologic doses of 1,25(OH)$_2$D partially corrected Ca malabsorption, inducing a small but non-significant increase in ^{32}P absorption (Table 4).

Table 3. Effects of 10 days of treatment with 25OHD on the intestinal absorption of Ca and Pi in normal subjects and CRF patients

n	daily dose	^{45}Ca fx before	^{45}Ca fx after	^{32}P fx before	^{32}P fx after
Normal subjects					
5	1 mcg	0.228±0.020	<u>0.341±0.040</u>**	0.190±0.028	<u>0.322±0.055</u>**
CRF patients					
8	5 mcg	0.071±0.024	0.077±0.028	0.090±0.032	0.086±0.037
7	50 mcg	0.076±0.027	<u>0.178±0.033</u>**	0.087±0.057	0.093±0.062

Values given as mean±standard deviation.
Significance according to paired data Student's "t" test:
*p<0.01 **p<0.001

Table 4. Effects of 10 days of treatment with $1,25(OH)_2D$ on the intestinal absorption of Ca and Pi in normal subjects and CRF patients

n	daily dose	^{45}Ca fx before	^{45}Ca fx after	^{32}P fx before	^{32}P fx after
Normal subjects					
4	1 mcg	0.210±0.012	<u>0.283±0.022</u>*	0.193±0.012	<u>0.328±0.055</u>*
CRF patients					
10	5 mcg	0.062±0.022	<u>0.143±0.037</u>**	0.070±0.037	0.048±0.039

Values given as mean±standard deviation.
Significance according to paired data Student's "t" test:
*p<0.02 **p<0.001

DISCUSSION

This study demonstrates that the dissociation between the two absorption processes is not uncommon in different pathologic states characterized by negative effects on bone such as postmenopausal osteoporosis, nutritional or malabsorptive osteomalacia and CRF. The clinical data on the dissociation between Ca and Pi absorption is scarse. Recently, in patients with CRF a dissociation in recovery from Ca and Pi malabsorption after treatment with synthetic 1α-hydroxy vitamin D or after successful renal transplantation has been documented[23,25].

From the pathogenetic point of view, all three pathologic states here considered seem to be tied to altered vitamin metabolism, with documented low levels of circulating $1,25(OH)_2D$ in osteomalacia and CRF, although not yet confirmed in postmenopausal osteoporosis. If Ca and Pi malabsorption was solely due to an unavailability of active metabolites of vitamin D then the deficit in the intestinal transport processes should be parallel. In addition, the correction of this deficit with vitamin D metabolites should improve, in equal degrees, the absorption of the two ions. On the contrary, the dissociation in recovery from Ca and Pi malabsorption after treatment with pharmacologic doses of active vitamin D metabolites observed in patients with CRF, the apparent earlier deterioration of Ca compared to Pi absorption with declining age in postmenopausal women or with declining renal function in CRF patients, may suggest the presence of separate regulatory mechanisms in the two transport processes, only partially dependent on vitamin D metabolites.

REFERENCES

1. D. Schachter and S.M. Rosen, Active transport of Ca^{45} by the small intestine and its dependence on vitamin D. Amer. J. Physiol. 196:357 (1959).
2. D. Schachter, E.B. Dowdle and H. Schenker, Active transport of calcium by the small intestine of the rat. Amer. J. Physiol. 198:263 (1960).
3. D.V. Kimberg, D. Schachter and H. Schonker, Active transport of calcium by intestine: effects of dietary calcium. Amer. J. Physiol. 200:1256 (1961).
4. D. Schachter, L'osteomalacie, in: "Vitamin D and the Intestinal Transport of Calcium and Phosphate", D. Hioco, ed., Masson, Paris (1976).
5. R.H. Wasserman and A.N. Taylor, Some aspects of the intestinal absorption of calcium with special reference to vitamin D, in: "Mineral Metabolism - An Advanced Treatise", C.L. Comar and F. Bronner, eds., Academic Press, New York (1969).
6. J. Harmeyer and H.F. De Luca, Calcium-binding protein and calcium absorption after vitamin D administration. Arch. Biochem. 133:247 (1969).

7. C. Gennari, Action de la vitamin D sur l'absorption digestive du calcium radio-actif chez l'homme, in: "Les Hormones et le Calcium", H.P. Klotz, ed., Expans. Scient. Franc., Paris (1971).
8. C. Gennari, Pathologie de l'absorption intestinal du calcium at du phosphore chez l'homme, in: "Proceedings of IV Congrés Latin de Rhumatologie", Masson, Paris (1980).
9. S.J. Birge, W.A. Peck, M. Berman and G.D. Whedon, Study of calcium absorption in man: a kinetic analysis and physiologic model. J. Clin. Invest. 48:1705 (1969).
10. R.H. Wensel, C. Rich, A.C. Brown and W. Volwiler, Absorption of calcium measured by intubation and perfusion of the intact human small intestine. J. Clin. Invest. 48:1768 (1969).
11. C.F. Cramer, Progress and rate of absorption of radiophosphorus through the intestinal tract of rats. Can. J. Biochem. Physiol. 39:499 (1961).
12. S. Kowarski and D. Schachter, Effects of vitamin D on phosphate transport and incorporation into mucosal constituents of rat intestinal mucosa. J. Biol. Chem. 244:211 (1969).
13. R.H. Wasserman and A.N. Taylor, Intestinal absorption of phosphate in the chick: effect of vitamin D_3 and other parameters. J. Nutr. 103:586 (1973).
14. A. Caniggia and C. Gennari, L'absorption digestive du radiophosphate chez l'homme, in: "Les Tissus Calcifiés", G. Milhaud ed., Sedes, Paris (1968).
15. A. Caniggia and C. Gennari, Absorption du phosphate radio-actif chez l'homme et sa régulation, in: "Phosphate et Métabolisme Phosphocalcique", D.J. Hioco, ed., Expans. Scient. Franc., Paris (1971).
16. R.H. Wasserman and R.A. Corradino, Vitamin D, calcium and protein synthesis. Vitam. Horm. 32:43 (1973).
17. R.H. Wasserman, A.N. Taylor and C.S. Fullmer, Vitamin D-induced calcium-binding protein and the intestinal absorption of calcium, in: "The Metabolism and Function of Vitamin D", D.R. Fraser, ed., The Biochemical Society, London (1974).
18. R. Wilkinson, Absorption of calcium, phosphorus and magnesium, in: "Calcium Phosphate and Magnesium Metabolism", B.E.C. Nordin ed., Churchill Livingstone, Edinburg (1976).
19. E.M. Short, H.J. Binder and L.E. Rosenberg, Familial hypophosphataemic rickets: defective transport of inorganic phosphates by intestinal mucosa. Science 179:700 (1973).
20. R. Wootton and J. Reeve, The relative merits of various techniques for measuring radiocalcium absorption. Clin. Sci. 58:287 (1980).

21. D.H. Marshall and B.E.C. Nordin, A comparison of radioactive calcium absorption tests with net calcium absorption. Clin. Sci. 61:477 (1981).

22. K. Farrington, M.N. Mohammed, S.P. Newman, Z. Varghese and J.F. Moorhead, Comparison of radioisotope methods for the measurement of phosphate absorption in normal subjects and in patients with chronic renal failure. Clin. Sci. 60:55 (1981).

23. M. Peacock, A.M. Davison and G.S. Walker, The effects of plasma phosphate on the action of $1\alpha OHD_3$ in haemodialysis patients. Adv. Exp. Med. Biol. 81:559 (1977).

24. D.H. Marshall and B.E.C. Nordin, Kinetic analysis of plasma radioactivity after oral ingestion of radiocalcium. Nature 222:797 (1969).

25. K. Farrington, Z. Varghese, S.P. Newman, K.Y. Ahmed, O.N. Fernando and J.F. Moorhead, Dissociation of absorptions of calcium and phosphate after successful cadaveric renal transplantation. Brit. Med. J. 1:712 (1979).

TOPICS ON BONE

BONE REMODELLING AFTER RENAL TRANSPLANTATION (RT)

Vittorio Bonomini, Carlo Feletti, Antonio Di Felice, and Andrea Buscaroli

Institute of Nephrology - St. Orsola University Hospital
Bologna - Italy

With the recovery of the excretory and endocrine renal functions after successful Renal Transplantation (RT), renal bone disease also tends to disappear. Nonetheless, several new biochemical changes to the calcium-phosphorus metabolism (e.g. hypercalcemia, hypophosphatemia) may appear while bone histology may remain altered or show new lesions. Apart from scattered reports in the literature, the new bone remodelling that invariably occurs after RT has not been sufficiently investigated, above all as a possible source of overt clinical bone disease.

The aim of this paper is to correlate the clinical, biochemical and histological findings in 42 transplanted patients (76 biopsies) in an attempt to define : the basic bone histology after RT, its pathophysiology and correlation with immunosuppressive therapy, and its clinical tie ups.

PATIENTS AND METHODS

This study selects 42 patients (26 males, 16 females; age: 22-47 years) out of the 223 RT carried out from 1969 to 1982. They alone fulfilled the following criteria: a) normal graft function (serum creatinine ≤ 1.5 mg%); b) a follow up of 2-5 years after transplantation; c) repeated bone histology; d) uniformity of immunosuppressive therapy. The immunosuppressive schedule consisted of steroids and azathioprine. After transplantation each patient received methylprednisolone intravenously in a scalar dose from 1 gr to 125 mg within the first 10 days. Subsequently, prednisone was given orally in a dose of 1 mg/Kg/day reduced to 0.5-0.7 mg/Kg/day over a period of 30 days. It was then progressively tapered until 20 mg/day at 6 months and 10 mg/day at 12 months after transplantation. This maintenance dose was continued indefinitely. The dose of azathioprine was 100-150 mg/day. Acute rejection was treated with 3 i.v. pulses of methylprednisolone 0.5-1.0 g each.

Bone biopsies were taken under local anesthesia from the iliac crest, 5 cm behind the anterior superior iliac spine. Details on inclusion and staining techniques have already been reported (3). Bone histology was evaluated using both static (micromorphometry), and dynamic (double tetracycline labelling) methods. Bone histomorphometry was performed by the Merz-Schenk method (4,5). The following parameters, whose significance has been reported in detail elsewhere (3), were measured: volumetric density of bone, surface density of bone, specific surface (structural parameters); total resorption surface, active resorption surface and osteoclast index (bone resorption parameters); volumetric density of osteoid, total osteoid surface, active osteoid surface (bone formation parameters). 25 healthy subjects (16 males, 9 females; age: 20-45 y) were taken as controls for the normal range of histomorphometric parameters. 9 patients were given a double tetracycline label, receiving two three-day courses of oxytetracycline (1 mg/day) separated by a 12 day drug free interval (3-12-3 label). The appositional rate, i.e. the distance between two separate labels, was determined.

The histological results were correlated with the biochemical findings: serum calcium, phosphate, alkaline phosphatase (by a Technicon autoanalyzer); parathyroid hormone (COOH terminal fragment) and 25 hydroxy-cholecalciferol by radio immunoassay (Immunonuclear Corporation). The renal threshold for phosphate (TmP/GFR) was determined by the nomogram of Walton and Bijvoet (6) and GFR was determined by creatinine clearance. Radio-calcium absorption was measured in the fasting state after oral administration of 20 µCu of 47Ca dissolved in 80 mg of CaCl2 carrier. Plasma radioactivity was followed over the next 2 hours and the data, analysed according to Marshall and Nordin (7), were expressed as fractional absorption.

RESULTS

The main histological lesions revealed by bone biopsy suggest dividing the patients into 3 groups.

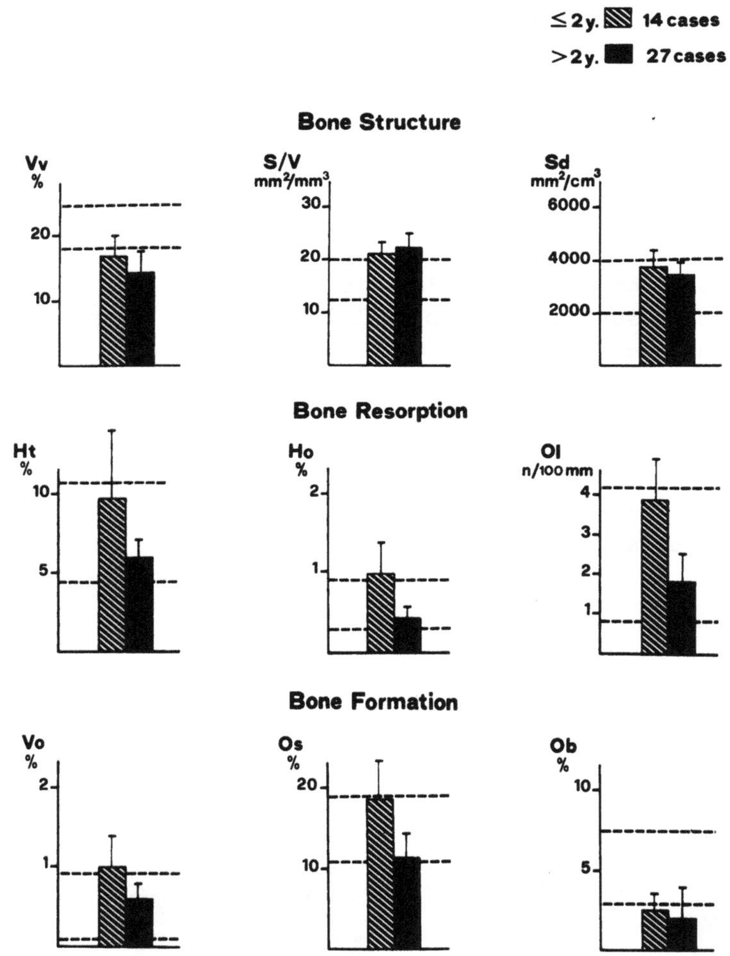

Fig. 1. Histomorphometry in post-transplant osteopenia, up to and after 2 years from surgery. For histomorphometric symbols, see Results.

Group I (Osteopenia)

27 patients presented a reduction in trabecular bone volume compared with the control group (Fig.1). Bone morphometry showed a decrease in volumetric density of bone (Vv),increasing with time, and associated with an increase in specific surface (S/V),inversely related to the mean trabecular diameter. The decrease in bone volume correlates with the amount of steroid dosage (Fig.2). In 14 cases where bone biopsies were sequentially obtained before and after transplantation,the percentual bone mass decrease per year was 33.5% in the 1st year, 8.7% in the 2nd year, and 11.9% in the 3rd year,whereas mean prednisone dosage per year dropped from 22,500 gr in the 1st year,to 8,300 and 3,250 gr in the 2nd and 3rd years respectively.

Bone resorption parameters,i.e. total resorption surface (Ht), active resorption surface with osteoclasts (Ho) and osteoclast index (OI) remained in the high normal range or slightly increased in the first 2 years,decreasing thereafter to normal low values (Fig. 1).

Among bone formation parameters,osteoid surface covered by osteoblasts (Ob) was always below normal; osteoid volume (Vo) and total osteoid surface (Os) were slightly increased in the first 2

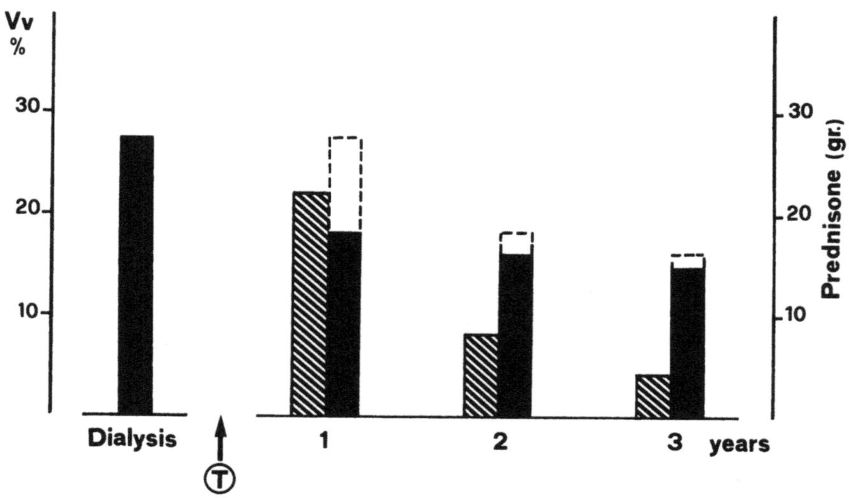

Fig. 2. Mean steroid dosage/year (□) and bone mass (■) in post-transplant osteopenia. (14 patients).

years, and then decreased to normal (Fig.1). Double tetracycline labelling performed in 9 patients 2-3 years after transplantation showed a reduction in the rate of bone apposition, with the mean thickness of osteoid seams ($\bar{S}$) being normal or low (Fig.3).

Post transplant osteoporosis had no clinical expression. In some cases a slight increase in PTH in the first two years, decreasing thereafter, was found, when alkaline phosphatase was in the lower normal range. The intestinal absorption of 47 Calcium was found to be reduced shortly after transplantation, then progressively increased to reach the normal range after 2-3 years.

Group II (Persisting osteitis fibrosa)

After 2 years from transplantation 5 patients still presented hypercalcemia, hypophosphatemia, reduction in renal phosphate threshold and persistingly high PTH levels. Bone morphometry showed an increase in bone resorption (active resorption surface, osteoclast index), increase in bone formation (osteoid volume, osteoid surface covered by osteoblasts) and presence of endosteal fibrosis (Eof). Bone mass was normal in 3 cases and increased in 2 (Fig.4).

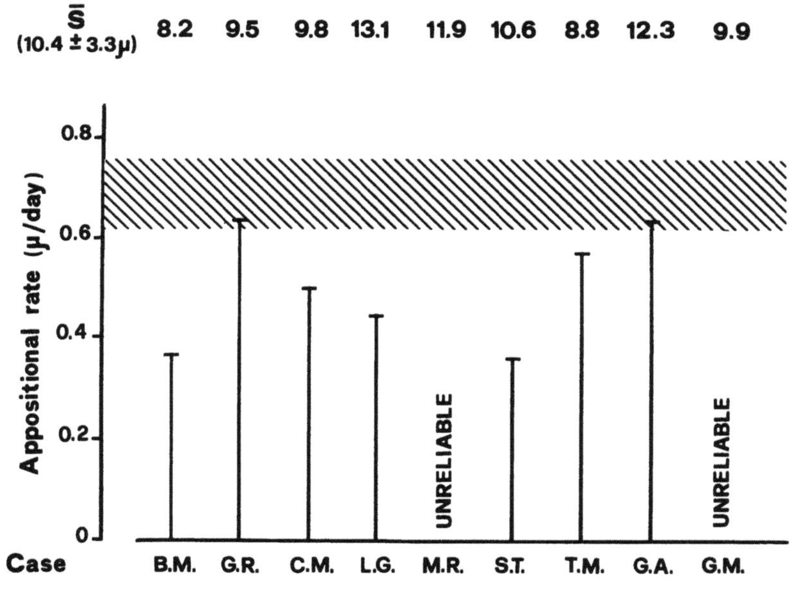

Fig. 3. Bone formation in renal transplantation. Double tetracycline labelling (3-12-3). $\bar{S}$ = mean thickness of osteoid seams.

In one patient,severe hypercalcemia (13.5 mg/dl) was associated with a progressive impairment in graft function (serum creatinine from 1.1 to 2.3 mg/dl),not related to immunological or infectious causes. Subtotal parathyroidectomy with removal of 2 hyperplastic glands (2.5 and 3.7 cm),induced a normalization of calcium levels with subsequent recovery of renal function. Prior to transplantation, all these patients had been on low protein diet for 3-5 years,and regular dialysis treatment was started when residual renal function was under 2 ml/min.

Group III (Osteomalacia)

10 transplant patients with chronic hypophosphatemia (serum phosphate $\leq$ 2.5 mg/dl after over 2 years) not related to PTH,underwent bone biopsy. Hypophosphatemia was associated with a low TmP/GFR in 7 cases (1.73$\pm$0.26 mg/dl; normal range 2.20-4.20 mg/dl), normal TmP/GFR in 3 cases (3.1, 3.8, 2.9 mg/dl respectively).Serum PTH was normal (0.93$\pm$0.2 ng/ml; upper normal limit 1.5 ng/ml) in all patients. Bone morphometry documented an increase in osteoid volume and total osteoid surface in hypophosphatemic patients, if compared to 17 normophosphatemic patients with the same age of

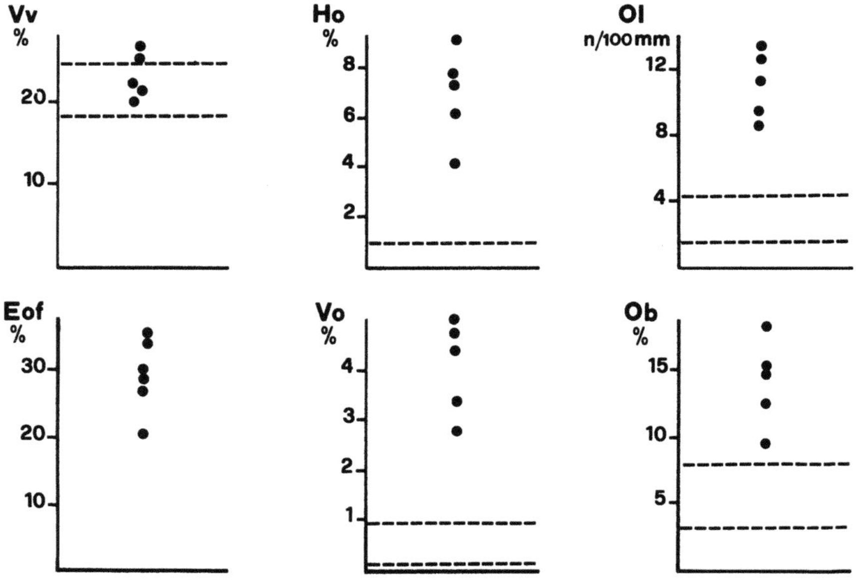

Fig. 4. Histomorphometry in persistent hyperparathyroidism after renal transplantation. For histomorphometric symbols, see Results.

graft. Bone mass and osteoid seams covered by osteoblasts were below normal in both groups (Fig.5). A delay in calcification rate, as measured by double tetracycline labelling,was observed in 7 cases (0.5 ± 0.4 µ/day; normal range: 0.8-1.1 µ/day).

DISCUSSION

The present poor knowledge of bone remodelling after RT may be explained by the inadequacy of previous studies,on the one hand,and by the intrinsic difficulties of the subject itself,on the other. The latter include: 1) the variability of basic bone lesions and their frequent subclinical course; 2) the lack of clinico-morphological studies; 3) the heterogeneity of patients' clinical histories before and after transplantation. Clearly in order to investigate the bone remodelling that occurs after RT,one needs selected,homogeneous material (clinical criteria) and bone biopsies repeated before and after transplantation with static and dynamic evaluation of the lesions (morphological criteria). Isolated reports (1,2)

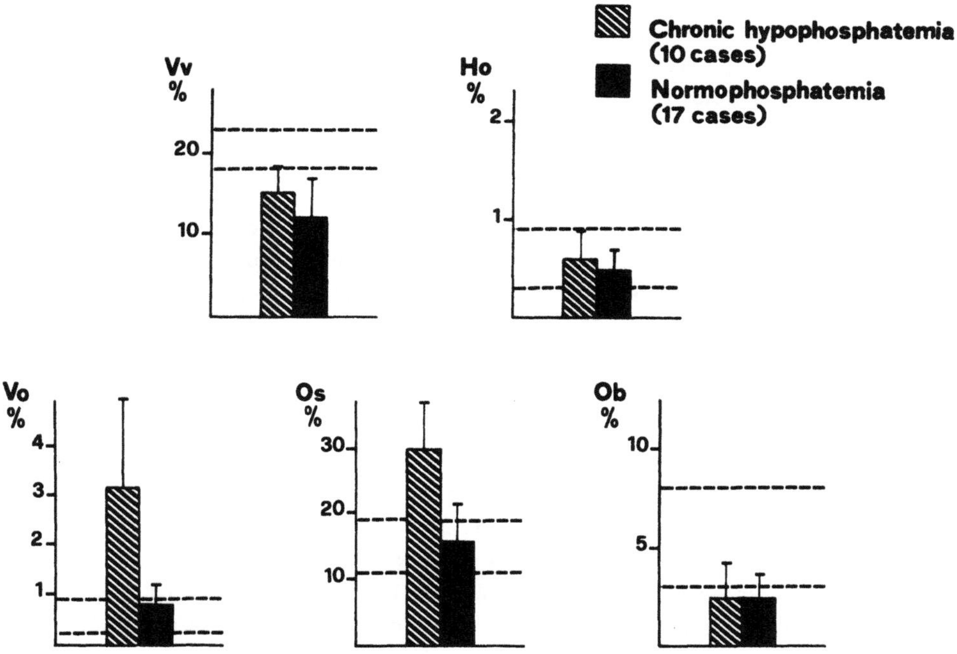

Fig. 5. Histomorphometry in chronic hypophosphatemia after renal transplantation. For histomorphometric symbols, see Results.

have in the past stated that successful RT generally leads to a gradual steady improvement in renal bone disease: in most cases osteomalacia tends to clear up after 1 year,whereas osteitis fibrosa may take longer to heal. But,in spite of this progressive tendency to recover,the bone may actually not be normal and a subclinical bone pathology may occur (8). Repeated bone biopsy checks show three basic lesions with various combinations: osteopenia,persistent osteitis fibrosa,osteomalacia.

Osteopenia is a reduction in bone mass when compared with a healthy control group of corresponding age and sex,which is inconceivable without a negative balance in bone remodelling. Now all transplanted patients necessarily receive steroids and it is well known that a steroid-induced osteopenia exists. This is due to: a) a direct inhibition of bone formation (decrease in bone collagen synthesis by pre-existing osteoblasts and in the conversion of precursor cells to functioning osteoblasts) and/or b) an indirect stimulation of bone resorption (owing to secondary hyperparathyroidism induced by steroid-related decreased intestinal Calcium absorption) (9, 10, 11). However,the pathophysiology of post-transplant osteopenia is more complicated and seems to follow a pattern comprised of two phases (Fig.1): <u>phase I</u> (less than 2 years): decrease in bone formation with bone resorption still high; <u>phase II</u>: (after 2 years): decrease in bone formation with a normal or low rate of resorption. A condition of low bone turnover thus sets in owing principally to a contraction in the active osteoblast pool, which mainly consists of flat cells lining the bone trabeculae. There is a strong correlation between this behaviour shown by histology on the one hand and biochemical and radiokinetic studies on the other: in phase I,PTH may still be high and intestinal Ca absorption still impaired; in phase II,PTH is normal,intestinal Ca absorption improved,and alkaline phosphatase is within the lower normal limit. The central role played by steroids in the development of renal transplant osteopenia and the dose-dependent mechanism find confirmation in results. The percentage reduction in bone mass varied with time,mainly according to the steroid dosage. A more rapid and marked reduction in bone mass is found in the first year after transplantation when the total yearly dosage of prednisone is higher (Fig.2). That other immunosuppressive drugs (such as azathioprine) should play a similar role is likely in theory, although difficult or impossible to confirm in practice.

When osteitis fibrosa persists after RT,the main causes are

autonomous hyperparathyroidism or delayed involution of hypertrophied parathyroid glands. This condition seems related to a persistent chronic stimulation of the parathyroid glands due to the disturbance of the calcium-phosphorus metabolism occurring in uremia,which is not sufficiently controlled by pharmacological and dialysis treatment before transplantation. This typically occurs in patients who started dialysis too late (12). The most evident hallmark of this histological condition is hypercalcemia which can induce a functional impairment of the graft,not related to immunological vascular or infectious factors,and which may recover after subtotal parathyroidectomy (13).

Osteomalacia,which is a defect in bone mineralization due to a delayed calcification rate,has been found after renal transplantation associated with chronic persistent hypophosphatemia not related to PTH hypersecretion (14, 15). It remains to be established whether the defect in mineralization indicates incomplete healing of preexisting uremic lesions or de novo lesions. It is a fact that, when radiology and densitometry reveal a generic condition of post transplant osteopenia,only bone biopsy is able to distinguish between osteoporosis (reduction in bone mass) osteomalacia (defect in mineralization) or a combination of both. Without bone biopsy, therefore,no clinical assessment is possible. This cannot be overstressed in view of the likely "risk state" that these lesions may represent in the bone.

REFERENCES

1. R.N.P. Carrol, E.D.Williams, T.Aung, E.Yeboah and R.Shackman: The effects of renal transplantation on renal osteodystrophy. Proc. EDTA 10:446 (1973).
2. A.M. Pierides, A.H. Ellis, K.M. Peart, W.Simpson, P.R.Vedall and D.N.S. Kerr: Assessment of renal osteodystrophy following renal transplantation. Proc. EDTA 11:481 (1974).
3. G.C. Bortolotti, C. Feletti, M.P. Scolari and V. Bonomini: Subclinical bone pathology after kidney transplantation (KT) in man. Calcif. Tissue Res. Supp. 22:486 (1977).
4. C. Feletti and V. Bonomini: Effect of calcitonin on bone lesions in chronic dialysis patients. Nephron 24:85 (1979).
5. R.K. Schenk and W.A. Merz: A quantitative histological study on bone formation in human cancellous bone. Acta Anat. 76:54(1970).

6. R.K.Schenk and W.A.Merz: A quantitative histological study on bone resorption in human cancellous bone. Acta Anat. 74:44 (1969).
7. R.J.Walton and O.L.M.Bijvoet: Nomogram for derivation of renal threshold phosphate concentration. Lancet ii:309 (1975).
8. D.H.Marshall and B.E.C.Nordin: Nature 222:797 (1969).
9. H.M.Frost and A.R.Villanueva: Human osteoblastic activity III. The effect of cortisone on lamellar osteoblastic activity. Henry Ford Hosp. Med. Bull. 9:97 (1961).
10. J.Jowsey and B.L.Riggs: Bone formation in hypercortisolism. Acta Endocr. 63:21 (1970).
11. C. Bressot, P.J. Meunier, M.C. Chapuy, E. Lejeune, C. Edouard and A.J. Darby: Histomorphometric profile,pathophysiology and reversibility of corticosteroid induced osteoporosis. Metab. Bone Dis. and Rel. Res. 1:303 (1979).
12. V. Bonomini, L. Baldrati, C. Feletti, S. Stefoni and A. Vangelista: Long-term early dialysis in Uremia:pathobiology of patients treated for 10 years or more. Edited by C.Giordano and E.Friedman, Wichtig, Milan, p. 133 (1981).
13. S.N. Chatterjee, R.M. Friedler, T.V. Berne, S.B. Oldham, F.R. Singer and S.G. Massry: Persistent hypercalcemia after successful renal transplantation. Nephron 17:1 (1976).
14. J.F. Moorhead, K.Y. Ahmed, Z. Varghese, M.R. Wills, R.A.Baillod and G.L. Tatler: Hypophosphatemic osteomalacia after cadaveric renal transplantation. Lancet ii:694 (1974).
15. R.W. Rosenbaum, K.A. Hruska, A. Korkor, C. Anderson and E. Slatopolsky: Decrease phosphate resorption after renal transplantation: evidence for a mechanism independent of calcium and parathyroid hormone. Kidney Int. 19:568 (1981).

INORGANIC PHOSPHATE, PYROPHOSPHATE AND THE DIPHOSPHONATES ACTIVATE BONE (CALVARIA) GLUTAMINASE

R.M. Biltz, E.D. Pellegrino, J.M. Letteri, and L.M. Pinkus

Department of Medicine, Georgetown University Medical Center, Washington, D.C.; SUNY, Stony Brook and Nassau County Medical Center, East Meadow, New York

Inorganic phosphate (P_i), pyrophosphate (PP_i) and its synthetic analogues, dichloromethanediphosphonate (Cl_2MDP) and 1-hydroxyethane-1, 1-diphosphonate (EHDP) compete for sites in bone mineral affecting the formation and dissolution of apatite.[1] The diphosphonates may also affect the metabolism of bone and cartilage cells and possibly other tissues by interacting with enzymes or proteins which bind phosphate or phosphorylated intermediates. Available data indicate that Cl_2MDP increases the production of CO_2 from acetate, leucine, citrate and palmitate; stimulates the synthesis of collagen, proteoglycans and glycogen; increases alkaline phosphatase activity and inhibits lactate formation in cultured calvaria cells.[2,3]

A role for glutamine in bone metabolism was suggested by its active transport into calvaria and degradation to glutamate and ammonia in a reaction catalyzed by mitochondrial phosphate-dependent glutaminase.[4] The activity of this enzyme, which may regulate the utilization of glutamine in bone cells, is influenced by the concentrations of phosphate and phosphorylated intermediates in the mitochondria. Consequently, it was of interest to determine if the diphosphonates could stimulate the degradation of glutamine in bone and the activity of the phosphate-dependent glutaminase in bone extracts.

METHODS AND PROCEDURES

Calvaria were carefully dissected from newborn rats. Homogenates for enzyme studies (10-15% w/v) were prepared by pulverizing the calvaria with mortar and pestle at 4°C. The buffer employed contained sucrose (250 mM) and phosphate (25 mM), pH 8. Glutaminase (EC3.5.1.2) was determined by measuring glutamate formation.[5] Assays were performed at 37° in a total volume of 0.3 ml containing glutamine (20 mM), homogenate (0.1-0.7 mg protein) with the addition of P_i, PP_i, Cl_2MDP and EHDP as indicated. The reaction was stopped at 4° by the addition of 20µl of 82% trichloroacetic acid and the precipitated protein was separated by centrifugation for 1 min. at 13,500g. The glutamate contained in 100-200 µl aliquots of supernatant was determined. The diphosphonates were provided by W. Hedglin, Procter & Gamble Co., Cinti. Ohio.

For metabolic studies using intact calvaria; specimens were preincubated for 60 min. at 37° in Erlenmeyer flasks (25 ml) containing 2 ml of basal salt solution (BSS) consisting of 125 mM NaCl, 0.75 mM NaH_2PO_4, 1.2 mM KH_2PO_4, 5.4 mM KCl, 0.81 mM $MgSO_4$, 1.5 mM $CaCl_2$ and 22 mM $NaHCO_3$, pH 7.4. The gas phase was 5% CO_2 -95% O_2. The tissues were then transferred to fresh medium containing glucose (5.5 mM), and glutamine (2 mM), with the addition of P_i, PP_i, Cl_2MDP, and EHDP. The incubations were continued for 90 min. with constant agitation and terminated at 4° by the addition of 50 µl of 82% trichloroacetic acid. Bone and precipitated protein were removed by centrifugation and the medium was analyzed for ammonia and glutamate with glutamate dehydrogenase.[5]

Activation of Glutaminase in Bone Homogenates

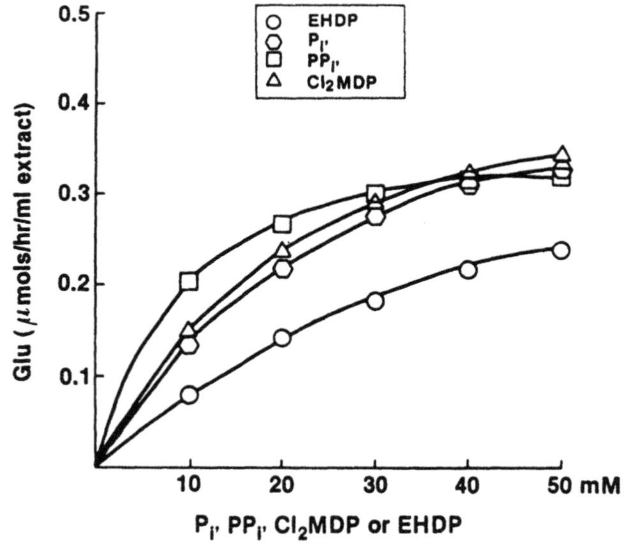

Figure 1. Phosphate, pyrophosphate and diphosphonate (Cl_2MDP and EHDP) activation of glutaminase in bone homogenates. Incubations contained 20 mM glutamine, 3 mM potassium phosphate (pH 8.0) and other compounds as indicated.

PP_i with an estimated K_a of 10 mM was the most potent activator of the bone glutaminase and EHDP (K_a of 50 mM) was the least potent. P_i and Cl_2MDP exhibited a K_a of 25 mM and 15 mM, respectively. The maximum velocity obtained at saturating concentrations of each activator was not significantly different for P_i, PP_i and Cl_2MDP, whereas EHDP was somewhat less effective as an activator of phosphate-dependent glutaminase in bone homogenates.

Activation of Glutaminase in Intact Calvaria

The addition of Cl_2MDP to BSS (containing 2 mM P_i) increased glutamate (and ammonia) production (Figure 2). The stimulation by Cl_2MDP was greater than that obtained in response to additional P_i, which was greater than the response to PP_i. EHDP was only slightly effective at the lowest concentrations tested and did not elicit a concentration dependent response. These results suggest that Cl_2MDP is a more effective activator of glutamine degradation in bone than EHDP and that Cl_2MDP may act synergistically with P_i and PP_i to stimulate metabolism of glutamine in bone.

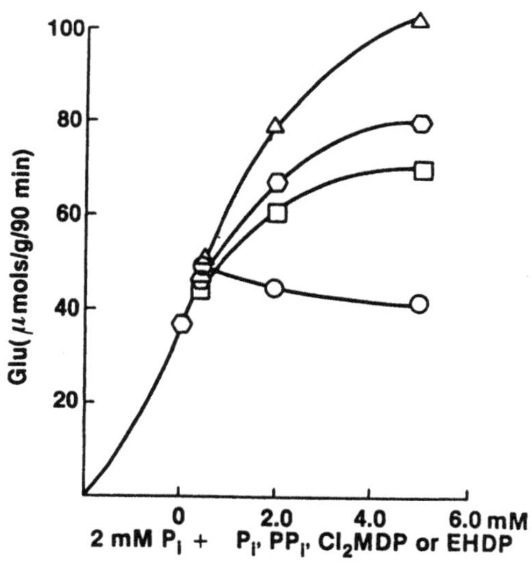

Figure 2. Intact calvaria, when incubated in a bicarbonate buffered salt solution (pH 7.4) at 37° under 95% O_2-5% CO_2, degraded glutamine to form glutamate and ammonia. Cl_2MDP was the most effective activator of bone glutaminase: $Cl_2MDP > P_i > PP_i >$ EHDP.

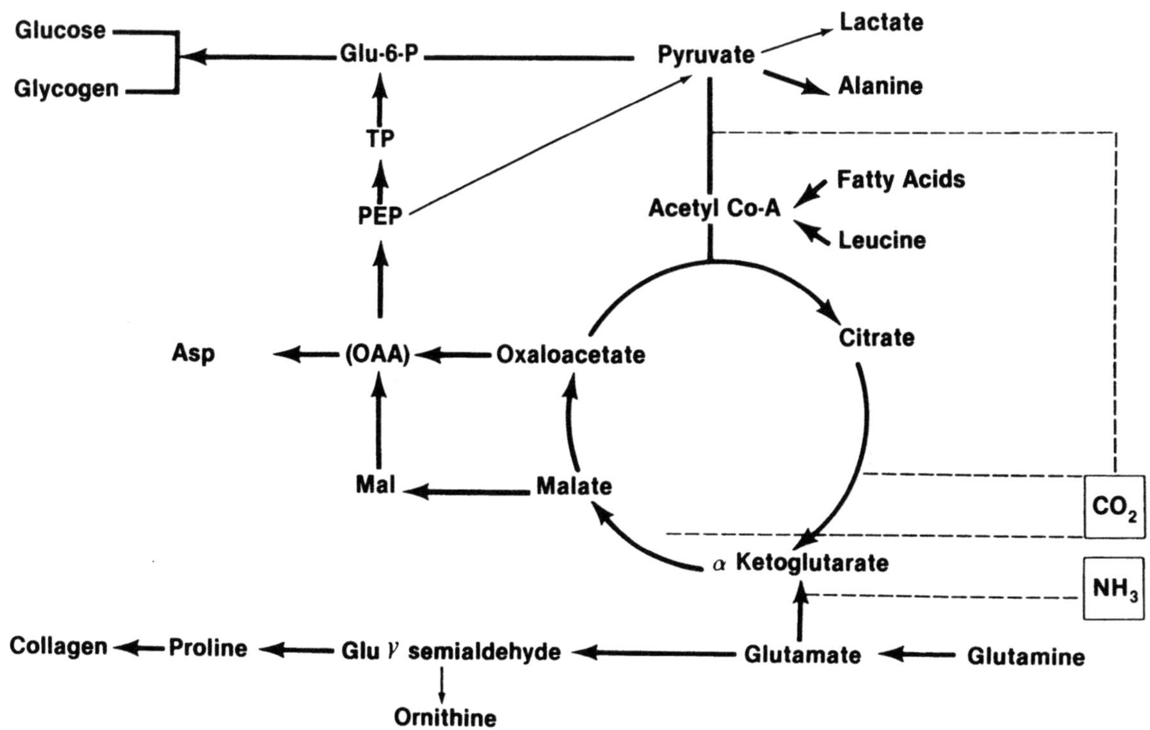

Figure 3. Possible effects of diphosphonates on bone metabolism and their relationship to the utilization of glutamine. Activation of the glutaminase gives rise to glutamate, α-ketoglutarate and other amino acids which lead ultimately to the synthesis of collagen and other important macromolecules of the cell. Glycolysis might be suppressed and the oxidation of fatty acids, acetate, leucine and citrate stimulated through the utilization of Krebs cycle intermediates (α-ketoglutarate, malate and oxaloacetate).

DISCUSSION

Glutamine is utilized as a preferred source of nitrogen for the biosynthesis of purine and pyrimidine nucleotides, glucosamine 6-P and other amino acids which lead to the synthesis of proteins, nucleic acids and complex polysaccharides. We have shown that glutamine is a precursor of aspartate, alanine, proline and ornithine in bone.[4] It would appear from the present study that the diphosphonates may affect the metabolism of bone, cartilage and possibly other tissues by activating the mitochondrial phosphate-dependent glutaminase. The effects of the diphosphonates (particularly Cl_2MDP) on bone metabolism could, therefore, be attributed in part to a persistent increase in glutamine metabolism (Fig. 3). Substrates (α-ketoglutarate, malate and oxaloacetate) derived from glutamine might have the effect of stimulating the tricarboxylic acid cycle. α-Ketoglutarate is a required co-factor in the hydroxylation of proline in collagen. In addition, glutamine reduces lactate formation from glucose in compact bone from young rats (unpublished observations). Bone, as compared with other tissues, may contribute significantly to ammonia production from blood-derived glutamine.[4] However, a role for the ammonia generated from glutamine remains to be established. We may only assume, at this point, that the uptake and metabolism of glutamine in bone is predominately a function of osteoblasts or osteoblast-like cells.

REFERENCES

1. H. Fleisch, R.G.G. Russell, and M. D. Francis, Diphosphonates inhibit hydroxyapatite dissolution in vitro and bone resorption in tissue culture and in vivo, Science 165: 1262 (1969).

2. H. Fleisch and R. Felix, Diphosphonates, Calcif. Tiss. Intl. 27:91 (1979).

3. R. Felix and H. Fleisch, Increase in fatty acid oxidation in calvaria cells cultured with diphosphonates, Biochem. J. 196:237 (1981).

4. R. M. Biltz, J. M. Letteri, E. D. Pellegrino, A. Palekar, and L. M. Pinkus, Glutamine metabolism in bone, Mineral Electrolyte Metab. 9:125 (1983).

5. E. Bernt and H. U. Bergmeyer, Glutamate; UV assay with glutamate dehydrogenase, and NAD, in: "Methods of Enzymatic Analysis," H. U. Bergmeyer, ed., Academic Press, New York (1974).

EFFECT OF CALCIUM-SODIUM EXCHANGE AND CALCIUM CHANNEL INHIBITION ON CALCIUM RELEASE FROM BONE IN AN IN-VITRO BONE PERFUSION SYSTEM

Peter J. Somerville and Michael Kaye

Division of Nephrology
Montreal General Hospital
1650 Cedar Avenue
Montreal, Quebec, Canada

INTRODUCTION

The regulation of calcium release from bone is likely to be at least in part, dependant on cellular activity. In recent years it has been shown that the intracellular calcium concentration is important in regulating the activity of many cells from a wide range of tissues including those of the endocrine system and bone. There are several mechanisms involved in regulating cell calcium including calcium sodium (Ca-Na) exchange, calcium-magnesium sensitive ATPase and calcium transport via slow calcium channels[1]. Thus it is possible that by regulating intracellular calcium, some of these mechanisms could also regulate the cell mediated component of the transfer of calcium from bone to the extracellular fluid.

We have recently developed an in vitro bone perfusion system[2] which has enabled us to examine the effect of various agents on calcium release and we have used this model to study mechanisms which may regulate calcium release using inhibitors of Ca-Na exchange or the slow calcium channel. Various pharmacological agents which could influence these processes were added to the perfusing fluid of the bone perfusion model and calcium release was determined by measuring the amount of ^{45}Ca, previously given to the intact animal, appearing in the effluent. Our results suggest that both Ca-Na exchange and transport via the slow calcium channel have a role in the regulation of calcium release from bone.

METHODS

The bone perfusion system which uses isolated perfused rat

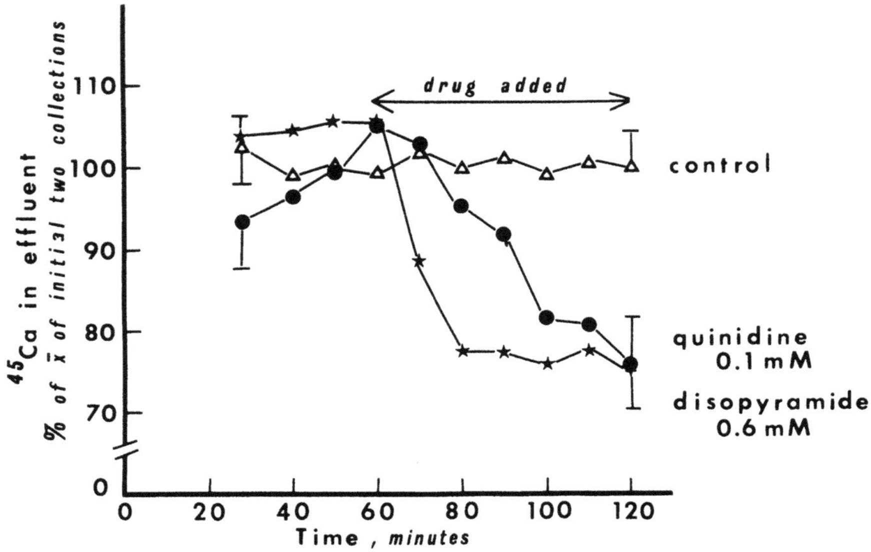

Fig. 1 Amount of ^{45}Ca in effluent coming from rat tails perfused with an aqueous buffer to which quinidine or disopyramide was added during the second hour of the two hour study. The effluent was collected every 10 minutes and the results are expressed as a percentage of the mean of the first two collections. The open triangles represent the controls, the closed circles the quinidine group and the stars the disopyramide group. Each point represents the mean of 7 or 8 experiments except for the disopyramide group, where N = 14. The vertical bars represent the S.E.M.

tails has been described in a recent publication[2]. In brief, rats weighing about 170 gm are given 75 μCi of ^{45}Ca subcutaneously a week before use. On the day of the experiment, the tail is removed, placed in a heated chamber and perfused with a Krebs-Ringer bicarbonate solution via the ventral artery at a pressure of about 100mm Hg. The perfusate is heated to 37.5°C, equilibrated with 95% O_2, 5% CO_2 gas mixture and the pH is adjusted to between 7.35 and 7.4. The pH stability was verified following the addition of any pharmacological agent.

In the studies to be described, the tails were initially perfused for a two hour "wash out" and stabilization period, experiments were then commenced and lasted for a further two hours. During the two hour experimental period, the phosphate concentration was zero whereas it was 3.5mg/dl during the wash-out period. Previous studies have shown that a zero phosphate perfusate resulted in a constant ^{45}Ca release from bone over the two hours.

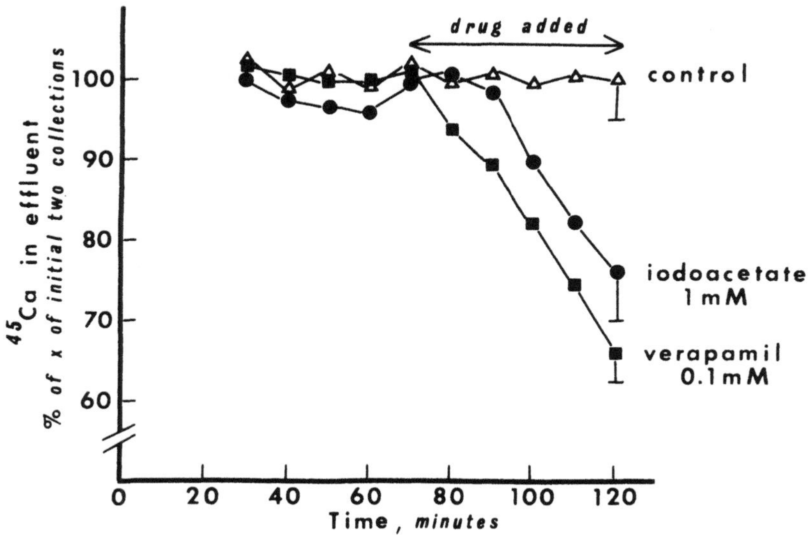

Fig.2 Similar format to Fig.1. In this instance, the circles represent vanadate, the squares ouabain and the stars choline Cl which was used to replace sodium chloride such that the final sodium concentration was 50mM. (N=6 except for choline when N=10).

The pharmacological agents were added to the perfusate during the second hour of the two hour experimental period. The ^{45}Ca concentration in the effluent was measured every ten minutes and compared to that in control experiments in which no agent was used. In order to show that a particular agent is having a direct effect on ^{45}Ca release from bone rather than indirectly by diverting perfusate flow away from bone, we added a bolus of ^{85}Sr labelled microspheres, 15 μm in diameter, to the perfusate at the end of each experiment. The bone was then separated from the soft tissue and each was counted in a gamma counter.

Biochemical and radioactive measurements were carried out as described previously[2]. Results are expressed as mean ± the standard error of the mean (S.E.M.) and Students t-test was used to determine the significance of differences between the control and treated groups.

RESULTS

Figure 1 shows the effect on ^{45}Ca release of using perfusate containing disopyramide or quinidine during the second

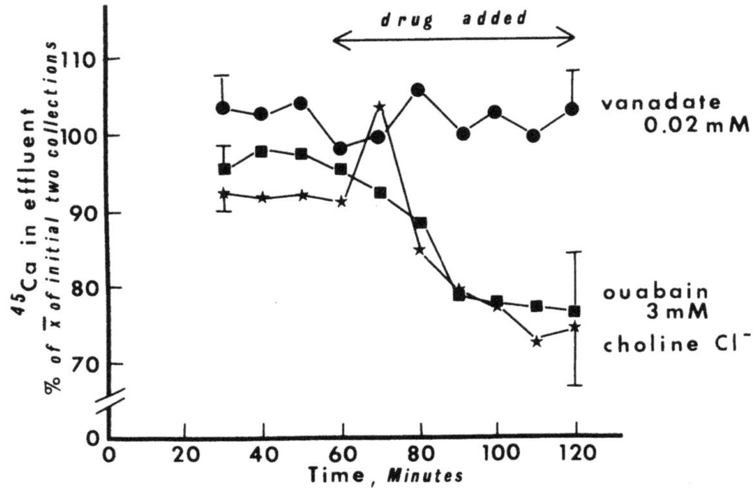

Fig.3 Format similar to Figs. 1 and 2. The closed circles represent iodoacetate and the squares, verapamil. The control group is the same as that shown in fig.1 (N=6 - 8).

hour. Both agents significantly inhibited ^{45}Ca release compared to the control group (open triangles) in which no drug was added and the calcium release remained constant.

Figure 2 shows the results of three additional studies carried out to examine the effect of inhibition of Ca-Na exchange on ^{45}Ca release. Two inhibitors of Na-K ATPase were used, vanadate and ouabain. In the third instance, the sodium chloride in the perfusate was replaced by choline chloride such that the final sodium concentration was 50mM. The rationale for this manoeuvre was that if extracellular Na is important in the calcium release phenomenon, then its replacement with an equimolar concentration of the monovalent cation choline should reduce calcium release. Our results show some evidence for this. The data points for the choline group are shown by stars and although there was an increase in calcium release in the initial ten minute collection following the change from sodium to choline, by the end of the experiment the amount of ^{45}Ca in the choline group was significantly less than the control group, 75 ± 7.8% compared with 100 ± 5.5% respectively ($p < 0.05$). It should be pointed out however that the four baseline points in the choline group were somewhat lower than the controls, even though the experimental conditions were identical during this period, thus diminishing the strength of this difference. In the case of the two Na-K ATPase inhibitors, vanadate had no effect whereas ouabain,

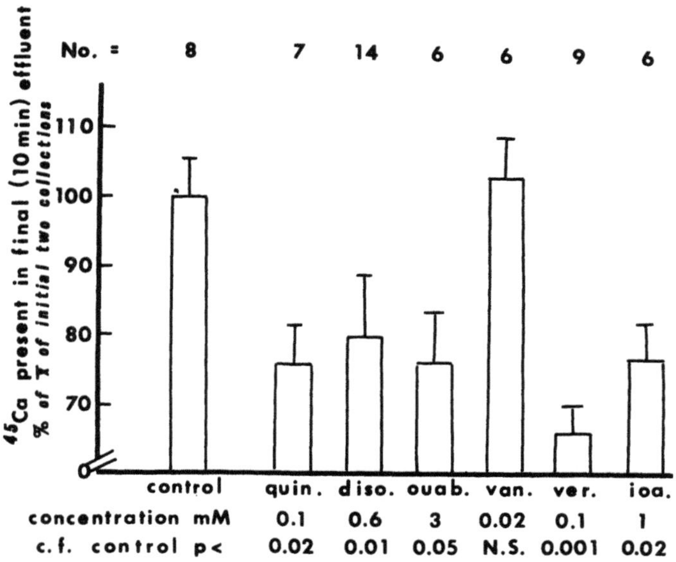

Fig.4 This shows ^{45}Ca concentration in the effluent collected during the final 10 minute period plotted for the control and the various inhibitors of calcium transport. Data from the same studies shown in Figs. 1 - 3.

albeit at a much higher concentration significantly inhibited ^{45}Ca release, compared to the control group ($p < 0.05$).

Figure 3 shows the results of some further experiments in which the effect of adding either the calcium channel blocking agent verapamil, or the non-specific metabolic inhibitor iodoacetate, to the perfusion fluid. The control group (open triangles) is the same as that shown in figure 1. It can be seen that the verapamil caused a marked inhibition of calcium release. A similar but less pronounced effect was seen with the non-specific metabolic inhibitor iodoacetate showing that ^{45}Ca release in this model is able to be inhibited in a non specific manner, little different from the more specific inhibitor verapamil.

In figure 4, a summary of the results of some of the experiments previously shown in figures 1 to 3 has been presented in a different manner. In this figure, the mean ^{45}Ca concentration in the effluent collected during the final ten minutes of each experiment is plotted to permit comparison with the others and the control. It can be seen that the ^{45}Ca release in the vanadate perfused group was not significantly different from the control group, whereas in all the other experimental groups ^{45}Ca release was significantly less than the control. This difference was greatest in the case of verapamil and a difference was still present when this agent was used in a concentration one order of magnitude lower i.e. 0.01mM (data not shown).

In all the studies described, (except in the case of quinidine 0.1mM) none of the pharmacological agents used caused a significant reduction in the flow of perfusate to the bone of the tail as determined by the distribution of ^{85}Sr microspheres between bone and soft tissue.

DISCUSSION

In the earlier studies using this model, we have shown that the tail remains viable during the time of an experiment and that more than 95% of the ^{45}Ca present in the tail at the beginning of an experiment is associated with the bone rather than the soft tissue component[2]. Thus a change in the amount of ^{45}Ca appearing in the venous effluent represents a change in ^{45}Ca release from bone. Most of the drugs used in the studies described have the potential for altering blood flow through tissues. However, except in the case of quinidine, the flow studies using the radioactive microspheres indicate that effects on ^{45}Ca release was not the result of diversion of perfusate away from bone. Although quinidine did result in decreased flow of perfusate to the bone, compared to control studies, this was not the case with disopyramide which is thought to act on cells in a manner very similar to quinidine[3]. Thus we have assumed that this is not the mechanism by which quinidine inhibits calcium release.

We believe that the inhibitory effect on ^{45}Ca release of the agents studied is due to some change in "bone cell" function rather than a direct physico-chemical action on bone, for several reasons. Firstly, the chemical nature of the substances is quite diverse making it unlikely that they would all have an effect of decreasing bone crystal solubility. Secondly, complete inhibition of cell function using the non specific inhibitor iodoacetate in the perfusate, caused a decrease in calcium release similar to that seen with verapamil. Thirdly, when two diphosphonates, EHDP and Cl_2 MDP were added to the perfusate in a manner similar to the experiments described above, no change in ^{45}Ca release was noted (data not shown). These agents have been shown to inhibit bone crystal disolution[4] although it is acknowledged that they may have additional effects on bone cell metabolism.

In a recent paper, Kreiger and Tashjian, using a 48 hour bone culture preparation, have presented evidence that parathyroid hormone stimulated calcium release is mediated via a Na-Ca exchange mechanism[5]. Our results (fig.2) showing that either the addition of ouabain to the perfusate or the replacement of NaCl in the perfusate with choline chloride inhibits ^{45}Ca release, are in accord with their hypothesis. Ouabain, by reducing sodium transport out of the cell, would be expected to reduce the normal Na gradient across the plasma membrane, which creates a favourable situation for Na to diffuse into the cell in exchange for Ca extrusion. The mechanism by which the antiarrhythmic drugs, quinidine and disopyramide, inhibit the ^{45}Ca release is less clear but may also involve inhibition of Ca-Na exchange. These two drugs belong to the same pharmacological class in terms of their electrophysiological action on heart muscle[3]. Quinidine has been shown to inhibit sodium entry into cardiac muscle cells possibly by blocking the fast sodium channel[6] and it has also been shown to inhibit sodium transport by epithelial cells[7], perhaps by the same mechanism. It has also been found to inhibit ^{45}Ca release in a fetal bone culture system, and in this latter paper the authors considered that the drug was acting as a membrane stabilizing agent[8]. Diphenylhydantoin, another antiarrhythmic with some similarities to quinidine[3], has also been shown to inhibit bone resorption in tissue culture by two groups of workers[9, 10]. Thus, there is good evidence that these antiarrhythmic agents inhibit Ca release from bone and a mechanism which could be common to all three is inhibition of Na-Ca exchange. Our results do not however explain the precise mechanism at the cell level. It was not clear why vanadate failed to inhibit ^{45}Ca release (fig.2), as it is a powerful inhibitor of Na-K ATPase[11] at concentrations lower than the one used in our study. The drug affects other enzyme systems including Ca-Mg stimulated ATPase[12] and this may be the explanation.

Our studies using the calcium channel blocking agent verapamil (fig.3) show that this agent, which is thought to affect cell calcium in a manner different from the quinidine like drugs[13], also inhibits calcium release from bone. Whereas quinidine[7] or Na-Ca exchange inhibition with ouabain[5] might be expected to result in an increase in intracellular calcium, verapamil would be expected to lower intracellular calcium, thus the mechanism of its inhibition of ^{45}Ca release is probably different from the other agents used in our studies. Perhaps it reduces ^{45}Ca available to be released into the perfusate. Some support for this hypothesis comes from a recent paper by Lerner and Gustafson[14] who have shown that verapamil inhibits both unstimulated and 1 α OHD_3 stimulated bone resorption in a tissue culture. These workers used verapamil in concentrations similar to that in our report and concluded that this agent was exerting its effect by lowering intracellular Ca.

In conclusion, in an isolated bone perfusion system, we have used two different manoeuvres to inhibit release of previously labelled ^{45}Ca from bone into the perfusate. The effect on calcium release was rapid, occuring within thirty minutes of exposure of the bone to the drug, consistent with an effect on membrane or intracellular transport processes. These results do not describe in detail the mechanism of calcium release, nor do they show which bone cells are being inhibited, although the time course of the effect would be more in keeping with a decrease in cell transport rather than inhibition of bone resorption.

ACKNOWLEDGEMENTS

The authors thank Mrs M. Foldiak and Ms B. Barber for their technical assistance and G.D. Searle and Co. for a generous supply of disopyramide. This study was supported by the medical Research Council of Canada, Grant MA 5996.

REFERENCES

(1) R. P. Rubin "Calcium and cellular secretion". Plenum Press New-York (1982)

(2) P. J. Somerville and M. Kaye. "Studies on the action of inorganic phosphorus on calcium transport in isolated rat tails used as an organ perfusion system". Kidney Internat. 22:348-354 (1982)

(3) O. Hauswirth and B. N. Singh, "Ionic mechanisms in heart muscle in relation to the genesic and pharmacological control of cardiac arrhythmias. Pharmacol. Rev. 30:5-63 (1979)

(4) H. Fleish and R. Felix, "Diphosphonates". Calcif. Tiss. Internat. 27:91-96 (1979)

(5) N. S. Kreiger and P. H. Tashjian, "Parathyroid hormone stimulates bone resorption via a Na-Ca exchange mechanism. Nature. 287:843-845

(6) P. Ducouret, "The effect of quinidine on membrane electrical activity in frog auricular fibres studied by current and voltage clamp. Brit. J. Pharmacol. 57:163-184 (1976)

(7) J. A. L. Arruda and S. Sabatini, "Effect of quinidine on Na, H and water transport by the turtle and toad bladders. J. Memb. Biol. 55:151-147 (1980)

(8) J. W. Dietrich, G. R. Mundy and L. G. Raisz. "Inhibition of bone resorption in tissue culture by membrane stabilizing drugs". Endocrinology. 104:1644-1648 (1979)

(9) T. J. Hahn, C. R. Scharp, C. A. Richardson, L. R. Halstead, A. J. Kahn and S. J. Teitlebaum. "Interaction of diphenylhydantoin (phenytoin) and phenobarbital with hormonal mediation of fetal rat bone resorption in vitro". J. Clin. Invest. 62:406-414 (1978)

(10) U. Lerner and L. Hanstrom. "Influence of diphenylhydantoin on on lysosomal enzyme release during bone resorption in vitro". Acta Pharmacol. 47:144-150 (1980)

(11) L. C. Cantley, L. Josephson, R. Warner, M. Vanagisawa, C. Lechene, G. Guidotti. Vanadate is a potent (Na,K) ATPase inhibitor found in ATP derived from muscle".

J. Biol. Chem. 252:7421-7423 (1977)
(12) T. B. Simons. "Vanadate - a new tool for biologists". Nature. 281:337-338 (1979)
(13) B. N. Singh, E. N. Vaughan-William. "A fourth class of anti-dysrhythmic action? Effect of verapamil on ouabain toxicity, on atrial and ventricular intracellular potentials and on other features of cardiac function". Cardio-vasc. Research. 6:109-119 (1972).
14) U. Lerner and G. T. Gustafson. "Inhibition of 1 hydroxy Vitamin-D_3 stimulated bone resorption in tissue culture by the calcium antagonist verapamil". Eur. J. of Clin. Investig. 12: 185-190 (1982)

PHOSPHATE-RESTRICTED DIETS versus CALCITONIN IN THE PREVENTION OF OSTEODYSTROPHY IN EXPERIMENTAL RENAL DISEASE

Angela D'Angelo, Ermanno Bonucci, Paola Ballanti, Antonia Fabris, Sandro Giannini, Paolo Ferrarese, Paolo Vassanelli and Giuseppe Maschio

I Clinica Medica, Universitá di Padova; V Cattedra Anatomia Patologica, Universitá di Roma; Cattedra Nefrologia Medica, Universitá di Verona; and Cattedra Chirurgia Sperimentale, Universitá di Padova - Italy

INTRODUCTION

Restriction of dietary phosphate intake is beneficial in preventing the development of secondary hyperparathyroidism and bone disease in experimental renal failure in the dog (1-3). If associated with vitamin D administration, this dietary regimen can prevent both pathologic bone resorption and osteomalacia in the same experimental model (3). In rats with surgically-induced renal failure, the administration of phosphate-deficient diets (0.03% phosphate) is followed by anorexia, hypophosphatemia, growth arrest, stunting, and severe rickets (4,5). On the other hand, growth failure is also commonly observed when the same animals are given high-phosphate diets (1.58 % phosphate) (6).

This study was undertaken with the purpose of evaluating the effects of different dietary phosphate contents - a low-phosphate diet, containing 0.09% phosphate, and a normal phosphate diet, containing 0.5 % phosphate - with or without calcium supplementation, on the development of bone lesions in various groups of rats with the same degree of surgically-induced chronic renal failure.

Furthermore, the potential "protective" effect of calcitonin administration was studied in an additional group of rats with renal failure kept on a normal phosphate intake.

MATERIAL AND METHODS

In seventy-seven male Sprague-Dawley rats,each weighing between 250 and 300 grams,chronic renal failure was induced by unilateral nephrectomy and removal (ligation and cautery) of the outer poles of contralateral kidney,leaving the animals with approximately one quarter of one kidney. All operations were performed through a flank incision,after the animals were anesthetized with ether.

Immediately after surgery,the rats were divided into four groups receiving different experimental isocaloric (about 400 Kcal per 100 grams) diets,containing 0.5 % phosphate,1.5 % calcium,and 24 % protein as bovine fibrin (Group 1, 19 rats); 0.09 % phosphate, 0.5 % calcium,and 20 % protein (Group 2, 21 rats); 0.09 % phosphate,2.0 % calcium,and 20 % protein (Group 3, 16 rats); 0.5 % phosphate,1.5 % calcium,and 24 % protein (Group 4, 21 rats).
The animals in Group 4 were also given 1 U MRC of salmon calcitonin (SANDOZ) twice a week for about 3 months.

All diets contained a similar sodium content and were fully fortified with vitamins. All rats had free access to tap water. Throughout the study period,all animals received and consumed an equal amount of food,approximately 12 g/day.

Control blood samples for creatinine,phosphate and calcium were obtained immediately prior to beginning the diets. After 90 to 160 days,all rats were killed and samples of blood were obtained for creatinine,phosphate and calcium evaluation. The samples were analyzed on an Autoanalyzer (Technicon).

The tibiae,two lumbar vertebrae,and two ribs (including the osteo-chondral junction) were immediately dissected and soaked in 4 % paraformaldehyde,buffered at pH 7.2 with phosphate buffer. While immersed in paraformaldehyde,the bone specimens were cut lenghtwise to improve fixative penetration,and were left soaked for 12 to 24 hours. Semithin sections were stained with Azur II - Methylene blue and with von Kossa method.

The statistical analysis of the data was performed by means of Student's "t" test and chi-square.

RESULTS

Table I summarizes the serum parameters in the four groups of rats prior to beginning the diets and at the end of the study period. All rats had basal serum creatinine values (about 1 mg/dl) which were nearly two and a half times higher than those found in controls (about 0.4 mg/dl). The basal values of serum phosphate and calcium were not statistically different in the various groups.

The increase in serum creatinine was statistically significant in all groups,the highest increment being observed in rats on normal phosphate intake (groups 1 and 4).

Serum phosphate concentration appeared to be significantly decreased in rats on low phosphate intake (groups 2 and 3),and showed a slight increase or no change in the other groups.

The serum levels of both creatinine and phosphate were significantly lower in groups 2 and 3 as compared to group 1 at the end of the study period. No significant change was observed between groups 1 and 4(Table I).

There was no significant change in the mean weight gain (6.41 %) in the four groups. The weight's changes were not correlated to serum creatinine nor to the lenght of administration of the diets.

Table I. Serum concentrations (mg/dl) of creatinine,phosphate and calcium in the 4 groups of rats at the beginning (A) and the end (B) of the study period. Values are given as means ± S.D.
t = Student's "t" test - NS = not significant.

		CREATININE mg/dl				PHOSPHATE mg/dl				CALCIUM mg/dl			
		A	B	t	p	A	B	t	p	A	B	t	p
GROUP 1		0.98	2.10	6.95	<0.001	5.20	6.60	2.54	<0.02	9.40	9.52	0.18	NS
(19)	±	0.24	0.66			1.32	2.00			2.18	1.90		
GROUP 2		1.01	1.40	3.08	<0.005	4.90	3.50	4.14	<0.001	9.50	9.59	0.15	NS
(21)	±	0.21	0.54			1.18	1.00			1.84	1.81		
GROUP 3		1.03	1.50	3.78	<0.001	5.05	3.70	2.92	<0.01	9.38	9.64	0.37	NS
(16)	±	0.19	0.46			1.20	1.40			1.91	2.00		
GROUP 4		0.99	1.90	6.60	<0.001	5.15	6.00	1.88	NS	9.48	9.55	0.11	NS
(21)	±	0.25	0.58			1.14	1.72			2.08	1.98		

1) Significance of creatinine values in B : Group 1 vs Group 2 : t = 3.68 p<0.001
" " " 3 : t = 3.06 p<0.005
" " " 4 : t = 1.02 p NS

2) Significance of phosphate values in B : Group 1 vs Group 2 : t = 6.29 p<0.001
" " " 3 : t = 4.87 p<0.001
" " " 4 : t = 1.02 p NS

The mortality rate in the various groups could not be assessed as all rats were killed prior to developing end-stage renal failure.

Being the ultrastructural investigation still in progress, only the histological findings are reported. The percent appearance of normal bone,osteomalacia,and associated osteomalacia and pathologic bone resorption is reported in Table II.

Mild to severe osteomalacia was present in 42 % of rats in group 1,in about 30 % of those in groups 2 and 3,and in only 14 % of those treated with calcitonin. Severe osteomalacia,however,was more frequently observed in rats in group 1,whereas other groups usually had mild defective mineralization.

Osteomalacia was characterized by a variable amount of uncalcified osteoid tissue,so that its degree ranged from mild to severe. Often,the osteoid borders were more numerous and wider in the endosteal surface of the compact bone of the tibiae than in spongy bone of the tibial metaphyses and of the ribs and vertebrae. Ribs and vertebrae were less affected than tibiae. The uncalcified osteoid tissue was often bordered by active osteoblasts (fig. 1).

Histological signs of hyperparathyroidism,such as increased number of osteoclasts and Howship's lacunae,were associated to osteomalacia in about 26 % of rats in group 1,in about 9 % of those in group 2,and in less than 5 % of those in group 4 (Table II and fig. 2).

Table II. Bone histology in the four groups of rats.

	GROUP 1 (19)		GROUP 2 (21)		GROUP 3 (16)		GROUP 4 (21)	
	N	%	N	%	N	%	N	%
NORMAL BONE	6	31.58	13	61.90	11	68.70	17	80.90
OSTEOMALACIA	8	42.10	6	28.58	5	31.30	3	14.20
OSTEOMALACIA HYPERPARATHYROIDISM	5	26.32	2	9.52	-	-	1	4.90

Statistical evaluation of the differences between bone histology in the four groups:

Group 1 vs group 2 : chi-square 4.68 p NS

" " " 3 : chi-square 6.96 $p < 0.05$

" " " 4 : chi-square 10.12 $p < 0.01$

The statistical analysis,performed by means of the chi-square,showed a significant connection between different treatments and bone histology,whether taken as a separation between normal and pathologic bone (chi-square 10.8, p less than 0.02),or as a distinction between normal bone,osteomalacia,and associated osteomalacia and hyperparathyroidism (chi-square 13.9, p less than 0.05).

The level of significance between groups 1 and 3 was mainly influenced by the lack of hyperparathyroidism in rats in group 3 (Table II).

The level of significance between groups 1 and 4 was largerly influenced by the high percentage of normal bone in rats treated with calcitonin (Table II).

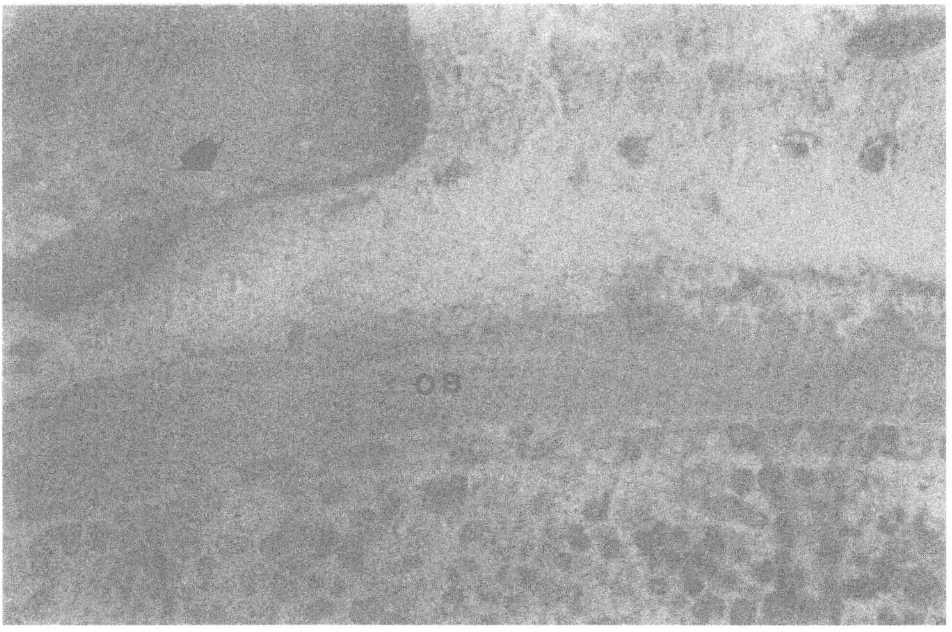

Figure 1. Thick osteoid border (OB) lined by active osteoblasts along a bone trabecula of the tibia metaphysis from a rat in group 1. Evidence of bone resorption on upper left (arrow). Azur II and Methylene blue, x 120.

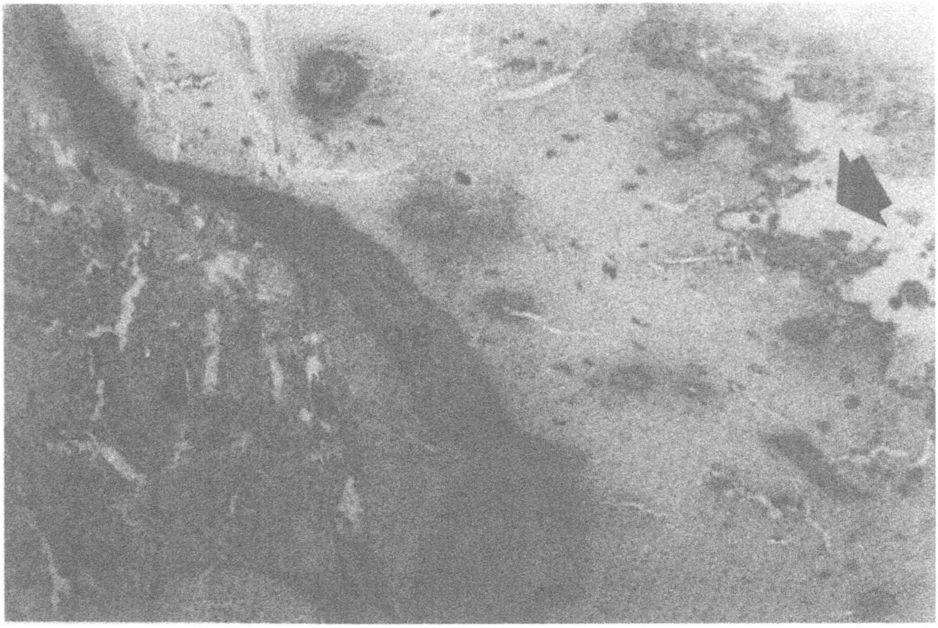

Figure 2. Compact bone of the tibial diaphysis from a rat in group 1. Presence of a wide osteoid border (OB) on the endosteal surface and of bone resorption (arrow) on the periosteal surface. Azur II and Methylene blue, x 32.

DISCUSSION

Our data show that a moderate dietary phosphate restriction can significantly reduce the morphologic appearance of bone pathology in rats with surgically-induced renal failure. In comparison with rats fed a normal phosphate diet,those moderately phosphate-restricted had a significantly higher percentage of normal bone, a significantly lower frequency of osteomalacia (despite a mild phosphate depletion),and a very low incidence of osteoclastic bone disease.

The calcium content of low-phosphate diets did not affect significantly bone pathology.

The most surprising results,however,were obtained in those rats whose normal diet (0.5 % phosphate) was regularly integrated with the administration of salmon calcitonin. The large majority of these animals with established chronic renal failure had normal bone,and the frequency of osteomalacia and hyperparathyroidism was negligible when compared to that observed in the other groups.

The role of calcitonin in the pathogenesis of renal osteodystrophy is still poorly understood (7),and the "protective" effect of this hormone against renal bone disease is controversial (8,9, 10).

Surprisingly,most clinical studies were conducted in dialysis patients,who usually have severe bone pathology. As it could have been predicted,contrasting results were obtained (11,12,13).

In our opinion,if the major effect of calcitonin is that of inhibiting the parathormone-mediated bone resorption,then it should be administered in early renal failure,in order to prevent,rather than to treat,pathologic bone resorption.

Our rats with established renal failure,regularly treated with salmon calcitonin,were virtually free of osteoclastic bone disease in spite of their normal dietary phosphate intake. In addition,calcitonin administration resulted in the lowest incidence of osteomalacia among the various groups.

These results show a new role for calcitonin in the prevention of renal bone disease. The clinical applicability of these data is currently investigated in randomized patients with early renal failure.

In our study,no specific attempt to evaluate the progression of renal failure under different dietary treatments was made. The increase in serum creatinine concentration,however,was significantly lower in rats fed low-phosphate diets than in those on regular phosphate intake,thus supporting the view that phosphate restriction can effectively prevent functional renal deterioration.

REFERENCES

1) SLATOPOLSKY E.,CAGLAR S.,PENNELL J.P.,TAGGART D.D.,CANTERBURY J. M.,REISS E.,BRICKER N.S.: On the pathogenesis of hyperparathyroidism in chronic experimental renal insufficiency in the dog. J.Clin.Invest. 50,422-499,1971.

2) SLATOPOLSKY E.,CAGLAR S.,GRADOWSKA L.,CANTERBURY J.,REISS E., BRICKER N.S.: On the prevention of secondary hyperparathyroidism in experimental chronic renal disease using "proportional reduction" of dietary phosphorus intake. Kidney Intern. 2,147-151,1972.

3) RUTHERFORD W.E.,BORDIER P.,MARIE P.,HRUSKA K.,HARTER H.,GREENWALT A.,BLONDIN J.,HADDAD J.,BRICKER N.,SLATOPOLSKY E.: Phosphate control and 25-hydroxycholecalciferol administration in preventing experimental renal osteodystrophy in the dog. J.Clin. Invest. 60,332-341,1977.

4) SALUSKY I.,KLEINKNECHT C.,BROYER M.,GUBLER M.-C.: Prolonged renal survival and stunting with protein-deficient diets in experimental uremia. J.Lab.Clin.Med. 97,21-30,1981.

5) LAOUARI D.,KLEINKNECHT C.,COURNOT-WITMER G.,HABIB R.,BROYER M.: Importance of anorexia in the preservation of renal function due to deficient phosphorus diets. Third Intern.Congr.Nutrition and Metabolism in Renal Disease,Abstract Book,n.89,1982.

6) KLEINKNECHT C.,SALUSKY I., BROYER M.,GUBLER M.-C.: Effect of various protein diets on growth,renal function,and survival of uremic rats. Kidney Intern. 15,534-541,1979.

7) FELETTI C.,DOCCI D.,CAPELLI M.,BONOMINI V.: Pathophysiology of endogenous calcitonin in chronic uremia. Min.Electrol.Metab. 6, 174-181,1981.

8) HEYNEN G.,KANIS J.A.,OLIVER D.,LEDINGHAM J.G.G.,RUSSELL R.G.G.: Evidence that endogenous calcitonin protects against renal bone disease. Lancet 2,1322-1326,1976.

9) KANIS J.A.,EARNSSHAW M.,HEYNEN J.,RUSSELL R.G.G.,WOODS C.G.:The possible role of calcitonin deficiency in the development of bone disease due to chronic renal failure. Calcif.Tissue Res. 22, suppl.,147-153,1977.

10) HABENER F.,SCHILLER A.L.: Pathogenesis of renal osteodystrophy: a role for calcitonin ? New Engl.J.Med. 296,1112-1113,1977.

11) FELETTI C.,BONOMINI V.: Effect of calcitonin on bone lesions in chronic dialysis patients. Nephron 24,85-88,1979.

12) FARRINGTON K.,VARGHESE Z.,MOORHEAD J.F.: Human calcitonin in the treatment of renal osteodystrophy. J.Labor.Clin.Med. 96, 299-306,1980.

13) CUNDY T.,KANIS J.A.,HEYNEN G.,PATON S.,EARNSHAW M.,WOODS C.G.: Deterioration of renal bone disease in patients treated with salmon calcitonin. Clin.Endocrinol. 16,29-37,1982.

CHANGES FOLLOWING PARATHYROIDECTOMY IN HEMODIALYZED PATIENTS

Y. Berland*, S. Charhon**, M. Olmer* and P.J. Meunier**

*Service de Nephrologie, Hopital de la Conception

13 005 Marseille, **Inserm U 234, Lyon, France

INTRODUCTION

Secondary hyperparathyroidism (HPT) remains a frequent complication of chronic renal failure (CRF) despite a better understanding of the factors responsible for its development (1). A prolonged survival of the patients by dialysis results in a growing number of uremics who present with severe HPT responsible not only for major bone lesions but also for an impairment of different vital functions (2). The metabolites of vitamin D such a 1,25 dihydroxycholecalciferol that can play a preventive role in renal osteodystrophy at an early stage of chronic renal failure (3) are inconsistently effective and difficult to handle during severe HPT (4). Thus, treatment by parathyroidectomy (PTX) appears sometimes to be required (5).

Several recent publications have revealed pathological fracture and the development of osteomalacia (OM) after PTX (7-7-8). We report our experience of PTX on biochemical and bone histology.

METHODS

Six patients with chronic renal failure, 3 females and 3 males, aged 28 to 56 years undergoing hemodialysis from 5 to 132 months have had a PTX: sub-total PTX in two cas3s and a total PTX with autotransplant in the forearm in the other four. PTX was done because the serum levels of parathormone (PTH) were high and the patients had asthenia, bone pain, pruritus, intense thirst. None of the patients received calcium or vitamin D therapy during the three months prior to PTX. All but one had an oral intake of aluminium hydroxyde. No patient had received glucocorticoid or anticonvulsant therapy. The dialysis was conducted using deionised water for 3 patients and softened water for the other 3 patients; the respective concentrations of calcium and magnesium were 1.75 mmol/l and 0.75 mmol/l.

Before each bone biopsy, the patients had received 600 mg of dimethyl-chlortetracycline during two days and then during four days after a free interval of 12 days. Transiliac bone biopsies were done with a trocar having a 7.5 mm internal diameter just before the PTX and repeated 12 to 16 months afterwards according to each patient. The biopsy samples were fixed in 70% alcohol then embedded in methylmetacrylate. Non consecutive 8 μ-thick sections were carried out and stained by Goldner's and solochrome cyanine R stains. Twenty μ sections served for analysis of tetracycline labels in fluorescent light.

All parameters and areas were measured by linear intersecte and point counting techniques with the calibrated merz grid (9-10). The static parameters evaluated included: 1) Trabecular bone volume (T.B.V.): the percentage of the spongy bone space occupied by trabecular bone (including osteoid tissue), 2) Relative osteoid volume (R.O.V.): the percentage of the trabecular bone which consists of osteoid, 3) Relative osteoid surface (R.O.S.): The percentage of the trabecular surfaces covered by osteoid, 4) Thickness index of osteoid seams (T.I.O.S.): ratio R.O.V./O.S. x 100 (11-12), it validly estimate the true thickness of osteoid seams, 5) Resorption surface (R.S.): The percentage of the total trabecular surfaces scalloped by Howship's lacunae including surfaces with and without osteoclasts, 6) Osteoclast number per square mm of spongiosal tissue, 7) Fibrotic surface: Only a qualitative estimate of the fibrosis was attempted +, ++, +++, and 8) Osteoblastic surface (O.S.). The percentage of the total trabecular surface lined by PLUMP osteoblasts. The dynamic parameters examined included: 1) Double labeled surface: The percentage of the trabecular surface showing double tetracycline labels, 2) Double labeled osteoid surface: The percentage of the osteoid surface showing double tetracycline labels, 3) Total labeled surfaces: The percentage of the trabecular surface showing single or double tetracycline labels, 4) Calcification Rate (C.R.): The rate at which mineral is deposited in the osteoid, calculated as the ratio of the separation between tetracycline labels (μm) and the time between the mid points of tetracycline administration (15 days). Expressed in μm/day, uncorrected for the section obliquity, and 5) Bone formation rate at tissue level: Which gives the amount of mineralized bone being made per unit surface area of trabecular bone per day: Total labeled surface x C.R. ($\mu m^3/\mu\ m^2$/day).

A staining by aurin tricarboxylic acid (aluminon) (14-15) has been performed on 7 μ non consecutive sections. This staining gives aluminium a bright red stain.

On the day the biopsy was done, blood samples were withdrawn from the measurements of calcium, phosphorus, alkaline phosphatases (AP), PTH (radioimmunoassay identifying the C-terminal fragment and of aluminium (atomic absorption spectrophotometry).

The results are expressed in form of mean±SE or mean±SD for the histomorphometric parameters. The statistical study has used student's t test for a comparison of the two mean results.

RESULTS

The clinical signs of hyperparathyroidism, asthenia in particular, disappeared after PTX; 4 patients expressed a sensation of general well-being and 2 of the patients returned to their sports activities. The results of the evolution of biological parameters are given in Table 1. Before PTX, calcemia was low in 2 cases, normal or elevated in the other patients. A phase of sevre hypocalcemia was observed in 5 cases immediately after PTX; only one of the two patients who had not undergone total PTX was clear from such a severe state. At the time the second biopsy was performed, only one patient had a relatively low serum calcium level (2.17 mmol/l), the other patients having a calcemia maintained within normal values between 2.30 and 2.66 mmol/l by treatment with calcium (Ca CO_3) and vitamin D metabolites (1-α hydroxycholecalciferol). Simultaneously, hyperphosphatemia was controlled by aluminium hydroxyde using doses that were equivalent before and after PTX. The serum levels of AP and PTH decreased considerably in all the patients after PTX, 70±14% and 82±12%, respectively.

The histomorphometric results are represented in Table 2. Before PTX, all the patients demonstrated histomorphometric evidence of severe HPT as shown by both the increase in the resorption parameters (number of osteoclasts/mm^2 and extension of the resorption surfaces) and in the bone apposition parameters (osteoid volume, osteoblastic surfaces and tetracycline labeled surfaces). The calcification rate was within the normal range or increased in all patients. Two patients (1 and 4) however, demonstrated a relative delay of bone mineralization. In these two male patients, the thickness index of osteoid seam was increased (normal range: 18.8 ± 4.7) (16) and the calcification rate was inferior to the normal plus 2 S.D.: 0.96 μm/day (17). Bone aluminium staining did not reveal bone aluminium deposit except in patient 4. In this case, aluminium was mainly deposited at the interface between calcified and osteoid tissue but also inside the calcified bone along the cementic line. After PTX, there was a reduction in cellularity with a decrease in the number of osteoclasts from a mean value of 3.91±2.20/mm^2 to 0.45±0.29 ($p<0.05$), a decrease of the resorption surface (55±12% from the initial value), as well as a reduction in the osteoblastic surface from 22.53±12.80% to 7.26±5.83% ($p<0.05$), (Fig. 1). The decrease of PTH on the one hand, and the reduction of osteoclasts ($r = 0.77$) and of osteoblastic surfaces ($r = 0.83$) on the other hand, were related. The bone formation rate at the tissue level was decreased in all the patients on average by 74.4± 8.7%. The calcification rate reduced in 4 patients, remained within normal values (Fig.2). The thickness index os osteoid seams was never increased (Fig.3). Thus, none of our patients developed

TABLE 1 BIOCHEMICAL VARIABLES AND THERAPY BEFORE (a) AND AFTER (b) PTX

	PATIENT 1		PATIENT 2		PATIENT 3	
	a	b	a	b	a	b
SERUM VALUES						
CALCIUM (mmol/l)	2.18	2.48	2.56	2.30	2.17	2.66
PHOSPHORUS (mmol/l)	1.45	1.50	3.03	2.13	1.63	1.05
ALKALINE PHOSPHATASE (U.I.)	857.0	100.0	404.0	80.0	132 .0	76.0
PTH (μleq/ml)	1000.0	11.5	2250.0	84.0	400.0	170.0
ALUMINIUM μg/l	23.0	9.0	11.0	18.0	42.0	34.0
THERAPY †						
Ca CO_3 (g/day)	No	2.85	No	1.78	No	-
25 OH VIT D_3 (μg/day)	No	71.0	No	6.65	No	50.0
1αOH VIT D_3 (μg/day)	No	0.54	No	0.54	No	-
ALUMINIUM HYDROXYDE (g/day)	8.0	2.0	0	0.0	6.0	6.0

† Mean dosage/day between PTX and the second biopsy.

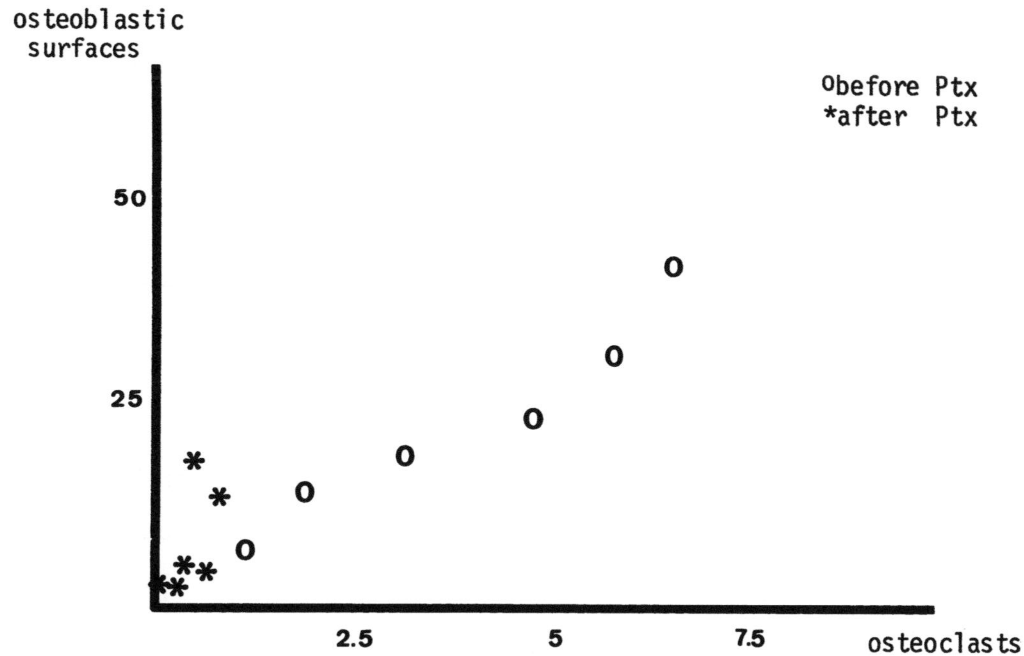

Figure 1: Osteoblastic surfaces (%) and osteoclast number per mm^2 of spongiosal tissue before and after PTX.

TABLE 1 BIOCHEMICAL VARIABLES AND THERAPY BEFORE (a) AND AFTER (b) PTX - (Continued)

	PATIENT 4		PATIENT 5		PATIENT 6	
	a	b	a	b	a	b
SERUM VALUES						
CALCIUM (mmol/l)	2.42	2.13	2.35	2.60	2.51	2.17
PHOSPHORUS (mmol/l)	1.67	1.54	1.88	1.70	0.62	1.13
ALKALINE PHOSPHATASE (U.I.)	260.0	115.0	488.0	120.0	792.0	178.0
PTH (μleq/ml)	860.0	160.0	660.0	160.0	960.0	165.0
ALUMINIUM μg/l	109.0	30.0	49.0	Not Done	30.0	25.0
THERAPY †						
Ca CO_3 (g/day)	No	2.15	No	0.20	No	No
25OH VIT D_3 (μg/day)	No	18.75	No	18.2	No	No
1αOH VIT D_3 (μg/day)	No	0.20	NO	0.46	No	1.0
ALUMINIUM HYDROXYDE (g/day)	4.0	6.0	6.0	6.0	2.0	4.0

† Mean dosage/day between PTX and the second biopsy.

osteomalacia as defined by an increased thickness of index of osteoid seams and a decreased calcification rate.

DISCUSSION

At the tissue level, PTH increases the bone remodeling by increasing the number of new basic multicellular units (B.M.U) (9). Firstly, PTH increases the number of osteoclasts and consequently, the resorption surfaces and secondly, because of the coupling between resorption and formation (19-20), PTH increases the osteoblastic surfaces and osteoid surfaces. Thus, marked increase in bone formation, noted in severe secondary hyperparathyroidism, is responsible for the development of osteosclerosis as frequently seen in chronic renal failure. At the cell level, the bone formation is also increased as demonstrated by the increased calcification rate found in uremics (6). In our experience, PTX is associated with a marked reduction in the cell population involved in bone remodeling (osteoclasts and osteoblasts.

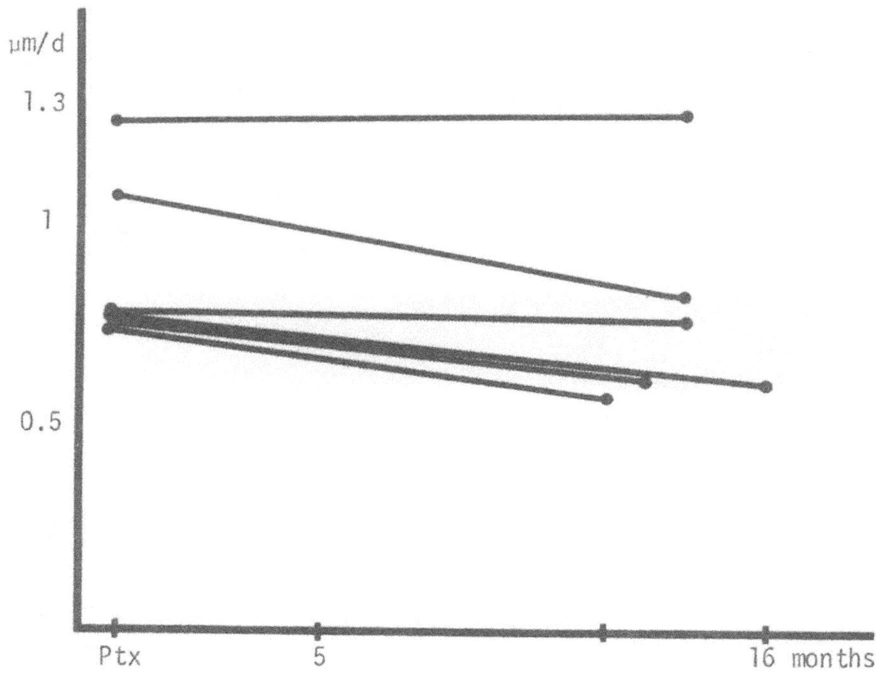

Calcification Rate (C.R.)

Figure 2: PTX incidence on C.R. (normal range cross-hatched).

Both bone resorption and bone formation are thus reduced at the tissue level. At the cell level, bone formation is also found to be reduced by PTX as shwon by the decrease in the thickness of osteoid seams and the calcification rate. Such a depression of bone formation has been found in the rat afte thyroparathyroidectomy (21). In our patients, the calcification rate remained within normal range after PTX, thus excluding osteomalacia as it has recently been reported by several authors (6-7-8). The descrepancy between our results and those reporting the development of osteomalacia after PTX could arise from different factors possibly involved in the mineralization process affecting individual patients. In some observations found in literature (7), the reduction of parathyroid hormone secretion could have been excessive creating a hypoparathyroid state and consequently an osteomalacia (18-22). In contrast, all our patients except for one, still had increased serum PTH indicating the maintenance of a secretion of PTH. Furthermore, hypophosphatemia after PTX was not prolonged. It has also been suggested that aluminium intoxication could be responsible for the development of osteomalacia (23-24). Only one of our patients showed aluminium bone deposits at the time of PTX;

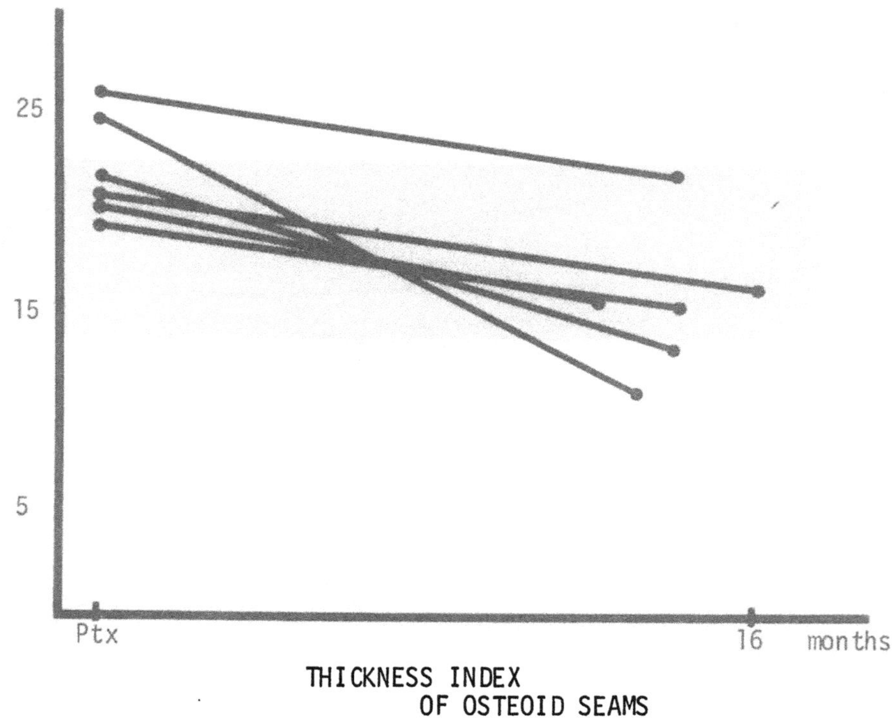

Figure 3: PTX incidence on T.I.O.S. (normal range cross hatched).

however, this patient did not demonstrate morphological or dynamical evidence of osteomalacia on the second bone biopsy. This, could be due to the treatment of the dialysis water by reverse osmosis, introduced a few months after the PTX (25). Whether osteomalacia reported after PTX is directly related to the reduction of PTH secretion or is the result of associated pathological conditions remains unclear. It is, however, interesting to note that in our patients, PTX was accompanied with a reduction in plump osteoblasts and in double tetracycline labels. Since osteoblasts appear to be involved in the mineralization process, PTX could thus favor the development of osteomalacia under certain particular conditions such as aluminium intoxication.

In opposition to the PTX, medical treatment specially with vitamin D metabolites gave diverging results. The 1-α hydroxycholecalciferol (26-27-28)) and the 1,25 dihydroxycholecalciferol (27-29-30) are effective on osteitis fibrosa and on bone resorption. However, the 25-hydroxycholecalciferol appears to be superior on bone mineralization (26-31). Our biological and bone histomorphometric results are concordant with those obtained by Teitelbaum (32) and Frost (33) by rising calcifediol ($25OHD_3$). However, if Frost observes a decrease in the bone formation in the group of patients with "active bone", the mineralization rate remains high. We could thus believe that this medical treatment is better than PTX. But during severe HPT, the calcemia is normal or even high and the prescription of vitamin D metabolites easily exposes to hypercalcemia.

REFERENCES:

1. J.W. Coburn, Renal osteodystrophy, Kidney Internat. 17:677-693, 1980.
2. S.G. Massry, D.A. Goldstein, The search for uremic toxin (s) "X" "x" = PTH, Clin. Nephrol. 11:181-189, 1979.
3. M.D. Healy, H.H., Malluche, D.A. Goldstein, F.R. Singer, S.G. Massry, Effects of long-term therapy with calcitriol in patients with moderate renal failure, Arch. Int. Med. 140:1030-1033, 1980.
4. J.C. Prior, E.C. Cameron, H.S. Ballon, D.S. Lirenman, M.V. Moriarty, J.D.E. Price, Experience with 1,25 dihydroxycholecalciferol therapy in hemodialysis patients with progressive Vit D_2 treated osteodystrophy, Am. J. Med. 67:583-587, 1979.
5. J.A. Diaz-Boxo, W.T. Geissinger, P.J. Walker, J.T. Chandler, C.D. Farmer, K.L. Holt, P. Wolfe, Total parathyroidectomy and autotransplantation, Clin. Nephrol. 16:276-282, 1981.
6. R.S. Weinstein, Decreased mineralization in hemodialysis patients after subtotal parathyroidectomy, Calcif. Tis. Int. 34:16-20, 1982.
7. A.J. Felsenfeld, J.M. Harrelson, R.A. Gutman, S.A. Wells, M.K. Drezner, Osteomalacia after parathyroidectomy in patients with uremia, Ann. Intern. Med. 96:34-39, 1982.

8. J. Zingraff, T. Drueke, J. Gueris, P. Jungers, J. Crosnier, Severe osteomalacia after subtotal parathyroidectomy in chronic uremic patients. Kidney Internat. 14:204, Abst., 1978.
9. P.J. Meunier, C. Bressot, Endocrine influences on bone cells and bone remodeling evaluated by clinical histomorphometry. Endocrinology of calcium metabolism, Edited by John A. PARSONS. Raven Press, New York, 445-465, 1982.
10. P.J. Meunier, P. Courpron, Iliac trabecular bone in 236 controls. Representativeness of iliac samples in bone morphometry. Ed. Z.F.G. Jaworski Univ. Ottawa. Press Ottawa: 100-105, 1976.
11. P.J. Meunier, C. Edouard, C. Bressot, J.N. Valat, P. Courpron, , P. Zech, Histomorphometrie osseuse dans l'insuffisance renale aigue et chronique, J. Urol. Nephrol. 81:931-940, 1975.
12. P.J. Meunier, C. Edouard, P. Courpron, F. Toussaint, Morphometric analysis of osteoid in iliac trabecular bone methodology, Dynamical significance of the osteoid in iliac trabecular bone methodology. Dynamical significance of the osteoid parameters. In: Vitamin D and problems related to uremic bone disease. Ed. by A.W. Norman, K. Schaefe, H.G. Grigoleit, D.V. Herrath, E. Ritz, Walter de Groyter, Berlin: 149-155, 1975.
13. F. Melsen and L. Mosekilde, Tetracycline double-labeling of iliac trabecular bone in 41 normal adults, Calcif. Tiss. Res. 26:99-102, 1978.
14. N.A. Maloney, S.M. Ott, A.C. Alfrey, N.L. Miller, J.W., Coburn, D.J. Sherrard, Histological quantitation of aluminium in iliac bone from patients with renal failure, J. Lab. Clin. Med. 99:206-216, 1982.
15. M.R. Buchanan, B.U. Ihle, C.M. Dunn, Haemodialysis related osteomalacia: A staining method to demonstrate aluminium. J. Clin. Pathol. 34:1352-1354, 1981.
16. P.J. Meunier, C. Edouard, P. Courpron, Morphometric analysis of trabecular resorption surfaces in normal iliac bone, In: Bone morphometry, Ed. Z.F.G. Jaworski, 156-160 University of Ottawa Press, Ottawa, 1976.
17. P.J. Meunier, P. Courpron, C. Edouard, C. Alexandre, C. Bressot, P. Lips, B.F. Boyce, Bone histomorphometry in osteoporotic states, In: Osteoporosis II, Ed. V.S. Barrel; 27-47 Grune and Stratton, New York, 1978.
18. S.L. Teitelbaum, M.A. Bengfeld, J. Freitag, K.A. Hruska, E. Slatopolsky, Do parathyroid hormone and 1,25 dihydroxyvitamin D modulate bone formation in uremia? J. Clin. Endocrinol. Metab. 51:247-251, 1980.
19. A.M. Paritt, The coupling of bone formation to bone resorption: A critical analysis of the concept and of its relevance to the pathogenesis of osteoporosis. Metab. Bone. Dis. and Rel. Res. 4:1-6, 1982.

20. G.A. Howard, B.L. Bottemiller, D.J. Baylink, Evidence for the coupling of bone formation to bone resorption in vitro. Metab. Bone Dis. Rel. Res. 2:131-135, 1980.
21. J. Wergedal, M. Stauffer, D. Baylink, C. Rich, Inhibition of bone matrix formation, mineralization and resorption in thyroparathyroidectomized rats, J. Clin. Invest. 52:1052-1058, 1973.
22. M.K. Dresner, F.A. Neelon, J. Jowsey, H.E. Lebovitz, Hypoparathyroidism: A possible cause of osteomalacia, J. Clin. Endocrinol. Metab. 45:114-122, 1977.
23. G. Cournot-Witmer, J. Zingraff, J.J. Plachot, F. Escaig, R. Lefevre, P. Boumati, A. Bourdeau, M. Garabedian, P. Galle, R. Bourdon, T. Drueke, S. Balsan, Aluminium localization in bone from hemodialysed patients: Relationship to matrix mineralization, Kidney Internat. 20:375-385, 1981.
24. H.A. Ellis, Aluminium and osteomalacia after parathyroidectomy, Ann. Intern. Med. 96:533-534, 1982.
25. M.K. Ward, H.A. Ellis, T.G. Feest, I.S. Parkinson, D.N.S. Kerr, J. Herrington, G.L. Goode, Osteomalacic dialysis osteodystrophy: Evidence for a water-bone aetiological agent, probably aluminium, The Lancet. 1:841-845, 1978.
26. A. Fournier, P. Bordier, J. Gueris, J.L. Sebert, P.M. Ferriere, J. Bedrossian, H.F. De Luca, Comparison of 1-α-hydroxycholecalciferol in the treatment of renal osteodystrophy: Greater effect of 25-hydroxycholecalciferol on bone mineralization, Kidney Internat. 15:196-204, 1979.
27. P. Bordier, J. Zingraff, J. Gueris, P. Jungers, P. Marie, M. Pechet, H. Rasmussen, The effect of 1-αOHD_3 and $1\alpha 25$ OH_2D_3 on the bone in patients with renal osteodystrophy, Am. J. Med. 64:101-107, 1978.
28. H.E. Nielsen, F. Melsen, M.S. Christensen, H.E. Hansen, P. Rodbro, A. Johannsen, 1α-hydroxycholecalciferol treatment of long-term hemodialyzed patients. Effects of mineral metabolism, bone mineral content and bone morphometry, Clin. Nephrol. 8:429-434, 1977.
29. A.M. Pierides, H.A. Ellis, W. Simpson, J.H. Denar, M.K. Ward, D.N.S. Kerr, Variables response to long-term $1\alpha OHD_3$ in hemodialysis osteodystrophy, Lancet 1:1092-1095, 1086.
30. K.Y. Ahmed, M.R. Wills, Z. Varghese, E.A. Meinhard, J.F. Moorhead, Long-term effects of small doses of 1,25 dihydroxycholecalciferol in renal osteodystrophy, Lancet 1:629-632, 1978.
31. J.B. Eastwood, T.C.B. Stamp, H.E. de Wardener, P.J. Bordier, C.D. Arnaud, The effect of 25-hydroxyvitamin D_3 in the osteomalacia of chronic renal failure, Clin. Sci. Mol. Med. 52:499-508, 1977.
32. S.L. Teitelbaum, J.M. Bone, P.M. Stein, J.J. Gilden, M. Bates, V.C. Boisseau, L.V. Avioli, Calcifediol in chronic renal insufficiency skeletal response, JAMA, 235:164-167, 1976.

33. H.M. Frost, D.L. Griffith, W.S.S. Jee, D.B. Kimmel, R.P. Mc Candlis, S.L. Teitelbaum, Histomorphometric changes in trabecular bone of renal failure patients treated with calcifediol. Metab. Bone Dis. and Rel. Res. 2:285-295, 1981.

MINERALS, PARATHYROID HORMONE AND BLOOD PRESSURE

SERUM IONIZED CALCIUM AND DIETARY CALCIUM IN HUMAN AND EXPERIMENTAL HYPERTENSION

David A. McCarron

Division of Nephrology
Oregon Health Sciences University
Portland, OR 97201

INTRODUCTION

Calcium and its binding protein, calmodulin, exert multiple effects that serve to regulate blood pressure in humans. From experimental work in various organ systems and cell types that are integrated to control cardiovascular function, it is evident that calcium and the calcium-calmodulin complex are essential components of diverse physiologic processes that modulate arterial pressure. The abnormal peripheral resistance that underlies essential hypertension is principally a reflection of altered vascular smooth muscle basal tone and reactivity. As such, the vascular smooth cell is prototypical of calcium's influence on blood pressure control.[1]

While the cation's role at a cellular level may be well accepted, recognition that modification of a subject's calcium status may be a factor in the pathogenesis and/or treatment of hypertension is a recent development. As with any new area of clinical and basic research, many more questions are emerging than the initial data can answer.[2] This review will summarize the current status of data from three areas of calcium metabolism that have recently been associated with human and experimental hypertension. First, the relationship between serum calcium concentrations and level of blood pressure will be assessed. Second, the association between dietary exposure to calcium and either level of blood pressure or risk of developing hypertension will be discussed. As a final consideration, the interaction among serum calcium concentrations, dietary exposure to the cation and level of blood pressure will be addressed.

Serum Calcium

Human Studies. The initial report that serum ionized calcium values of a well-defined population of hypertensives were different from those of normotensives was based upon observations from our program.[3] As a group, the serum ionized calcium concentrations were lower in the 23 hypertensive subjects, averaging 2.09 mEq/L compared to 2.17 mEq/L. These data were collected in a Clinical Research Center study under a prospectively designed protocol. Only new, untreated hypertensives free of secondary causes were entered into the study. Samples, averaging 2.09 mEq/L compared to 2.17 mEq/L. These data were collected in a Clinical Research Center study under a prospectively designed protocol. Only new, untreated hypertensives free of secondary causes were entered into the study. Samples were gathered between 8 and 9 a.m. while the subjects were still fasting. A control group matched for age, race, sex and weight served as the comparison population. Serum Ca^{2+} was measured on a calcium specific electrode which adjusted the samples for pH 7.4. With the exception of serum phosphorous, there were no other significant differences in the two groups' serum chemistries including electrolytes, albumin, and total proteins. Even though the differences between the normals and hypertensives were statistically significant, the values for serum Ca^{2+} exhibited a substantial amount of overlap. The feature that distinguished the hypertensives from the normals was an absence of values at the upper end of normal, and an over-representation of values at the low end. Serum total calcium concentrations were not different between the two groups.

Resnick et al subsequently reported values for serum Ca^{2+} in hypertensive subjects categorized by their renin status and compared them to serum concentrations of a normal group that was not subdivided.[4] They noted that serum Ca^{2+} was significantly lower only in those individuals with low renin levels. Hypertensives with elevated renin levels exhibited higher ionized calcium values than did the normals. This was not a prospective evaluation of the subjects and did not define a matched control population so that age, race, sex and body weight influences cannot be excluded. The data was gathered by re-analyzing available serum samples from previous protocols. The effect, therefore, of prolonged storage on the serum samples was not controlled for either. Nevertheless, in this report a subset of hypertensives did have low free serum calcium concentrations which paralleled their renin-volume status.

In a protocol evaluation of calcium metabolism in essential hypertension, Strazzullo et al were unable to distinguish hypertensives from normals based upon serum ionized calcium concentrations.[5] Serum total calcium levels, though, were lower in the subjects with high blood pressure. These investigators studied 55 matched individuals in both groups. Blood pressure values were not reported and entry criteria may have allowed for inclusion of borderline hypertensives. The authors acknowledged that this factor likely accounted for their not detecting a decrease in the mean serum ionized calcium values of the hypertensives.

All three of these investigative teams have identified additional metabolic abnormalities consistent with a general perturbation of calcium metabolism. These have included increased parathyroid hormone concentrations[5,6] and urinary cyclic AMP excretion,[5,6,7] as well as lower serum phosphorus levels.[3,6] Paradoxically, each of these research programs has documented increased urinary calcium excretion in the face of enhanced PTH function, suggesting an end-organ resistance.[4,5,6]

In the single cross-sectional analysis of serum Ca^{2+} and blood pressure levels in 977 individuals, Fogh-Andersen et al reported a weak positive correlation between the two parameters.[8] However, their observations are of limited comparative value as they studied only subjects who were 45 years old and included at least 70 individuals who were receiving antihypertensive medications. It is noteworthy that those subjects who were receiving thiazide diuretics had serum Ca^{2+} values that were normal. Previous observations in such a population have demonstrated an increased serum Ca^{2+} concentration.[9] The authors' failure to identify such an effect in their subjects suggest that these hypertensives may have indeed started with lower values.

In well-defined populations with appropriate control groups for comparison, mean serum ionized calcium levels are decreased in hypertensives. The observation is consistent with associated disturbances involving the calcium-PTH axis, also reported in subjects with fixed increases in their arterial pressures.

In population studies that have assessed total serum calcium values, uncorrected weak positive correlations with blood pressure levels have been reported. Kasteloot and Geboers reported positive correlations between blood pressure and serum total calcium (systolic, r=0.10; diastolic, r=0.06) in 9,321 men.[10] Their data was collected under uncontrolled conditions and did not provide appropriate corrections for serum albumin, age and body mass index. When the latter data was added to the analysis, the correlations were not evident. In a similar report, Robinson et al noted that when corrected for albumin, age and weight significant correlations did not exist between arterial pressure and the serum total calciums of 22,764 men who were screened.[11]

Fogh-Anderson et al have appropriately noted that because of the positive correlations between serum total calciums and serum albumin concentrations as well as the relationship between serum albumin and intravascular volume, it would be anticipated that total calcium values might be weakly correlated with blood pressure.[8] A hallmark of established hypertension is a reduction of intravascular volume, predictably resulting in a weak positive correlation between levels of arterial pressure and total serum calcium.

The importance of reductions in serum ionized calcium values in hypertensives must be distinguished from these spurious reports of increased serum total calcium concentration. The former reflect potentially meaningful alterations in calcium metabolism while the latter may simply reflect correlations with other co-variates of blood pressure in adults. Failure to properly correct for these co-variables will predictably produce statistically significant but clinically irrelevant positive correlations. Furthermore, in the studies that have characterized differences in serum Ca^{2+} between hypertensives and normals, no differences in total calciums have been noted.[2,4]

Animal Studies. Similar to the reports in humans, observations in experimental models of hypertension have characterized lower serum ionized calcium values in the hypertensive animal. Wright et al first described such abnormalities in the spontaneously hypertensive rat (SHR).[12] In the first longitudinal study of the SHR's calcium metabolism, McCarron et al documented that reduced serum ionized calcium concentrations were a persistent defect present from early adolescence and the developmental phase of hypertension through older age and the "fixed" phase.[13]

In a second report, Toraason and Wright demonstrated that serum Ca^{2+} was not only reduced in the SHR but also the DOCA rat model of salt-dependent hypertension.[14] Additional reports in the SHR by Chen et al[15] and Sterns et al[16] have confirmed the previous findings that extracellular free Ca^{2+} is decreased in the SHR. The latter group have characterized the difference as early as five weeks of age before hypertension is established. Preliminary observations in the Milan[17] and New Zealand[18] strains of genetically hypertensive rats have indicated that significant reductions in serum calcium concentrations exist in those laboratory models also. In the New Zealand rat, the data has been limited to serum total calcium values and not to measurements of ionized fractions.

Consistent with the observations in humans, the SHR also possesses a variety of additional abnormalities of calcium metabolism. These include elevated PTH levels,[13] abnormal renal handling of calcium[13, 15] possible disturbances of intestinal transport of Ca^{2+} [19] and multiple defects of Ca^{2+} flux rates,[20] distribution and binding in vascular smooth muscle cells.[21] The vascular and PTH abnormalities are evident before blood pressure is significantly elevated. Treatment of the hypertension does not necessarily correct the vascular smooth muscle cell's disturbances of calcium metabolism.[22]

Dietary Calcium

Humans Studies. In spite of numerous efforts to define the relationship between diet and hypertensive cardiovascular disease, until very recently little data existed for nutrients other than sodium. Specifically, no information was available relative to calcium intake and blood pressure. Prior to our index report,[23] the postulated association between dietary calcium was based solely on the indirect observation that urinary calcium excretion was positively correlated with blood pressure in large population surveys.[10] Investigators extrapolated these findings to conclude that subjects with high blood pressure must eat more calcium. The possibility that the excessive urinary calcium excretion was a reflection of the previously reported inappropriate renal leak[6] of calcium was not considered.

Subsequently, several published reports have documented that dietary calcium in fact is less in subjects with high blood pressure. Our initial report of a prospective evaluation of newly diagnosed essential hypertensives (N=46) noted that they consumed significantly less dietary calcium (668 mg/day) than normal individuals (N=44) (886 mg/day.)[23] Those findings were based on a diet recall survey in these two demographically matched populations. No other nutrient, of the 17 assessed, was reduced in the hypertensives when compared to the normal subjects. Total calcium intake was not the only parameter that distinguished the high blood pressure group. Fewer hypertensives (8/46) reported a greater than 1 gm calcium intake than did the normals (18/46). Median intake from non-fluid milk sources (cheese, yogurt, ice cream) of dairy calcium (21 mg/day) was also significantly less (normals = 225 mg/day).

To address further the association between calcium intake and blood pressure in the United States, we turned to a data base from the National Center for Health Statistics (NCHS). The Health and Nutrition Examination Survey I (HANES I) was carried out between 1972 and 1974 by the National Center. It was designed to provide a representative cross-sectional assessment of demographic, socioeconomical, anthropromorphic, nutritional and health characteristics of the U.S. population. Over 21,000 Americans between ages 1 and 74 participated in the survey. Access to this data to interested investigators is provided by the NCHS. We identified 12,411 individuals between ages 20 and 74 who denied any history of hypertension, chronic diseases or intentional dietary modification.[2] As would be predicted, approximately 10% of this population was hypertensive (>160/95 mmHg), though undiagnosed previously. In this representative population of "free-living" Americans, reduced dietary calcium consumption was most consistently identified in those subjects with hypertension from those with normal pressure or borderline blood pressures.[2] This difference in calcium intake in the hypertensive subjects was independent of effects of age, race and sex. Those subpopulations at greatest risk also tended to exhibit the lowest exposure to dietary calcium. Overall, hypertensives reported 572±17 mg/day of calcium, while the normotensives reported 695±7 mg/day, an 18% reduction. That figure is comparable to that reported in our initial survey.

In an analysis of data gathered for the NIH-sponsored Lipid Research Clinic trial, Ackley et al reported on a population of 5,050 men and women drawn from a predominantly white upperclass community.[24] In their subjects, calcium intake from dairy products was significantly and negatively associated with both systolic and diastolic blood pressure. This inverse correlation was more evident in the male subjects. After controlling for age, obesity and alcohol consumption, the relationship was not altered. These investigators concluded that some component of dairy products, probably calcium, exerts a protective effect against hypertension.

In our own continuing assessment of the HANES I data, we have analyzed further the association between reported dietary calcium intake and the blood pressure profile of the United States in the mid-1970's. In our initial summary of that data we suggested that younger women (>55 years) were relatively protected against excessive hypertensive cardiovascular disease in spite of their remarkably low levels of calcium consumption.[2] In contrast, and consistent with our understanding of osteoporosis, older females (>54 years) appeared then to incur an excessive risk from the same level of calcium intake. The same age effect was apparent in the male segment, though, not as evident as what was seen in the women.

For Figures 1 and 2, we have utilized the entire database for subjects included in our first publication of the HANES Data. The computer identified males and females and then subdivided by age (18-54, 55-74). They were further categorized by their dietary intake of calcium (mg/day). The mean systolic blood pressure for each 75 mg/day increments of dietary calcium was then calculated for the respective age and sex groups.

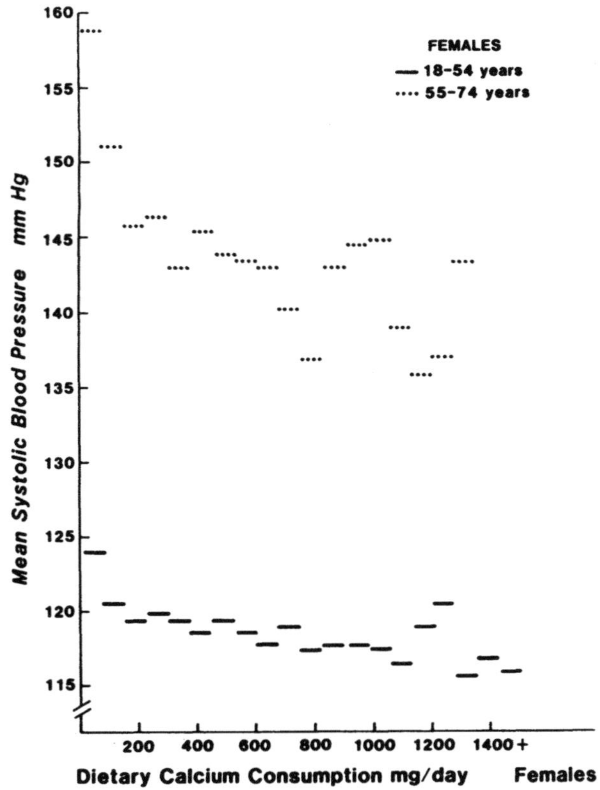

FEMALES
Figure 2.

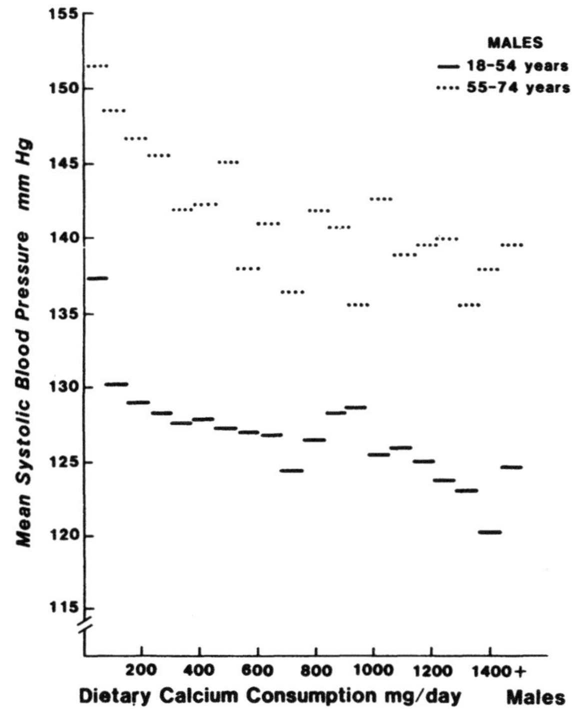

MALES
Figure 1.

"Mean Systolic Blood Pressure of Subjects 18-54 and 55-74 Years of Age, Based on Dietary Calcium as Reported in HANES I Survey"

In Figure 1, we have portrayed the relationship among systolic blood pressure, calcium intake and age for females in the HANES I survey. As previously suggested for younger females, blood pressure appears to vary little based upon reported levels of calcium consumed. The reverse is evident for older women (>54 years) in whom there is a clear and dramatic increase in mean systolic blood pressure for those individuals reporting less than the recommended daily allowance (800 mg).

The comparable data for males in the HANES I survey is depicted in Figure 2. In distinction to females, younger males exhibited an increase in their blood pressure profile at calcium intake levels less than 400 mg/day, as well as a suggestion that a lowering effect on blood pressure occurred in those younger males consuming more than 1,200 mg/day. In the older (>55 years) subset, the risk of elevating one's systolic blood pressure occurred in those individuals eating less than 800 mg/day. It is important to note that the blood pressure profile of women over the age of 55 years exceeds that of the men in the HANES I database. These observations are consistent with the postulate that emergence of hypertension in the older female segment of the U.S. population is, in part, another manifestation of the failure of the post-menopausal female to adequately protect her calcium balance.

These recent findings, which associate a lower intake of dietary calcium with a higher blood pressure, are significant because they suggest a relationship that cuts across the entire society, fitting with the demographics of hypertensive-cardiovascular disease in the United States. From the studies currently available, the critical level of calcium intake below which the risk to the population increases, appears to be 750-800 mg/day. By virtue of factors not yet fully delineated, younger women are afforded additional protection down to levels approaching 450-500 mg/day.

Several intervention studies in humans have assessed the effect of supplemental calcium in the diet on blood pressure. Belizan studied 59 individuals between 18 and 35 years of age, all of whom were healthy and normotensive.[25] The subjects (29 females and 28 males) were administered either placebo or 1,000 mg of calcium per day for 22 weeks. Significant reductions in both systolic and diastolic blood pressure were observed in both sexes. The greater decline (5-9%) was seen in the diastolic pressures.

In a second experiment, the same investigative group reported on the blood pressure response of non-hypertensive, pregnant subjects who were provided with either 1,000 mg or 2,000 mg of supplemental calcium per day throughout their gestational period.[26] Both doses were associated with lower blood pressures in the second trimester when compared to placebo. However, only those women receiving the 2,000 mg/day demonstrated a sustained reduction of their blood pressure through to term.

We have recently presented the preliminary results of the Oregon Hypertension Program's intervention trial of oral calcium for the treatment of mild to moderate hypertension.[27] In this ongoing study, we provided 1,000 mg/day of elemental calcium at bedtime to normal subjects (n=32) and matched hypertensives (n=48). This was a randomized, double-blind, cross-over protocol. Each subject's calcium response is compared to his or her own placebo response. Both the calcium phase and placebo period was eight weeks with a four-week washout period between Phase 1 (Ca^{2+} or placebo) and Phase 2. At the time of our initial report, 30 normals and 28 hypertensives had completed the protocol. Compared to the normals, the calcium significantly lowered blood pressure (systolic, diastolic, MAP) in the patients with hypertension. Using the criteria of a 10 mmHg reduction in blood pressure as a clinically meaningful response, 13/28 patients were categorized as responders. In this 45% of the hypertensives who responded, systolic blood pressure decreased from 152 mmHg to 131 mmHg and diastolic pressure declined from 96 mmHg to 87 mmHg. In those individuals who failed to change their blood pressure with the calcium, there was no significant alteration in either systolic or diastolic pressures. While approximately 20% of the normals demonstrated a significant lowering of their pressures, overall, the normals' blood pressures did not change significantly.

These three trials of oral calcium supplementation in both normals and hypertensives have demonstrated a significant effect of the nutrient, calcium, on arterial pressure. The level of blood pressure reduction observed exceeds that reported previously for any single nutrient intervention trial. Specifically, the effect is greater than that noted in any comparable trial that modified either sodium or potassium intake.

Animal Studies. Within the past five years, a number of investigators have demonstrated an effect of dietary calcium intake on blood pressure in laboratory animals.[13,15,28] The reported effects are consistent with those observed in the human studies. Calcium supplementation in the SHR lowers blood pressure in the younger animal.[13,28] More importantly, it reverses the "fixed" hypertension of the adult animal.[13] As first noted from our laboratory, the introduction of a 4% calcium diet in our adolescent SHR dampened the rise in their pressures, but it was only at the time of skeletal maturity (24-26 weeks of age) that the animals significantly lowered their arterial pressures. Ultimately, the older SHR (>45 weeks of age) fed the higher calcium diet lowered its blood pressure to values approaching 160 mmHg (systolic) compared to 200 mmHg in the normal diet animal.

The salutory effect of calcium on the SHR's presumed genetic hypertension is modified by the time at which it is introduced. When administered to the young SHR (five weeks old) for five weeks, it does not significantly lower blood pressure.[16] However, the peak pressure that develops in an adult SHR is lower, the earlier the calcium supplementation is provided.[29] Increasing dietary calcium at the time of weaning (four weeks of age) results in a lower maximum systolic pressure in the young adult animal and a greater attentuation of pressure in the older SHR, than when the calcium is added to the diet at 10 weeks of age.[29]

The adult SHR's pressure in the "fixed" phase of its hypertension can be modified by short-term dietary intervention. Table 1 depicts the mean arterial pressure (± SEM) of 24- to 26-week-old SHRs after two weeks on either a low-calcium (0.01%) or a supplemented (4%) intake. The animals had been raised on a standard 1% calcium diet before the switch.

Table 1. Mean Arterial Pressure (±SEM) of 24- to 26-Week-Old SHRs

	4%	0.01%
MAP (mmHg)	165±5.1	214±4.5†
Weight (gm)	375±9	379±21
(N=)	8	8

† $p<.001$

As is apparent, within two weeks, modifying the SHR's exposure to calcium will significantly lower the pressure of the 4% animal and increase that of the calcium-restricted SHR. With only two weeks of dietary calcium manipulation it is possible to spread the SHR's blood pressure by 49 mmHg ($p<.001$).

The blood pressure of the normotensive Wistar-Kyoto rat is similarly affected by the level of dietary calcium. Chronically supplementing the WKY beginning in adolescence will lower peak adult pressures and attenuate further the "normal" pressures in the older WKY.[30] A modest reduction of dietary calcium (0.5% vs. 0.25%) will produce a chronic increase of the WKY's blood pressure. As with the SHR, it is possible to induce significant changes in the adult WKY's blood pressure within two weeks of either increasing or restricting its calcium intake. Table 2 shows the effects of such a manipulation in the WKY. The protocol was identical to that described above for the SHR.

Table 2. Mean Arterial Pressure (±SEM) of 24- to 26-Week-Old WKYs

	4%	0.01%
MAP (mmHg)	148±3.3	156±3.3
Weight (gm)	388±14	404±10
(N=)	8	8

Within two weeks it is possible to affect an 8 mmHg difference in the mean arterial pressures of the WKY simply by altering the animals exposure to dietary calcium. Restriction of the nutrient for this limited period is sufficient to produce a "hypertension" in the WKY.

A similar effect on the pregnant WKY's blood pressure has been reported. Belizan et al have induced hypertension during gestation by restricting calcium consumption.[31] Adding calcium back to the diet reversed the increased pressures.

These consistent and reproducible observations in the SHR and the WKY indicate that the level of chronic dietary consumption of calcium significantly influences the developmental and maintenance phases of increased arterial pressures. The findings to date are consistent with marked protective effects of the nutrient, calcium, on blood pressure in the experimental setting. Although partly influenced by them, this vasodepressive action of calcium is, in part, independent of factors such as age, strain and level of arterial pressure prior to the introduction of the calcium supplement. The observation from the animal studies are consistent with data available from the human experiments reviewed earlier.

Interaction of Diet Ca^{2+}, Serum Ca^{2+}, and Blood Pressure

Acute Effects. The acute blood pressure effects of calcium administration to humans varies from the chronic effects. In two separate studies, Weideman and co-workers have demonstrated that the infusion of calcium into subjects with mild to moderate renal failure produces a pressor response.[31, 33] However, as the investigators have noted the level of hypercalcemia achieved does not predict the blood pressure response.

In a previous report, we have characterized the blood pressure response to acute hypercalcemia in normal subjects and successful renal transplant recipients. In spite of a marked increase in serum Ca^{2+} the normal individuals did not change their blood pressure.[34] In contrast, the transplant patients experienced a pressor effect from the calcium infusion. However, once again the concentration of serum Ca^{2+}, was not predictive of this blood pressure increase.

In a preliminary report of a similar study, carried out in hypertensives, the patients given an acute infusion of calcium experienced a transient, but significant rise in their blood pressure.[7] The increase in blood pressure occurred early in the infusion with a later reduction in blood pressure to baseline pressures by the end of the infusion at the time of maximal increase in the serum Ca^{2+} concentration. Again in this experiment, there was no change in the normals' blood pressure in spite of the induction of the same degree of hypercalcemia as that produced in the hypertensive subjects.

The acute effects on blood pressure of Ca^{2+} administration can be dissociated from the degree of hypercalcemia. In addition, a pressor response to acute hypercalcemia has not been observed in normal subjects. A pressor response has been induced only in patients with underlying hypertensive cardiovascular and/or renal disease. Hypertensives respond differently to acute hypercalcemia than they do to chronically administered calcium.

Animal Studies. In our initial report of calcium's salutory effect on the SHR's blood pressure, we noted that with diet supplementation, serum Ca^{2+} levels normalized 10 weeks before the attenuating effect on blood pressure was observed.[13] Temporally, the effects on serum Ca^{2+} and blood pressure were dissociated in the SHR. Stern et al in their preliminary report of calcium supplementation in the weanling SHR have noted a similar response.[16] Serum calcium increased within several weeks, without an evident effect on the animals' blood pressure.

As is described above, in both the adult SHR and WKY, the imposition of two weeks of either calcium supplementation or restriction will, respectively, lower or increase mean arterial pressure. Table 3 shows the concurrent effects on serum ionized calcium of these divergent dietary calcium interventions.

Serum ionized calcium values were relatively unchanged in both the SHR and the WKY regardless of whether they were calcium-restricted or supplemented. The one exception was the 4% SHRs which did increase their levels, though, not significantly. This observation from the laboratory further indicates that the blood pressure response to either chronic or acute manipulations of calcium balance do not necessarily parallel concurrent changes in extracellular ionized calcium.

Table 3. Serum Ionized Calcium (mEq/L)

Strain	Diet		
	1% (Pre)	4% (Post 2 Wks)	0.01% (Post 2 Wks)
WKY	2.29±0.06	2.27±0.04	2.26±0.04
SHR	1.98±0.09	2.24±0.1	1.95±0.13

SUMMARY

Serum ionized calcium and related biochemical parameters of calcium metabolism distinguish hypertensive humans and animals from their respective normotensive controls. These differences in serum calcium, though, should be viewed as possible markers of fundamental cellular abnormalities of calcium handling that contribute to the pathogenesis of increased smooth muscle tone and reactivity and a consequent increase in peripheral resistance. The differences in serum calcium should not be interpreted as directly contributing to the pathogenesis of the hypertension.

Dietary calcium modifies blood pressure in both humans and experimental animals. Humans with essential hypertension ingest significantly less calcium daily. Correcting this deficit will lower blood pressure in a significant percentage of adult hypertensives. The cardiovascular response to either acute or chronic modification of calcium exposure in both humans and animals can be dissociated from the concurrent effects on extracellular ionized calcium concentrations.

Collectively, the information available indicates that a continued commitment to elucidating the possible critical role of the nutrient, calcium, in the pathogenesis and treatment of hypertensive-cardiovascular disease may yield clinically and therapeutically relevant interventions. Protection of calcium balance and dietary intake may represent an effective preventive and/or therapeutic measure in the management of hypertensive-cardiovascular disease in humans.

ACKNOWLEDGEMENTS

The author's cited research in this review was supported in part by grants-in-aid from the American Heart Association, the Oregon Heart Association, the National Dairy Council and the M.J. Murdock Charitable Trust. I am grateful to Patricia Pingree-McCarron for editorial assistance and to Joni Utterback for preparation of the manuscript.

REFERENCES

1. H. Kuriyama, I. Yushi, H. Suzuki, K. Kitamura, T. Itoh, Factors modifying contraction-relaxation cycle in vascular smooth muscles, Am J Physiol. 243:H641 (1982).
2. D.A. McCarron, Calcium and magnesium nutrition in human hypertension, Ann Intern Med. 98:800 (1983).
3. D.A. McCarron, Low serum concentrations of ionized calcium in patients with hypertension, New Engl J Med. 307:226 (1982).
4. L.M. Resnick, J.H. Laragh, J.E. Sealey, M.H. Alderman, Divalent cations in essential hypertension, New Engl J Med. 309:888 (1983).
5. P. Strazzullo, V. Nunziata, M. Cirillo, R. Giannatasio, L.A. Ferrara, P.L. Mattioli, M. Mancini, Abnormalities of calcium metabolism in essential hypertension, Clin Sci. 65:13 (1983).
6. D.A. McCarron, P. Pingree, R.J. Rubin, S.M. Gaucher, M. Molitch, S. Kurtzik, Enhanced parathyroid function in essential hypertension: A homeostatic response to a urinary calcium leak, Hypertension 2:162 (1980).
7. D.A. McCarron, D.H. Ellison, Ca^{2+} infusion at varying Na^+ intakes in hypertensive humans: altered cardiovascular and renal response, Clin Res. 31:42A (1983).
8. N. Fogh-Anderson, L. Hedegaard, J. Thode, O. Siggaard-Anderson, Sex-dependent relation between ionized calcium in serum and blood pressure, Clin Chem. 30:116 (1984).
9. M.S. Stote, L.H. Smith, D.M. Wilson, et al, Hydrochlorothiazide effects on serum calcium and immunoreactive parathyroid hormone concentrations. Studies in normal subjects, Ann Intern Med. 77:597 (1972).
10. H. Kesteloot, J. Geboers, Calcium and blood pressure, Lancet i:813 (1982).
11. D. Robinson, A.R. Bailey, P.T. Williams, Calcium and blood pressure, Lancet ii:1215 (1982).

12. G.L. Wright, M.A. Toraason, J.J. Barbe, W. Crouse, The concentration of ionic and total calcium in plasma of the spontaneously hypertensive rat, Can J Physiol Pharmacol. 58:1494 (1980).
13. D.A. McCarron, N.N. Yung, B.A. Ugoretz, S. Krutzik, Disturbances of calcium metabolism in the spontaneously hypertensive rat, Hypertension 3:1162 (1981).
14. M.A. Toraason, G.L. Wright, Transport of calcium by duodenum of spontaneously hypertensive rat, Am J Physiol. 241:G334 (1981).
15. S. Chen, B. Eby, K. Lau, Mechanism of salutory effects of high-calcium diet on blood pressure in spontaneously hypertensive rats, Kidney Internat. 23:74A (1983).
16. N. Stern, D.B. Lee, F.W. Beck, V. Silis, L. Debtos, J.R. Sower, High calcium diet reverses abnormal calcium and PTH but does not prevent hypertension in young spontaneously hypertensive rats, Clin Res. 31:336A (1983).
17. Personal communication.
18. Personal communication.
19. G.L. Wright, G.O. Rankin, Concentrations of ionic and total calcium in plasma of four models of hypertension, Am J Physiol. 243:H365 (1982).
20. R.C. Webb, D.F. Bohr, Recent advances in the pathogenesis of hypertension: consideration of structural, functional and metabolic vascular abnormalities resulting in elevated arterial resistance, Am Heart J. 102:251 (1981).
21. M.A. Devynck, M.G. Pernollet, A.M. Nunez, P. Meyer, Analysis of calcium handling in erythrocyte membranes of genetically hypertensive rats, Hypertension 3:397 (1981).
22. M.J. Mulvany, N. Korsgaard, N. Nyborg, Evidence that the increased calcium sensitivity of resistance vessels in spontaneously hypertensive rats is an intrinsic defect of the vascular smooth muscle. Clin Exp Hyperten. 3:749 (1981).
23. D.A. McCarron, C.D. Morris, C. Cole, Dietary calcium in human hypertension, Science 217:267 (1982).
24. S. Ackley, E. Barrett-Connor, L. Suarez, Dairy products, calcium and blood pressure, Am J Clin Nutr. 38:457 (1983).
25. J.M. Belizan, J. Villar, O. Pineda, A.E. Gonzalez, E. Sainz, G. Garrera, R. Sibrian, Reduction of blood pressure with calcium supplementation in young adults, J Am Med Assoc. 249:1161 (1983).
26. J.M. Belizan, J. Villar, A. Zalazar, L. Rojas, D. Chan, G.F. Bryce, Preliminary evidence of the effect of calcium supplementation on blood pressure in normal pregnant women, Am J Obstet Gynecol. 146:175 (1983).
27. D.A. McCarron, H.J. Henry, C.D. Morris, Randomized, placebo-controlled trial of oral calcium in human hypertension, Clin Res. 32:37A (1984).
28. S. Ayachi, Increased dietary calcium lowers blood pressure in the spontaneously hypertensive rat, Metabolism 28:1234 (1979).

29. D.A. McCarron, Calcium, magnesium and phosphorus balance in human and experimental hypertension, Hypertension 4:III-27 (1982).
30. D.A. McCarron, Blood pressure and calcium balance in the Wistar-Kyoto rat, Life Sci. 30:683 (1982).
31. J.M. Belizan, O. Pineda, E. Sainz, L.A. Menendez, J. Villar, Rise of blood pressure in calcium-deprived pregnant rats, Am J Obstet Gynecol. 141:163 (1981).
32. P. Weidmann, S.G. Massry, J.W. Coburn, M.H. Maxwell, J. Atleson, C.R. Kleeman, Blood pressure effect of acute hypercalcemia, Ann Intern Med. 76:741 (1972).
33. C. Marone, C. Berretta-Piccoli, P. Weidmann, Acute hypercalcemia in man: role of hemodynamics, catecholamines, and renin, Kidney Internat. 20:92 (1981).
34. D.A. McCarron, R.S. Muther, S.B. Plant, S. Krutzik, Parathyroid hormone: a determinant of post-transplant blood pressure regulation, Am J Kidney Dis. 1:38 (1981).

THE RELATIONSHIP BETWEEN BODY PHOSPHATE AND BLOOD PRESSURE

Vito M. Campese, Yahya Saglikes, Kunitoshi Iseki and Shaul G. Massry

University of Southern California, Los Angeles, CA

Phosphate depletion alters the function of the cardiovascular system. Decreased myocardial performance has been described in phosphate depleted dogs (1) and humans (2). In the most severe cases of hypophosphatemia, congestive cardiomyopathy can occur (3). Phosphate supplementation reverse these abnormalities.

The effects of phosphate depletion on blood pressure regulation have been critically evaluated only recently. Some investigators have demonstrated an inverse correlation between serum phosphorus levels and blood pressure suggesting that decreased serum levels of phosphorus may be associated with increased blood pressure via unexplained mechanisms (4).

A large body of evidence, however, indicated that phosphate depletion may lead to a decrease in blood pressure. O'Connor et al. showed that mean arterial pressure (MAP) increased in 4 of 7 hypophosphatemic patients after phosphate repletion and attributed this increase to improvement in myocardial function (2). More recently, in our laboratory we have examined the possibility that phosphate depletion may affect other determinants of blood pressure regulation such as the activity of the sympathetic nervous system, the function of the renin-angiotensin system or the peripheral vascular response to pressor agonists (5).

The studies were conducted on Sprague-Dawley rats made hypophosphatemic by feeding with low phosphorus (0.03%) chow for 4-6 weeks and while they were awake, unrestrained and undisturbed. Phosphate depleted rats displayed lower serum phosphorus concentrations (3.4±0.2 mg/dl) and lower MAP (112±2.0 mmHg) than control rats fed with purina chow containing 0.74% phosphorus (8.9±0.4 mg/dl), ($p<0.01$), and 122±2.2 mmHg, ($p<0.01$), respectively). Phosphate depleted animals displayed a significant reduction in cardiac index (95±11 vs 140±7 ml/min/kg body weight, $p<0.01$) and a modest but significant rise in systemic vascular resistance (1.2±0.12 vs 0.9±0.04 mmHg ml/min/kg body weight, $p<0.05$), which evidently was not adequate to sustain normal blood pressure.

We then investigated the possibility that the inadequate rise in systemic vascular resistance in response to the decrease in cardiac index might be due to abnormalities in the function of the sympathetic nervous system and/or of the renin-angiotensin system. Baseline plasma levels of norepinephrine were increased in phosphate depleted rats (44±5.5 vs 27±3.4 ng/dl, $p<0.01$). Similarly, during the stress of forced immobilization, plasma norepinephrine levels were significantly ($p<0.01$) greater in phosphate depleted than in control rats, despite similar rise in MAP. Plasma renin activity was also significantly greater in phosphate depleted rats (21±5.9 vs 6.2±2.6 ng/ml/h, $p<0.05$), and increased appropriately after administration of isoproterenol. These data indicated that the inappropriately low rise in systemic vascular resistance in phosphate depleted rats could not be attributed to abnormality in the function of the sympathetic nervous system or the renin-angiotensin system.

We then tested the possibility that the inadequate rise in systemic vascular resistance in phosphate depleted rats might depend on decreased vascular response to agonists. Norepinephrine injected in bolus of 10, 30, 100 and 300 ng and angiotensin II in doses of 3, 10, 30 and 100 ng produced significantly lower ($p<0.01$) increments in MAP in phosphate depleted than in control rats. A dose of norepinephrine of 1.28±0.34 μg/min was required to produce a rise in MAP of 30 mmHg in phosphate depleted rats, whereas a dose of only 0.3±0.07 μg/min was required to produce the same rise in MAP in control animals. During the infusion of norepinephrine, cardiac index fell and systemic vascular resistance rose similarly in the two groups of rats. Cardiac index in normal rats was 140±7 ml/min/kg pre-infusion and 114±7.7 ml/min/kg after NE infusion. In PD rats, cardiac index was 95±11 pre and 84±7.2 ml/min kg post-infusion of NE. Systemic vascular resistance was 0.9±0.04 pre and 1.4±0.09 mmHg/ml/min/kg after NE infusion in normal rats and 1.2±0.12 and 1.7±0.14 mmHg/ml/min/kg, respectively in PD rats. Administration of norepinephrine in the perfusate of the hind-limb preparation produced less increase in the perfusion pressure in phosphate depleted than in control rats causing a significant ($p<0.05$) shift to the right of the dose-response curve. Other investigators have shown similar findings (6). These data taken together indicate that the reduction in MAP in phosphate depleted rats is due to a decrease in cardiac index and to an inadequate rise in systemic vascular resistance caused by a decrease in vascular response to agonists. The latter abnormality is independent of other hemodynamic influences since it can be demonstrated in the isolated hind-limb preparation.

Various mechanisms may be responsible for the reduced vascular response to agonists in phosphate depleted rats. These may include increased production of vasodepressor agents such as prostaglandins, receptor abnormalities and/or reduced availability of energy sources in vascular smooth muscle cells. Treatment with indomethacin 5 mg/kg injected subcutaneously did not affect the blood pressure response to norepinephrine. This observation practically excluded the possibility that the decrease in vascular response to agonists may be due to excessive production of vasodilating prostaglandins.

Since phosphate depleted rats manifest increased plasma levels of norepinephrine and of plasma renin activity, it is possible that the reduced pressor response to agonists may be due to down-regulation of receptors in the vascular wall. Since techniques to direct measure adrenergic receptors in blood vessels of the rat are not readily available, we measured these receptors in the cardiac muscle. Both the content and affinity of alpha and beta-receptors was similar in the myocardium of PD and control rats. These data suggest that the reduced vascular response to pressor agonists cannot be simply attributed to down-regulation of adrenergic receptors.

Since phosphate depletion is associated with reduction in energy stores in the myocardium and in skeletal muscles (7), it is theoretically possible that this abnormality may occur in smooth muscle cells and be responsible for reduced response to pressor agonists. To test this hypothesis, we measured the content of inorganic phosphorus, adenosine triphosphate (ATP), adenosine-diphosphate (ADP) and adenosine-monophosphate (AMP) in mesenteric vessels by the ashomatic method of Bessman et al (8). The content of ATP and AMP was significantly ($p<0.01$) reduced in PD rats. These data are in keeping with the notion that the decrease in vascular response to pressor agonists in phosphate depletion may be the result of reduced energy stores in vascular smooth muscle cells.

More recently, the effects of phosphate depletion on the development of hypertension have been evaluated by Chen et al (9) in spontaneously hypertensive rats (SHR). These authors were studying the mechanisms for the improvement in blood pressure induced in these rats by a high dietary calcium intake. They found that serum and urinary phosphorus and intestinal absorption of phosphorus were markedly reduced in SHR when they were fed a diet containing high (4.3%) calcium than when they ingested a normal (1.2%) calcium diet. Furthermore, when rats fed 4.3% calcium diet received intraperitoneal administration of sodium phosphate to sustain normal serum levels of phosphorus, the beneficial effect of high calcium diet on the development of hypertension was completely abolished.

Our data and those of Chen et al (9) clearly demonstrate that phosphate depletion can cause a reduction in MAP. This hemodynamic abnormality is due to both a reduction in cardiac index and to decreased vascular response to pressor agonists. The latter abnormality may be caused by reduced energy stores in vascular smooth muscle cells.

References

1. T.J. Fuller, W.M. Nichols, B.J. Brenner, J.C. Peterson, Reversible depression in myocardial performance in dogs with experimental phosphorus deficiency, J. Clin. Invest. 62: 1194 (1978).
2. L.R. O'Connor, W.S. Wheeler, J.E. Bethune, Effect of hypophosphatemia on myocardial performance in man, New Engl. J. Med. 297:901 (1977).
3. J.R. Darsee and D.O. Nutter, Reversible severe congestive cardiomyopathy in three cases of hypophosphatemia, Ann. Intern. Med. 89:867 (1978).
4. S. Ljunghall and H. Hedstrand, Serum phosphate inversely related to blood pressure, Brit. Med. J. 1:553 (1977).
5. V.M. Campese, Y. Saglikes, N. Brautbar, R. Barndt, S.G. Massry, Effect of phosphate depletion on blood pressure, Amer. Soc. Nephrol., 15th Ann. Meet., Chicago, Ill. 4A, (1982).
6. W. Kreusser, H. Scholz, W. Rascher, A. Schomig, R. Dietz, D. Klormann, E. Ritz, Circulatory response to pressor agents in phosphorus depletion, In: Regulation of phosphate and mineral metabolism, Ed. S.G. Massry, J.M. Letteri, E. Ritz, Adv. Exp. Med. Biol. 151:259 (1982).
7. N. Brautbar, R. Baczynski, C. Carpenter, S. Moser, P. Geiger, P. Finander, S.G. Massry, Impaired energy metabolism in rat myocardium during phosphate depletion, Am. J. Physiol. 242: F699 (1982).
8. S.P. Bessman, P.J. Geiger, T.S. Lu, Cho, F.R.B. McCabe, Separation and automated analysis of phosphorylated metabolic intermediates, Analytic Biochem. 59:533 (1974).
9. S. Chen, B. Eby, K. Lau, Mechanism for the salutary effects of high diet Ca on blood pressure in spontaneous hypertensive rats (SHR), Amer. Soc. Nephrol., 15th Ann. Meet., Chicago, Ill. 74A (1982).

INTERACTIONS BETWEEN MG AND BLOOD PRESSURE

Kai Lau and Claire Oasa

Division of Nephrology
Department of Internal Medicine
The University of Michigan
Ann Arbor, Michigan

INTRODUCTION

The relationship between magnesium and blood pressure has been sought, evaluated and studied in considerable depth both in the intact animal and at the level of the various organs involved. In the simplest form, three potential interactions are possible (Table 1). Although new insights have been gained regarding the acute effects of Mg loading or withdrawal on muscle cell excitability-contraction coupling, the contractile process and energy metabolism, present knowledge is still inadequate to establish the first form of interaction, viz. whether changes in Mg metabolism would produce sustained alterations in blood pressure in the intact but complex animal, endowed with all the physiologic counterregulatory and/or adaptive mechanisms. Bluntly put, the role of disturbances in Mg homeostasis, if any, has not been sufficiently defined in the pathogenesis and/or maintenance of hypertension.

Table 1. Interaction between Mg and Blood Pressure

1.	Changes in Mg Metabolism	⟶	Hypertension
2.	Changes in Mg Metabolism	⟵	Hypertension
3.	Changes in Mg Metabolism	⟷	Hypertension

Similarly, our current state of information does not permit us to establish the second form of interaction, viz. whether hypertension would lead to disorders of Mg metabolism.

In the succeeding paragraphs, an attempt will be made to update, in a summary fashion, the current concepts on the role of Mg in the function and structural integrity of the cardiac and vascular smooth muscle cells. The experimental and clinical data regarding the interaction between Mg and blood pressure will be reviewed, focusing on the first and second possibilities as outlined in Table I. A thesis will be developed pointing to the need for more data by vigorous studies designed specifically for defining the relationship between blood pressure and Mg.

CHANGES IN MG METABOLISM PRODUCING CHANGES IN BLOOD PRESSURE

Acute Changes

Results from animal work and clinical experience have fairly convincingly demonstrated a hypotensive effect in response to acute hypermagnesemia[1-6] (Fig. 1). Conversely, hypomagnesemia induced by acute hemodilution was associated with a slight increase in systemic

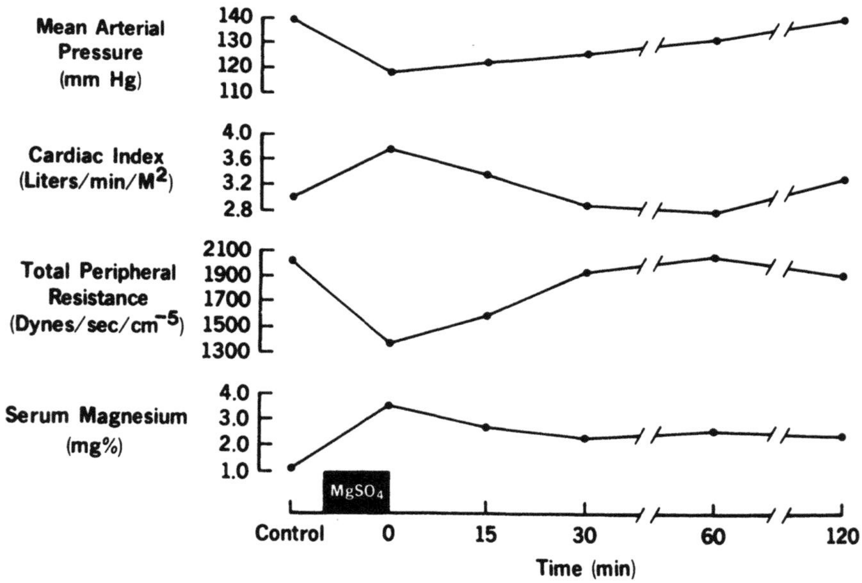

Fig. 1. Acute effects of hypermagnesemia on arterial blood pressure, cardiac index and peripheral resistance (Ref. 6).

or perfusion blood pressure,[7] although this effect was more equivocal in earlier studies by the same group,[8] unless there were concomitant hypokalemia[9,10] and/or metabolic alkalosis, hypo-osmolality and hypercalcemia,[8,9] or there was spinal block by procaine[11] (Fig. 2).

Mechanisms for the Hypotensive Effects of Acute Mg Infusion. First, examining the potential mechanisms, one can focus on four involved organs or systems, where interactions could take place: (1) Brain (vasomotor center); (2) Heart; (3) Sympathetic activity; (4) Peripheral "resistance" vasculature.

Brain. The available experimental data tend to argue against a major role of depression of the vasomotor center in mediating the antihypertensive effects of hypermagnesemia. First, perfusion of cerebral ventricles required very high Mg concentration (10mM) before there was a fall in vasomotor reflexes and arterial pressure[12]. Whether this is merely part of the generalized central anesthetic and depressant effect by Mg is not clear. Brain adenosine triphosphate (ATP) hydrolysis is known to be impaired with Mg anesthesia. Second, intracarotid injection of Mg produced a rise in blood pressure even after exclusion of vasomotor reflexes by evulsion of the cranial nerves IX through XII[13].

Heart. Tension development by the heart is a critical determinant of cardiac output and hence systemic blood pressure. Although there is an overwhelming amount of experimental evidence in

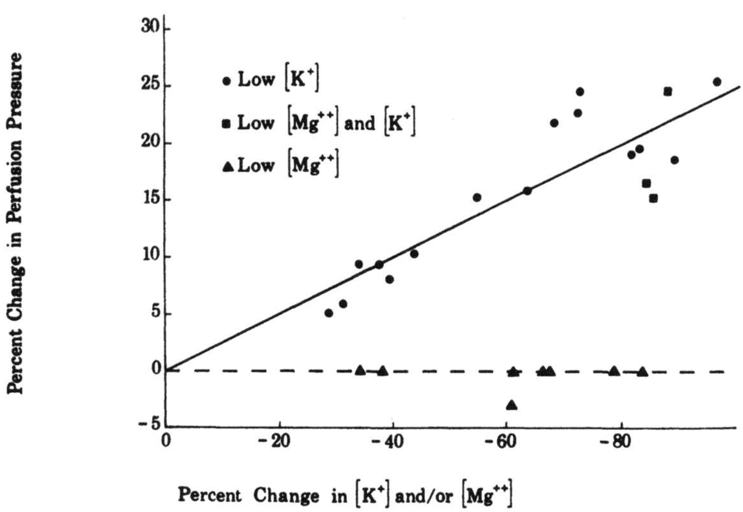

Fig. 2. Lack of effect of hypomagnesemia on the perfusion pressure of gracilis muscle at constant flow (Ref. 10).

various cardiac tissues indicating impairment of tension development by elevated Mg concentration in the perfusate or bathing media,[14-21] rather excessive concentrations of Mg (10 to 40 mM) were employed, making extrapolation to the intact animal in a more physiologic setting very difficult.

In both anesthetized dog[4] and conscious man[6], where more modest hypermagnesemia (between 1.5 and 4 mM) was produced and found to be antihypertensive, measured cardiac output or cardiac index were not depressed in these acute experiments. Furthermore, coronary hemodynamics and myocardial O_2 and CO_2 metabolism were not affected by this degree of hypermagnesemia. Transient fall in systemic blood pressure was attributed in these experiments to the significant reduction in peripheral vascular resistance observed. These whole animal data notwithstanding, the in vitro work is still important in elucidating the mode and mechanism whereby Mg interferes with the contractility of not only the cardiac but also the smooth muscle cell, the key component in maintaining the tone and reactivity of resistance vessels. The potential mechanisms for the depressant action of Mg on the heart include: (A) Inactivation of myofibrillar ATPase activity normally stimulated by Ca;[22,23] (B) Reduction of cellular Ca uptake by competitive displacement of Ca on the sarcolemmal binding sites;[16,18,24] (C) Reduction of Ca efflux from sarcoplasmic reticulum that normally takes place during activation by an action potential;[15,25] (D) Increases in Ca binding capacity of the sarcoplasmic reticulum;[15] (E) Membrane stabilization by increasing the resting potential and diminishing membrane permeability and excitability;[26] (F) Decreases in K efflux[16].

Similarly, even though increases in Mg concentration (3 to 5 mM) exert a depressant action on cardiac rhythm and conduction (prolonging P-Q conduction time, extending QRS complex and reducing heart rate),[27] these effects are seen at a time when the heart muscle is relatively unimpaired, the systole being vigorous until arrest (at 15 to 20 mM).[20,28] Thus, these events probably do not contribute to the reduction in blood pressure produced by Mg injection.

<u>Sympathetic Ganglia</u>. One major site of the antihypertensive action of Mg appears to be the neuromuscular blockade of the sympathetic ganglia (superior cervical, stellate and inferior mesenteric ganglia), since there is no effect on the conduction of impulses in pre- and post-ganglionic fibers.[13] In hypermagnesemic preparations, diminished sensitivity to acetylcholine and altered metabolism of acetylcholine (increased anticholinesterase and choline acetylase activity) have been implicated in the neuromuscular block.[29] Via the inhibition by acetylcholine, Mg could blunt the release of adrenal catecholemines and hence reduce the blood pressure. Data are not available to evaluate this possibility. In addition to ganglionic blockage, other factors must

be involved since in dogs and cats[11,13] and in frogs with ablated central nervous system,[30] blood pressure could still be reduced by Mg injection.

<u>Peripheral Resistance Vasculature</u>. The classical vasodilation accompanying Mg injection has been confirmed in virtually every peripheral vascular bed studied, and studies have now been extended to include vascular tone, contractility, reactivity, and the cellular mechanisms mediating smooth muscular relaxation and vasodilation.[25,31-33]

As previously mentioned, the associated reduction in peripheral vascular resistance[4,6] has been implicated in the fall in blood pressure produced by Mg infusion. In addition to basal tension or tone, vascular reactivity is also modified by changes in extracellular fluid Mg concentration[31] (Fig. 3). Thus,

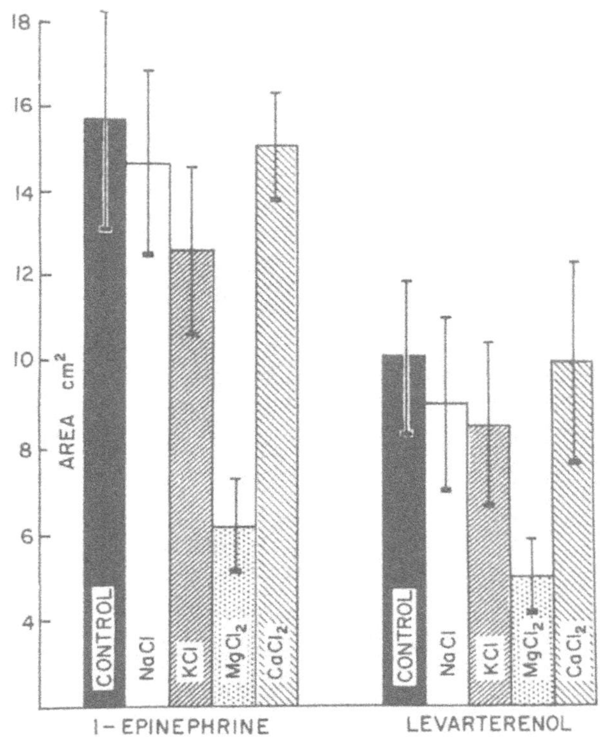

Fig. 3 Reduction in the increment in renal arterial pressure by $MgCl_2$ infusion to the renal artery (compared to control) in response to epinephrine and levarterenol. Data given as the area under the pressure curve (Ref. 35).

hypermagnesemia[34,35,36] depresses and hypomagnesemia[37] accentuates the response of isolated blood vessels, perfused arterioles and vascular beds to contractile agonists, including electrical stimulation, K and ouabain, angiotensin II, acetylcholine, and noreinephrine (Table 2). The relaxation of blood vessels induced by prostaglandin (PGE) and isoproterenol is attenuated by the absence of Mg. These vascular effects can be attributed to the rapid increases in tension development in muscle cell isolated from artery, arterioles and portal veins in response to reduced Mg concentrations and to decreases in spontaneous mechanical activity and baseline tension in a dose-dependent fashion in response to elevated Mg concentrations.[31]

As discussed earlier in reference to the cardiac muscle cells, the depressant effects of increases in extracellular fluid (ECF) Mg on vascular smooth muscle can be ascribed to one or more of the following mechanisms.

Cell Membranes. Increased ECF Mg can

(a) Produce competitive displacement of Ca from the sarcolemmal binding site, reducing influx of Ca.[18,27,31]

(b) Increase resting membrane potential and stabilize the membrane by reducing permeability and excitability.

(c) Reduce K efflux by mechanism independent of the Ca-Mg antagonism.

Myofibrillar Proteins. Increased Mg can

(a) Decrease myosin ATPase activity as stimulated by Ca[29] either directly by inactivation or indirectly by augmenting the sequestration of Ca by the myofibrils.[23]

Table 2. Inhibitory Effects of Elevated Mg in the Medium on Tension Development by Smooth Muscle in Rat Aorta (Ref. 37)

Vasoactive Agent	n	Developed Tension, Mg±SEM Control Response 1.2 mM $[Mg^{++}]_o$	4.0 mM $[Mg^{++}]_o$
Epinephrine	4	606.3 ± 63.9	303.7 ± 56.8[a]
Angiotensin	4	450.0 ± 25.0	200.0 ± 25.0[a]
KCl	6	861.2 ± 65.3	270.0 ± 76.4[a]
Serotonin	4	475.0 ± 12.5	312.5 ± 43.7[a]
Ouabain	6	295.8 ± 58.5	54.2 ± 23.8[a]

[a] Significantly different from control values in 1.2 mM Mg^{++}-Kregs-Ringer

(b) Compete with Ca for common binding sites present in troponin (and perhaps myosin), altering its conformation and interaction (with tropomyosin) and interfering with cross bridge formation between actin and myosin, the biochemical equivalent of contraction.

Sarcoplasmic Reticulum (SR). Increased Mg can

(a) Increase influx of Ca into SR by increasing the activity of the Mg-dependent ATP-driven Ca pump.[25,32]
(b) Decrease efflux of Ca from SR.[25]
(c) Compete with Ca for myofilament space binding sites that regulate contraction, shifting the force-Ca relationship (Fig. 4).

These competitive events could mediate the uncoupling by Mg of the action potential (which continues) from intestinal smooth muscle contraction (which stops) (38). Through these effects and possibly through the Mg-dependent cyclic AMP mediated Ca sequestration, ECF Mg and membrane Mg exert important regulatory role in the control of Ca uptake, content and distribution in muscle cells and hence modulate their contraction and relaxation, the latter processes being the critical determinants of vascular tone, peripheral vascular resistance and therefore systemic blood pressure.

The reversal of the hypotensive,[4] vasodilatory[36] and muscular relaxant effects[27,37] of Mg by increases in medium, perfused or arterial Ca is compatible with this formulation. To exert some of these effects, changes in Mg concentration must be in millimolar rather than micromolar range in contrast to Ca.[27] In addition, Mg penetration into cells is a slow process, and intracellular ionized Mg is well buffered by cytosolic proteins and metabolic pools. The

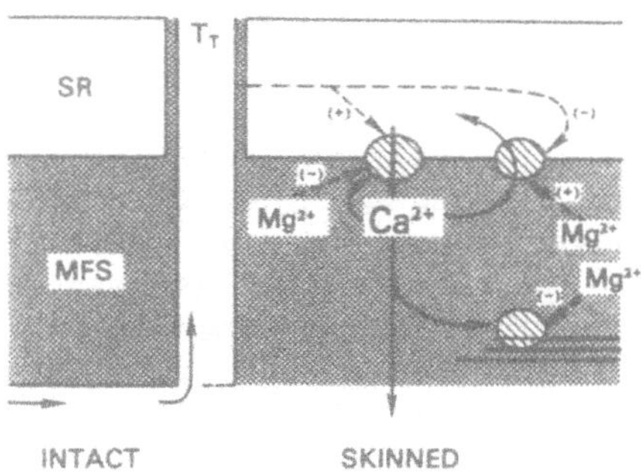

Fig. 4. Major sites of Ca^{++}-Mg^{++} interaction during activation of striated muscle. Mg^{++}, Ca^{++}, and depolarization can exert inhibitory (-) or stimulatory (+) effects on SR efflux channels, the SR active Ca transport system, or myofilament space (MFS) binding sites that regulate contraction.

acute rapid effects of hypermagnesemia therefore seem to be a consequence of interactions at the cytoplasmic and cytosolic membranes between Mg on the one hand and Ca, K and/or Na on the other hand. In brief, the bulk of data suggests that ganglionic blockade and membrane interference with Ca activation of muscle contraction play the most critical role in mediating the vasodilatory and antihypertensive effects of Mg loading. It should be pointed out that the magnitude of fall in blood pressure as produced by tolerable elevations in serum Mg is very modest[4,6] (Fig. 1). Although Mg is often used in the treatment of pre-eclampsia and eclampsia,[39,40] the reduction in blood pressure was not the primary indication and it was rarely achieved without specific antihypertensive agents.[39,40]

Chronic Effects of Mg

The hypotensive action of Mg infusion lasts only minutes[4,5,6] (Fig. 1). Although a sustained effect for up to 6 hours was implied in one early clinical study,[1] the lack of frequent serial monitoring precludes critical evaluation of the time course. There is a paucity of information regarding the chronic effects of Mg loading. To evaluate this issue, we fed a high Mg diet to adult spontaneous hypertensive rats (SHR) for 12 days and using the indirect tail cuff method compared their systolic blood pressure to that of similar rats fed a normal (0.04%) Mg diet. Over this period of time, the high and normal Mg groups gained comparable amounts of weight and experienced similar increases in blood pressure (168 to 187 torr vs 165 to 178 torr).[41] No alterations in the blood pressure could be found in rats orally loaded with Mg. Further augmentation of diet Mg to 0.50% for an additional 10 days failed to halt the progressive rise in blood pressure expected with age in these animals (22±4 vs 15±4 torr).[41] These preliminary data suggest that during chronic administration, the acute effects of Mg may be modified, offset or counterbalanced by some as yet undefined secondary adaptive changes.

The literature is similarly scant regarding the biochemical, physiologic or hemodynamic changes during chronic Mg administration. Increased Ca and PO_4 balance (primarily due to increases in net intestinal absorption) has been reported in adult rats fed a high Mg diet.[42,43] Whether these metabolic alterations would obscure an antihypertensive action by continued Mg loading cannot be determined without direct and specific studies.

Another possible explanation for the discrepancy between acute and chronic Mg loading is the fact that a hypertensive strain of rats was used in our experiments.[41] Preliminary data suggest blunted responsivity of the aortic smooth muscle in SHR to changes in medium Mg concentrations, when compared to normotensive Wistar Kyoto (WKY) control[31] (Table 3). Thus the expected increase in

Table 3. Influence of $[Mg^{++}]_o$ on Basal Tension in Aortas Isolated from WKY (control) and Spontaneously Hypertensive Rats (SHR)[a]

		Tension, mg ± SEM	
Rat	N	0 mM $[Mg^{++}]_o$	4.8 mM $[Mg^{++}]_o$
WKY	23	432.6 ± 33.6	-141.7 ± 14.5
SHR	23	127.0 ± 20.6[b]	-63.3 ± 13.8[b]

a Male rats 14-16 weeks old
b Significantly different from WKY controls ($p < 0.01$)

tension produced by the contraction of aortic smooth muscle when bathed in Mg free medium was only 30% of that in WKY. Conversely, the expected decrease in tension with high Mg medium was again only 40% of that in WKY, even though the basal contractile tension was higher in SHR.[31] Such differential sensitivity to acute alterations in medium Mg may explain the lack of effects with chronic Mg loading in SHR. Clearly, similar loading experiments in normotensive WKY rats will be helpful, as they are getting underway in our laboratory. Interestingly enough, the hypotensive action of hypermagnesemia is more pronounced in hypertensive subjects than the normal.[6]

The effect of chronic dietary Mg depletion on systemic blood pressure has been evaluated in one previous study.[44] In these young rats, Mg deficiency was associated with a significant reduction in tail cuff blood pressure (10 to 15 torr). Interpretation and extrapolation of these data are difficult since these Mg deprived rats were hypothermic and growth was arrested after 3 weeks of Mg deprivation, associated with structural and biochemical changes typical of Mg deficiency. It is therefore not possible to determine whether the effects on blood pressure were a direct result of decreased Mg balance.

In view of the fragmentory nature of information bearing on this issue, it is presently not feasible to define whether changes in Mg balance could lead to sustained changes in systemic blood pressure.

HYPERTENSION AFFECTIMG MG METABOLISM

The next issue of clinical and scientific interest relates to whether hypertension disturbs Mg homeostasis (Table 1). Little if any clinical or experimental data are available specifically evaluating this point. To vigorously document this point, it is necessary to examine Mg balance before and after hypertension is established. Unfortunately, if the SHR model is used, the growth and development associated with age would introduce other factors altering Mg absorption and excretion. The other approach is to compare Mg balance between hypertensive and normotensive subjects or rats, but to the best of our knowledge, this has not been performed or published. This latter approach of course could not define which precedes which, abnormality in Mg metabolism or hypertension, even if they were found to coexist.

Three indirect indices of Mg metabolism have, however, been examined. First, serum or plasma[49] Mg has been determined in hypertensive man[45-49] and rats.[50] Although an inverse correlation between blood pressure and serum Mg has been reported in normal elderly Danes,[51] conflicting results have been published in hypertensive subjects, including increases[45,46] no difference[49] or decreases.[46,47,48] It is not clear whether these divergent findings merely reflect patient heterogeneity with regard to renin profiling,[46] the presence of azotemia,[45] continuance or discontinuance of blood pressures treatment[47,49] and lean body weight or sex.[48] More importantly, the role of dietary intake of salt, vitamin D, Mg, and other related divalent ions was uncontrolled in these outpatient studies, making conclusions extremely difficult. Although increases in serum Mg were reported in a preliminary study of SHR, aged 11 to 17 weeks (1.54 vs 1.41 mg%),[50] this has not been confirmed by other studies, where low or normal values were found in the fasted hypertensive animals.[41] Clearly, the abnormality in serum Mg, if present in hypertension, is not settled.

Second, studies evaluating tissue content of Mg in hypertensive subjects also yielded similarly equivocal results. Post-mortem analysis of renal artery Mg content revealed no difference compared to normotensive subjects,[52] but information regarding the nature of the hypertension, prior treatment and clinical course culminating in deaths, is too scant to help evaluate these negative results. In a canine model of chronic renal vascular hypertension, arterial wall Mg was also found to be similar.[53] Similar to the hypomagnesemia and reduced Mg balance observed in mineralocorticoid-induced hypertension in man,[54,55] these structurally or hormonally induced models of hypertension may be quite different from the essential or genetic form.

Finally, one recent dietary survey suggests diminished intake of

Mg in hypertensive subjects (206 vs 261 mg/day).[56] The role of this dietary factor and the relevance of these data to the pathogenesis and maintenance of hypertension are obscure, especially when studies actually measuring urine and ingested Mg by duplicate portion techniques revealed no differences between hypertensive and normotensive women.[57]

It is obvious that existing data are too incomplete to evaluate whether essential hypertension is associated with abnormalities in Mg metabolism. Only balance studies in well-defined homogeneous patient populations could begin to shed light on this issue. Preliminary results from our laboratory using the SHR model suggest subtle intestinal malabsorption compared to the WKY control.[41] At comparable levels of ingested Mg, 40 week old SHR had mildly but significantly depressed net and fractional absorption of Mg (3.1 vs. 3.7 mg/day and 50 vs 61%, respectively). Although urine Mg excretion was not different, Mg retention (or balance) was significantly reduced in SHR (1.16 vs 1.93 mg/day). Similar results indicating diminished intestinal Mg absorption were found in the female SHR. The etiology of Mg malabsorption is unclear from these pilot studies. Likewise, the relationship between this abnormality and hypertension remains to be explored, although the lack of an attenuation in blood pressure during chronic Mg loading in these hypertensive rats[41] argues against a pathogenetic role of mild Mg deficiency. Accordingly only tentative conclusions can be drawn at present (Table 4).

In summary, although acute Mg loading depresses cardiac and smooth muscle cell functions and blocks neuromuscular transmission to produce a hypotensive effect,sustenance of these effects on a chronic basis remains to be established. Similarly, despite circumstantial and indirect evidence suggesting subtle abnormalities in Mg homeostasis in untreated essential or genetic hypertension, unequivocal data have yet to emerge. Until more interpretable results are available from balance studies in well defined groups, the cause and effect relationshiop between Mg deficiency and hypertension, if any, remains an unsettled issue.

ACKNOWLEDGEMENTS

The authors would like to thank Ms. C. Corson and Ms. E. Kabelka for secretarial assistance in the preparation of this manuscript. We also appreciate the technical assistance by Ms. B. Eby, J. Garno and D. Thomas in the experimental work. Thanks are also due to Dr. David Bohr for his generosity in loaning us the blood pressure machine. This work was supported by NIH Grant RO 1 AM 28035, and American Heart Association Grant 80-949. Dr. Lau is the recipient of a NIH RCDA K04 AM 00843.

Table 4. Tentative Conclusions Regarding Mg and Blood Pressure

1. Acute hypermagnesemia transiently decreases B.P., although the opposite effect of hypomagnesemia is more equivocal.
2. The hypotensive action of Mg is primarily mediated by sympathetic ganglionic blockade and peripheral vasodilatation.
3. The relaxant effect is due to depression by Mg on vascular smooth muscle tone, contractility and reactivity to agonists.
4. Most of these cellular actions of Mg are attributable to competitive interactions with Ca at the sarcolemmal membrane and in the sarcoplasmic reticulum.
5. By controlling Ca uptake, content and distribution in smooth muscle cells, Mg helps regulate vascular resistance and hence systemic B.P.
6. Chronic effects of Mg loading on B.P. are not demonstrable from preliminary studies in SHR, suggesting counterregulatory and/or offsetting adaptative changes.
7. Data on indirect indices of Mg metabolism in essential hypertension (serum, arterial and diet Mg) are conflicting, possibly due to patient heterogeneity.
8. Metabolic studies in SHR revealed intestinal Mg malabsorption and reduced Mg balance, but the relationship with hypertension is unclear.
9. The role of disturbances in Mg metabolism in the pathogenesis and/or maintenance of hypertension (and vice versa) await more studies for a full definition.

REFERENCES

1. K.D. Blackfan and B. Hamilton. Uremia in acute glomerular nephritis. Boston Med Surg J. 193(14):617-623 (1925).
2. S.J. Meltzer and J. Auer. Physiological and pharmacological studies of magnesium salts. III. The narcotizing effect of magnesium salts upon nerve fibers. Am. J. Physiol. 16:233-251 (1906).
3. S.A. Matthews and C. Brooks. On the action of magnesium sulfate. J. Pharmacol. & Exper. Therap. 2:87-99 (1910).
4. G.M. Maxwell, R.B. Elliott, and R.H. Burnell. Effects of hypermagnesemia on general and coronary hemodynamics of the dog. Am. J. Physiol. 208(1):158-161 (1965).
5. H.E. Hoff, P.K. Smith, and A.W. Winkler. The Relation of blood pressure and concentration in serum of potassium, calcium and magnesium. Am J. Physiol. 127:722-729 (1939).
6. W.J. Mroczek, W.R. Lee, and M.E. Davidov. Effect of magnesium sulfate on cardiovascular hemodynamics. Angiology. 28:720-724 (1977).

7. T.E. Emerson, J.B. Scott and F.J. Haddy. Effects of acute multiple changes in plasma electrolyte levels on dog blood pressure. Am J Physiol. 218:234-240 (1970).
8. F.J. Haddy, J.B. Scott, M.A. Florio, R.M. Daugherty, Jr., and J.N. Huizenga. Local vascular effects of hypokalemia, alkalosis, hypercalcemia, and hypomagnesemia. Am. J. Physiol. 204(2):202-212 (1963).
9. F.J. Haddy and J.B. Scott. Mechanism of the acute pressor action of hypokalemia, hypomagnesemia, and hypo-osmolality. Am Heart J. 83(5):655-661 (1973).
10. D.K. Anderson, S.A. Roth, R.A. Brace, D. Radowski, F.J. Haddy, and J.B. Scott. Effect of hypokalemia and hypomagnesemia produced by hemodialysis on vascular resistance in canine skeletal muscle. Circulation Research. 31:165-173 (1972).
11. W.J. Hoppe and T.E. Emerson. Effects of hemodialysis-induced hypokalemia and hypomagnesemia on blood pressure in dogs. Am Heart J. 88(2):198-204 (1974).
12. I. Leusen. The influence of calcium, potassium and magnesium ions in cerebrospinal fluid on vasomotor system. J. Physiol. 110:319-329 (1949).
13. J.B. Stanbury. The blocking action of magnesium on sympathetic ganglia. J. Pharmacol. & Exper. Therap. 93:52-62 (1948).
14. L.E. Ford and R.J. Podolsky. Intracellular calcium movements in skinned muscle fibres. J. Physiol. London. 223:21-33 (1972).
15. A. Fabiato and F. Fabiato. Effects of magnesium on contractile activation of skinned cardiac cells. J. Physiol. London. 249:497-517 (1975).
16. K.I. Shine and A.M. Douglas. Magnesium effects on ionic exchange and mechanical function in rat ventricle. Am. J. Physiol. 227:317-324 (1974).
17. W. Vierling, F. Ebner, and M. Reiter. The opposite effects of magnesium and calcium on the contraction of the guinea-pig ventricular myocardium in dependence on the sodium concentration. Arch. Pharmacol. 303:111-119 (1978).
18. G.A. Langer, S.D. Serena, and L.M. Nudd. Cation exchange in heart cell culture: correlation with effects on contractile force. J. Mol. Cell. Cardiol. 6:149-161 (1974).
19. M.R. Bristow, J.R. Daniels, R.S. Kernoff, and D.C. Harrison. Effect of D 600, practolol, and alterations in magnesium on ionized calcium concentration-response relationships in the intact dog. Circ. Res. 41:574-581 (1977).
20. J.B. Stanbury and A. Farah. Effects of magnesium ion on the heart and on its response to digoxin. J. Pharmacol. Exp. Ther. 100:445-453 (1950).
21. B.M. Paddle and N. Haugaard. Role of magnesium in effects of epinephrine on heart contraction and metabolism. Am J Physiol. 221(4):1178-1184 (1971).

22. J.P. Reuben, P.W. Brandt, M. Berman, and H. Grundfest. Regulation of tension in the skinned crayfish muscle fiber. J. Gen. Physiol. 57:385-407 (1971).
23. R.J. Solaro and J. Shiner. Modulation of Ca^{++} control of dog and rabbit cardiac myofibrils by Mg^{++}. Circ. Res. 39:8-14 (1976).
24. T. Kovacs and J.M. O'Donnell. An analysis of calcium-magnesium antagonism in contractility and ionic balance in isolated trabecular muscle of rat ventricle. Pfluegers Arch. 360:267-282 (1975).
25. E.W. Stephenson. Magnesium effects on activation of skinned fibers from striated muscle. Federation Proceedings. 40(12):2662-2666 (1981).
26. D.F. Bohr. Electrolytes and smooth muscle contraction. Pharmacological Reviews. 16:85-111 (1964).
27. K.I. Shine. Myocardial effects of magnesium. Am. J. Physiol. 237(4):H413-H423 (1979).
28. P.K. Smith, A.W. Winkler and H.E. Hoff. Electrocardiographic changes and concentrations of magnesium in serum following intravenous injection of magnesium salts. Am. J. Physiol. 126:720-730 (1939).
29. L. Engbaek. The pharmacological actions of magnesium ions with particular reference to the neuromuscular and the cardiovascular system. Pharm Review. 4:396-414 (1952).
30. V.G. Haury. The effect of intravenous injections of magnesium sulfate in the vascular system. J. Pharmacol. & Exper. Therap. 65:453-460 (1939).
31. B.M. Altura and B.T. Altura. Magnesium ions and contraction of vascular smooth muscles: relationship to some vascular diseases. Federation Proceedings. 40(12):2672-2679 (1981).
32. W. Hasselbach, E. Fassold, A. Migala, and B. Rauch. Magnesium dependence of sarcoplasmic reticulum calcium transport. Federation Proceedings. 40(12):2657-2661 (1981).
33. J.D. Potter, S.P. Robertson, and J.D. Johnson. Magnesium and the regulation of muscle contraction. Federation Proceedings. 40(12):2653-2656 (1981).
34. H.W. Overbeck, R.M. Daughtery, and F.J. Haddy. Response of the human upper extremity vascular bed to intrabrachial arterial infusions of magnesium sulfate and hypotonic sodium chloride solusions. The Physiologist. 9:258(abstract) (1966).
35. E.D. Frohlich, J.B. Scott, and F.J. Haddy. Effect of cations on resistance and responsiveness of renal and forelimb vascular beds. Am. J. Physiol. 203(3):583-587 (1962).
36. H. Viveros and G.G. Somjen. Magnesium-calcium antagonism in the contraction of arterioles. Experimentia. 24(5):457-459 (1968).
37. B.M. Altura and B.T. Altura. Magnesium and vascular tone and reactivity. Blood Vessels. 15:5-16 (1978).
38. N. Sperelakis. Contraction of depolarized smooth muscle by electric fields. Am. J. Physiol. 202:731-742 (1962).

39. L.C. Chesley and I. Tepper. Plasma levels of magnesium attained in magnesium sulfate therapy for preeclampsia and eclampsia. Surgical Clinics of North Am. 37:353-367 (1957).
40. C.E. Flowers, Jr. Magnesium sulfate in obstetrics. Am. J. Obst. & Gynec. 91(6):763-776 (1965).
41. C. Oasa, B. Eby, and K. Lau. Mg metabolism in spontaneous hypertensive rats: Effects of chronic Mg loading. Clinical Research. 31(4):abstract (1983).
42. I. Clark and L. Belanger. The effects of alterations in dietary magnesium on calcium, phosphate and skeletal metabolism. Calc. Tiss. Res. 1:204-218 (1967).
43. I. Clark. Effects of magnesium ions on calcium and phosphorus metabolism. Am J Physiol. 244(2):348-356 (1968).
44. Y. Itokawa, C. Tanaka, and M. Fujiwara. Changes in body temperature and blood pressure in rats with calcium and magnesium defiencies. J Applied Physiol. 37(6):835-839 (1974).
45. E.D. Frohlich. Plasma sodium, potassium, calcium, and magnesium concentrations in essential hypertension. Am. J. Med. Sci. 248:419 (1964).
46. L.M. Resnick, J.P. Nicholson, J.E. Sealey, and J.H. Laragh. Acute and long-term effects of calcium channel blockade on divalent ions, blood pressure and plasma activity. Clin Res. 30(2):253A (1983).
47. D.G. Albert, Y. Morita, and L.T. Iseri. Serum magnesium and plasma sodium levels in essential vascular hypertension. Circulation. 17:761-764 (1958).
48. F.K. Bauer, H.E. Martin, and M.R. Mickey. Exchangeable magnesium in hypertension. Proc. Soc. Expt. Biol. Med. 120:466-468 (1965).
49. R.H. Seller, O. Ramirez-Muxo, A.N. Brest, and J.H. Moyer. Magnesium metabolism in hypertension. JAMA, 191(8):118-120 (1965).
50. D.A. McCarron. Impaired nephrogenous cAMP response in the spontaneously hypertensive rat. Proceedings of the 15th Annual Meeting of the Am. Soc. Neph., p13A, 1982, Chicago.
51. B. Petersen, M. Schroll, C. Christiansen, and I.B. Transbol. Serum and erythrocyte magnesium in normal elderly danish people. Acta Med Scan. 201:31-34 (1977).
52. L. Tobian and J.T. Binion. Tissue cations and water in arterial hypertension. Circulation. 5:754-758 (1952).
53. G.M. Fischer, E.I. Mata, and J.G. Llaurado. Regional differences in magnesium, calcium, and zinc composition of arterial wall in normal and hypertensive dogs. Am Heart J. 75(6):784-789 (1968).
54. I.J. Mader and L.T. Iseri. Spontaneous hypopotassemia, hypomagnesemia, alkalosis and tetany due to hypersecretion of corticosterone-like mineralocorticoid. Am. J. Med. 19:976-988 (1955).

55. M.D. Milne, R.C. Muehrcke, and I. Aird. Primary aldosteronism. Quart. J. Med. 26:319-333 (1957).
56. D.A. McCarron, C.D. Morris, and C. Cole. Dietary calcium in human hypertension. Science. 217:267-269 (1982).
57. T. Thulin, M. Abdulla, I. Dencker, M. Jagerstad, A. Melander, A. Norden, B. Schersten, and B. Akesson. Comparison of energy and nutrient intakes in women with high and low blood pressure levels. Acta Med Scan. 208:367-373 (1980).

PARATHORMONE AND BLOOD PRESSURE IN THE SPONTANEOUSLY HYPERTENSIVE RAT

Johannes F.E. Mann, Jürgen Bommer, Willi Kreusser, Peter Klooker, Michael Rambausek and Eberhard Ritz

Department of Medicine, University of Heidelberg
6900 Heidelberg, Germany

In the present communication we report on the influence of parathormone deficiency on blood pressure development in genetic, spontaneously (SH) hypertensive rats. In our study, a group of SH rats were parathyroidectomized and fed a diet with high calcium content in order to assure normal serum calcium levels.
In a second experiment, normotensive, Wistar Kyoto (WK) rats were investigated under identical conditions. In a third experiment, parathyroidectomized WK rats and sham-operated WK rats were compared, when both groups were on a high dietary calcium intake.
In all rats, parathyroidectomy (PTX) (under the dissecting microscope),or sham-operation (SO) ,were done at 4 weeks of age. 5 days after surgery, hypocalcemia was present in all PTX-rats. All surgery was done under light ether anesthesia. The PTX group was then placed on a high dietary calcium intake and SO-rats continued on a normal diet. However, in the third experiment, SO-WK rats also received the diet with high calcium content. Two-three months after surgery, blood volume was determined by the Evans-blue dilution method. One week later, chronic arterial catheters were placed in the abdominal aorta via the femoral artery. The catheters were placed under the skin to exit at the neck. One day later, direct arterial blood pressure was monitored in the conscious, freely moving rats (1). With the high dietary calcium regime, serum calcium was normalized in all PTX-rats. Resting mean arterial blood pressure was 41 mmHg lower in PTX-SH-rats than in SO-

SH rats. Blood volume was significantly expanded after PTX in SH rats by 7.2%.

As compared to SH rats, mean arterial pressure was by more than 70mmHg lower in WK rats. Furthermore, mean arterial blood pressure was by 18 mmHg lower in PTX-WK than in SO-WK rats. Blood volume was greater in WK- than in SH rats, and was increased in PTX-WK rats by 10.7% as compared to SO-WK rats. When SO-WK- and PTX-WK rats were both on a diet with high calcium content, no changes for mean arterial blood pressure or blood volume could be detected.

Our data demonstrate that chronic parathormone deficiency may impede blood pressure development in eucalcemic SH rats. It is noteworthy that acute i.v. injection of parathormone induces a remarkable vasodilatation and a fall of arterial blood pressure (2). It is unknown, however, whether this acute pharmacological effect has any physiological relevance, since extremely high doses of parathormone have to be given in order to lower blood pressure in vivo. One explanation for our findings would be that parathormone has either a long-term vasoconstrictive action of its own or a permissive effect on the activity of other vasopressor hormones. Preliminary evidence from our laboratory indicates that plasma levels of angiotensin II and nor - epinephrine are unchanged after PTX (unpublished). However, the responsiveness of arterial resistance vessels has not been tested so far.

The expansion of blood volume following PTX points to increased vascular capacitance in the latter group. This argues against the contention that parathormone has a permissive effect on blood pressure by sodium- and volume retention.

Apart from parathormone we must consider high dietary calcium intake as a further variable. This point is important, since increased dietary calcium has been shown to lower blood pressure in SH rats (3). In the present experiment, we chose to supplement oral calcium to PTX-SH rats in order to assure normal serum calcium concentrations. Hypocalcemia may have its own effects on blood pressure (4). Although serum calcium concentration was not different between PTX- and SO-SH rats, calcium turnover and urinary excretion were obviously enhanced in the PTX group. The last experiment, in fact, showed that the high dietary calcium intake indeed may explain in part the differences in blood pressure we observed between groups. Further experiments will show, whether the effects of calcium and of parathormone on blood pressure can be dissociated from each other.

References

1. Mann, J.F.E., Phillips, M.I., Dietz, R., Haebara, H.: Am. J. Physiol. 234, H629-H637, 1978
2. Pany, P.K.T., Tenner, T.E., Yee, J.A., Yang, M.: PNAS 77, 675-678, 1980
3. Ayashi, S.: Metabolism 29, 1234-1238, 1979
4. Rambausek, M., Ritz, E., Rascher, W., Kreusser, W.: Adv. Exp. Med. Biol. 151, 619, 1982

TRIFLUOPERAZINE ATTENUATION OF PTH-INDUCED VASODILATION IN THE SPONTANEOUSLY HYPERTENSIVE RAT

David A. McCarron and James R. Grady

Division of Nephrology/Hypertension
Oregon Health Sciences University
Portland, Oregon 97201

ABSTRACT

Transmembrane Ca^{2+} fluxes and the Ca^{2+}-calmodulin binding have been implicated in PTH's acute vascular effects in experimental animals. To evaluate that postulate, we determined the influence of the calmodulin inhibitor, trifluoperazine (TFP), on the acute BP response to human PTH 1-34 of 18-week-old spontaneously hypertensive rats (SHR). Human PTH 1-34 was administered intravenously at doses of either 5 or 10 μg/kg. TFP 0.1 mg/kg was then given following recovery to baseline BP. Then hPTH 1-34 (5 μg/kg or 10 μg/kg) was again administered at both 1- and 30-minute intervals after TFP.

Human PTH 1-34 at both the 5 μg/kg ($p<.005$) and 10 μg/kg dose ($p<.001$) produced acute hypotension. The hemodynamic response was maximal at 1 minute and lasted up to 30 minutes. TFP significantly reduced the maximal (Δ MAP) hypotensive response for the 5 μg/kg ($p<.02$) and for the 10 μg/kg PTH dose ($p<.02$). When PTH was administered 30 minutes after TFP, the acute vasodepressive response was again inhibited in the SHRs who received the 5 μg/kg ($p<.02$) dose and in those who received the 10 μg/kg dose ($p<.01$). At the 10 μg/kg dose, TFP's inhibition of PTH-induced vasodilation not only impaired the 1-minute maximal response, but accelerated the return to baseline blood pressure. Human PTH's (1-34) vascular actions in the SHR appear to require the integrity of the Ca^{2+}-calmodulin system.

INTRODUCTION

When administered to a variety of species and/or injected into various organ systems, parathyroid hormone (PTH) and several of its analogs produce acute vasodilation.[1-6] The peptide lowers vascular resistance without significantly modifying cardiac output.[1,5] The cardiovascular actions of the hormone are specific since adrenergic, cholinergic and histaminergic blockade do not alter the peptide's vasodilating actions.[13] PTH's known effect on cellular Ca^{2+} fluxes[7-9], as well as the dependence of its vasodilation on the state of Ca^{2+} balance[10] in experimental animals, suggest that cytosolic Ca^{2+} and/or the calcium-calmodulin complex[11,12] contribute to cellular mechanisms that mediate the peptide's vasodepressive action. We addressed that hypothesis by measuring the effect of trifluoperazine (TFP),[11,13,14] a calmodulin inhibitor, on the vasodilatory response to acutely administered hPTH 1-34 in the spontaneously hypertensive rat (SHR).

METHODS

Eight male Aoki-Okamoto SHRs were raised on a synthetic rat chow (1% Ca^{2+} by weight) (Teklad, Madison, WI) until 18 to 20 weeks of age. The rats were anesthetized with intraperitoneal ketamine HCL (100 mg/kg Ketalar®) and PE_{50} polyethylene catheters were placed in the left jugular vein and left carotid arteries. Blood pressure was measured directly via Statham transducer on a Gilson MP5 physiograph.

Synthetic human PTH 1-34 (Peninsula Labs, San Carlos, CA) was reconstituted with Tris-HCL buffer containing 10% BSA to a strength of 100 µg PTH/ml and stored frozen in plastic vials. Aliquots were thawed as needed and dilutions made with 0.9% saline. Human PTH 1-34 was injected via the venous catheter in a dose of 5 µg/kg to four SHRs, and 10 µg/kg to the remaining four SHRs. The blood pressure was allowed to return to baseline at which time trifluroperazine (TFP), 0.1 mg/kg, was injected IV. One minute following the TFP, a repeat injection of hPTH 1-34 was given. Systolic, diastolic and mean blood pressures were recorded at 1-minute following each injection, and then at 3-minute intervals until it had returned to baseline. At 30 minutes a repeat injection of hPTH 1-34 was given and blood pressure was recorded in an identical manner. T statistics, analysis of variance and linear regression analysis were used in the statistical analysis of the data.

RESULTS

The mean (±SEM) weight of the SHRs was 326 grams ±6. Their opening mean arterial pressure (MAP) (±SEM) averaged 196±9 mmHg.

Both the 5 μg/kg (p<.005) and 10 μg/kg (p<.001) doses produced acute hypotension that was maximal at 1 minute and lasted up to 30 minutes (Tables 1 and 2). The SHR's maximal change in mean arterial pressure (Δ MAP) was -51±9 mmHg at 5 μg/kg (Table 1) and -80±5 mmHg at 10 μg/kg (Table 2).

When TFP was injected there was a transient (<1 minute) decrease in MAP (-25±2.8 mmHg, p<.001). Tables 1 and 2 show Δ MAP at 1,3,6,9,12 and 15 minutes after the various injections of PTH. Table 1 depicts the results using 5 μg/kg of hPTH (1-34), while Table 2 depicts the Δ MAP for the 10 μg/kg dose. TFP significantly reduced (p<.02) the maximal -Δ MAP response (-51.3±8.9 vs. -36.2±5.6 mmHg) for the 5 μg/kg dose given 1 minute after the TFP. For the 10 μg/kg PTH dose given 1 minute after TFP, the Δ MAP response (-80.0±5.0 vs. -51.2±4.3) was also significantly (p<.02) blunted. PTH-induced vasodilation 30 minutes after TFP was again diminished in the SHRs who received the 5 μg/kg dose (-51.3±8.9 vs. 33.7±8.8 mmHg, p<.02), as well as those who received the 10 μg/kg dose (-80.0±5.0 vs. -41.3±6.3 mmHg/ p<.01). With the 10 μg/kg dose of PTH, TFP's inhibition was greater (-51.2±4.3 mmHg at 1 minute vs. -41.3±6.3 mmHg at 30 minutes, p<.05) when the PTH was administered at the 30-minute interval than when given at the 1-minute interval. In addition at the 10 μg/kg dose of hPTH (1-34), TFP not only reduced the maximal Δ MAP response, but also accelerated the SHR's return to baseline blood pressures (p<.01).

TABLE 1

Vasodepressive Response To 5 μg/kg PTH
(Δ MAP - mmHg ± SEM)
Time Post-Injection

	1 Min.	3 Min.	6 Min.	9 Min.	12 Min.	15 Min.
PTH Alone	51.3±8.9	25±2.9	16.3±2.4	8.8±3.8	5.0±2.1	2.5±1.5
PTH 1 Min. After TFP	36.2±5.6	23±3.3	11.3±3.8	6.3±3.8	5.0±2.9	1.3±1.3
PTH 30 Min. After TFP	33.7±8.8	20±3.6	13.8±2.4	6.3±3.8	5.0±3.6	2.5±2.5

TABLE 2

Vasodepressive Response To 10 μg/kg PTH
(Δ MAP - mmHg ± SEM)
Time Post-Injection

	1 Min.	3 Min.	6 Min.	9 Min.	12 Min.	15 Min.
PTH Alone	80.0±5.0	65.0±8.4	39.0±8.4	31.2±8	20.0±4.6	6.3±4.8
PTH 1 Min. After TFP	51.2±4.3	18.8±4.3	15.0±4.1	8.8±2.4	5.0±3.6	2.5±2.5
PTH 30 Min. After TFP	41.3±6.3	23.0±2.3	16.0±3.8	9.2±4.0	5.0±2.1	2.5±1.5

DISCUSSION

In the SHR, human PTH 1-34 produces log dose-dependent vasodilation.[1] The hypotension is rapid in onset, and is maximal at 1 minute. Consistent with the peptide's known half life, the vasodilatory response persists from 15 to 30 minutes.[1] For PTH's vascular action the peptide's structural pre-requisites are similar to those required for its phosphaturic effects.[15] The first two amino terminal residues are required as well as maintenance of the tertiary structure of the 1-34 fragment. PTH principally lowers vascular resistance without significantly modifying cardiac output.[5] The hormone's effect on resistance appears to be specific, as other vasoactive substances and their agonists and antagonists do not modify the hypotensive response induced by the peptide.[16]

The current results demonstrate that the calcium binding protein inhibitor, TFP, reduces the vasodepressive actions of hPTH 1-34 in the SHR. Under the conditions of this experimental design, the inhibition was evident within 1 minute and demonstratable up to 30 minutes after the TFP. The Δ MAP response of the SHR to hPTH 1-34 was significantly reduced both at 1 minute and 30 minutes post-TFP. At the dose of 10 μg/kg of hPTH 1-34, there was significantly greater inhibition at 30 minutes than at 1 minute ($p<.05$). Not only was the maximal Δ MAP response at 1 minute reduced, but the rate of return to baseline blood pressure was accelerated.

In a variety of cell membranes PTH is known to enhance calcium fluxes.[7,8,9,17] Via such an ionophoric action, PTH may induce alterations in cytosolic calcium which mediate smooth muscle relaxation.[11,18] A non-peptide ionophore has been shown to produce comparable cardiovascular effects.[19] Acting as an ionophore, hPTH (1-34) would induce an increase in intracellular calcium. This effect of the peptide would be distinct from the more graded increase evoked by the Ca^{2+} influx via the membrane-inbedded slow channels.

Within the cell membrane Ca^{2+} is bound to phospholipids. The calcium ionophoric effect of PTH has been related to the hormone's activation of the phosphatidate-polyphosphoinositide pathway.[18] Following exposure to PTH there is an increase in phospholipid turnover.[18] As a result, membrane-bound calcium is released intracellularly.[20] Such a rapid influx of Ca^{2+} and rise in cytosolic calcium, has been postulated to increase Ca^{2+} binding to calmodulin.[11,12] The protein's ubiquitous distribution and highly conserved structure have been interpreted to suggest a fundamental role for it in the mediation of calcium's action in cellular regulation.[21] The cation and calmodulin have multiple cellular functions, including activation of adenylate cyclase and cyclic nucleotide phosphodiesterase, as well as various protein kinases.[21] Principally of interest here, is calmodulin's function as a transducer of Ca^{2+} regulation of the contractile apparatus of vascular smooth muscle cells.[22]

The Ca^{2+}-calmodulin complex modulates at least three intracellular events that control the state of smooth muscle relaxation. First, it activates both plasma and vesicle membrane pumps[11,12] that serve to restore cytosolic free Ca^{2+} to its basal level. Ca^{2+} efflux rates across membranes may ultimately exceed those of influx, and intracellular free Ca^{2+} is reduced.[11,12] Second, the Ca^{2+}-calmodulin complex stimulates the phosphorylation of the enzyme, myosin light-chain kinase (MLCK).[11,12] Normally, MLCK catalyzes the phosphorylation of the contractile protein, myosin light chain.[11,12] When phosphorylated, however, MLCK is significantly less active in catalyzing the crossbridge linking of the contractile proteins, actin-myosin, than is the non-phosphorylated form of MLCK.[11,12] Third, since Ca^{2+} binding to calmodulin is non-linear and increases after the initial cation sites are filled, the rapid rise of intracellular Ca^{2+} that follows an ionophoric action, as opposed to stimulation of Ca^{2+} fluxes through the slow channels, may actually result in a seemingly paradoxical fall in free Ca^{2+} intracellularly.[12] Thus, via reductions in cytosolic free Ca^{2+} by activating membrane pumps through phosphorylation of MLCK, and a subsequent reduction in its enzymatic rate constant, and/or acceleration of cation binding to calmodulin, PTH's calcium-ionophoric action may yield smooth muscle relaxation.

Trifluoperazine (TFP) selectively binds calmodulin at high-affinity, Ca^{2+}-dependent sites and inhibits its subsequent activity in test systems studied, for example, activation of phosphodiesterase.[13,14] TFP's use in the current experiment was predicated on this inhibition of the activity of the Ca^{2+}-calmodulin complex and the postulated mode of PTH's vascular actions. TFP and related phenothiazines, by binding calmodulin, prevent cation-complex formation and the consequent activation of intracellular enzyme systems, in this case ones which may be crucial to the expression of PTH's vasodilating effects. The results of this study are consistent with calmodulin's involvement in the SHR's vasodilating response to hPTH 1-34.

The SHR exhibits multiple abnormalities related to calcium metabolism including changes in the cation's distribution in the sarcolemina of vascular smooth muscle and in the myocardial sarcoplasmic reticulum. These may reflect a widespread alteration in cell membranes, specifically a change in their calcium binding ability.[23-25] Microsomal fractions have been shown to accumulate more calcium in the SHR than in controls.[26] These alterations in Ca^{2+} transport and membrane adherence may reflect several defects or one fundamental disorder of intracellular Ca^{2+} metabolism.

The specific sites of increased calcium binding are not known. Membrane phospholipid metabolism is also abnormal in the SHR and has been implicated in the animal's disordered membrane calcium kinetics.[27] In light of these disturbances of cellular calcium, the fact that TFP modified PTH's vascular actions in the SHR suggest that altered calcium binding protein may be a central defect in this animal model of human hypertension. The SHR's membrane-bound calmodulin may be, in part, responsible for the animal's identified defects in vascular smooth muscle cell membrane calcium metabolism, and the SHR's abnormalities in regulation of vascular resistance.

In summary, synthetic human PTH 1-34 produces an acute reduction in mean arterial pressure in the SHR. The SHR's vasodepressive response to hPTH (1-34) is partially inhibited by the calmodulin inhibitor, trifluoperazine. In the SHR, the cellular mechanisms mediating PTH-induced vasodilation are modified by the action of the calmodulin inhibitor, trifluoperazine.

ACKNOWLEDGEMENTS

Dr. Grady is a recipient of a National Kidney Foundation Fellowship and an N.L. Tarter Fellowship. Grants-in-aid from the American Heart Association and the M.J. Murdock Charitable Trust, as well as a Training Grant from the Oregon Affiliate of the American Heart Association, supported this research. We are indebted to Janet Dorow for technical assistance and to Joni Utterback for preparing the manuscript.

REFERENCES

1. D.A. McCarron, D.H. Ellison, and S.A. Anderson, Vasodilation mediated by human PTH 1-34 in the spontaneously hypertensive rat, Am. J. Physiol. 246(Renal Fluid Electrolyte Physiol 15):F96-F100 (1984).
2. G.A. Charbon, and P.F. Hulsteart, Augmentation of arterial and hepatic blood flow by extracted and synthetic parathyroid hormone, Endocrin. 95:621 (1974).
3. M.F. Crass, and P.K.T. Pang, Parathyroid hormone: a coronary artery vasodilator, Science 217:1087 (1980).
4. A. Lindner, J.A. Tremann, J. Plantier, W. Chapman, A.W. Farrey, G. Hanes, and G.M. Palmier, Effects of parathyroid hormone on the renal circulation in unanesthetized dogs, Min. Electrol. Metab. 1:155-165 (1978).
5. P.K.T. Pang, H.F. Janssen, and J.A. Yee, Effects of synthetic parathyroid hormone on vascular beds of dogs, Pharmacologist 217:213 (1980).
6. P.K.T. Pang, M. Yang, C. Oguro, J.G. Phillips, and J.A. Yee, Hypotensive actions of parathyroid hormone preparations in vertebrates, Gen. Comp. Endocrinol. 41:135-138 (1980).
7. A.B. Borle, Calcium metabolism at the cellular level, Fed. Proc. 32:1944-1950 (1973).
8. J.A. Parsons, R.M. Peer, and J.T. Polts, Initial fall of plasma calcium after intravenous injection of parathyroid hormone, Endocrin. 89:735-740 (1971).
9. H. Rasmassen, Calcium and cAMP stimuli-response coupling, Ann. NY Acad. Sci. 356:346-353 (1980).
10. S.A. Anderson, J.R. Grady, D.H. Ellison, and D.A. McCarron, Ca^{2+} balance and parathyroid hormone-mediated vasodilation in the SHR, Hypertens. 5:I-59-I-63 (1983).
11. H. Kuriyama, Y. Ito, H. Suzuti, K. Kitamura, and T. Itoh, Factors modifying contraction-relaxation cycle in vascular smooth muscle, Am. J. Physiol. 243:H641-H662 (1982).
12. H. Rasmussen, Cellular calcium metabolism, Ann. Intern. Med. 98:809-816 (1983).
13. R.M. Levin, and B. Weiss, Selective binding of anti-psychotics and other psychoactive agents to the calcium-dependent activation of cyclic nucleotide phosphodiesterase, J. Pharmac. Exp. Ther. 208:454 (1979).
14. R.M. Levin, and B. Weiss, Binding of trifluoperazine to the calcium-dependent activation of cyclic nucleotide phosphodiesterase, Molec. Pharmac. 13:690 (1977).
15. D.H. Ellison, and D.A. McCarron, Structural prerequisites of parathyroid hormone's hypotensive action, Am. J. Physiol. (in press).

16. P.K.T. Pang, T.E. Tenner, J.A. Yee, M. Yang, and H.F. Janseen, Hypotensive action of parathyroid hormone preparations on rats and dogs, Proc. Nat. Acad. Sci. 77:675-678 (1980).
17. R. Schleiffer, A. Berthelot, and A. Gainard, Action of parathyroid extract on arterial pressure and on contraction and $^{45}Ca^{++}$ exchanged in isolated aorta of the rat. Eur. J. Pharm. 58:163-167 (1978).
18. R.V. Farese, Phosphoinositide metabolism and hormone action, Endocrin. Rev. 4:78-95 (1983).
19. M.W. Osborn, F. Kouzelove, M.R. Cohen, and J.J. Wenger, Bromolasalocid (Ro 20-0006) anti-hypertensive ionophore, Fed. Proc. 42:191-195 (1983).
20. R.L. Rubin, Calcium-phospholipid interactions in secretory cells: a new perspective on stimulus-secretion coupling, Fed. Proc. 41:2181-2187 (1982).
21. L.J. VanEldik, J.G. Zendegui, D.R. Marshak, and D.M. Watterson, Calcium-binding proteins and the molecular basis for calcium action, Int. Rev. Cytol. 77:1-51 (1982).
22. C.B. Klee, and T.C. Vanaman, Calmodulin, in: "Advances in Protein Chemistry," Academic, New York (1982).
23. M.A. Devynck, M.G. Penollet, A.M. Muney, and P. Meger, Analysis of calcium handling in erythrocyte membranes of genetically hypertensive rats, Hypertens. 3:397-403 (1981).
24. Y.N. Postnov, and S.N. Orlov, Evidence of altered calcium accumulation and calcium binding by the membranes of adipocytes in spontaneously hypertensive rats, Pflügers Arch. 385:85-89 (1980).
25. Y.N. Postnov, S.N. Orlov, and N.I. Potodin, Decrease in calcium binding by red blood cell membranes in spontaneously hypertensive rats and essential hypertension, Pflügers Arch. 379:191-195 (1979).
26. R.C. Webb, and R.C. Bhalla, Altered calcium sequestration by subcellular fractions of vascular smooth muscle from spontaneously hypertensive rats, J. Molec. Cell Cardiol. 8:651-661 (1976).
27. S. Koutouzoo, P. Marche, J.F. Cloix, and P. Meyer, Phospholipid phosphorylation in erythrocyte of spontaneously hypertensive rats, Am. J. Physiol. 243 (Heart Circ Physiol 12):H641-H662 (1982).

EVIDENCE OF bPTH-(1-34) SENSITIVE ADENYLATE CYCLASE IN ISOLATED RABBIT RENAL CORTEX ARTERIOLES

J.J. Helwig[(1)], C. Judes[(2)], R. Schleiffer and A. Gairard
Laboratoire Leriche, Pav. Poincaré, Hospices Civils and Laboratoire Physiologie, (ERA CNRS 787), Fac. Pharmacie
Université Louis Pasteur, Strasbourg, France

INTRODUCTION

Current evidence suggest that parathyroid hormone (PTH), regulates Ca homeostasis by activating kidney and bone adenylate cyclase. In addition to this action, PTH has physiological effects, on the cardiovascular system. The synthetic 1-34 fragment of bovine PTH shows direct hypotensive action in the anesthetized dog (1). Extracted and synthetic PTH increases the arterial blood flow of renal and hepatic arteries (2). It has also been reported that PTH relaxes rat aortic strip *in vitro* to a slight but significant degree (3) and that parathyroid extract acts on arterial blood pressure, contraction and ^{45}Ca exchange in isolated rat aorta (4). The question that arises is whether or not PTH affects adenylate cyclase activity of isolated vascular and microvascular beds. It has also been just reported that bPTH-(1-34) stimulates adenylate cyclase in rat cerebral microvessels in much the same way as in the renal cortex (5). In a recent work (6) we described a successful method for isolating rabbit renal cortical and preglomerular arterioles characterized by their high renin content and the enrichment of the muscle-specific enzyme creatin-kinase. The present work examined the possible effect of bPTH-(1-34) on adenylate cyclase of such microvessels which play an important role in the renal and peripheral hemodynamic and glomerulo-tubular feed-back control.

---

1) Chargé de Recherches à l'INSERM
2) Chargé de Recherches au CNRS.

MATERIALS AND METHODS

[2,8 ^{3}H] cyclic AMP (31,5 Ci/mmol) and [α^{32}P] ATP (10-50 Ci/mmol) were purchased from New England Nuclear (Boston, MA). [Nleu^{8,18},tyr^{14}]-bovine parathyroid hormone (3-34)-amide [bPTH-(3-34)], lot R6149, was purchased from Bachem (Torrance, CA, USA) and bPTH-(1-34), lot 003052, from Peninsula laboratories Inc. (San Carlos, CA, USA).

Isolation of renal cortex arterioles

Renal cortical arterioles were prepared from rabbit (2,8 - 4 kg) according to the procedure of Helwig et al. (6). The isolated arterioles were suspended in 10 mM Tris-HCl buffer (pH 7.4) containing 3 mM-$MgCl_2$, 2 mM-EDTA and 0,25 M saccharose to give a protein concentration of 0,7-1,2 mg/ml. The arteriolar aggregates were dispersed using 5-10 seconds homogeneisation in a Elvehjem grinder. Protein concentration was determined with the method of Lowry et al. (7) with bovin serum albumin as standard.

Assay of adenylate cyclase in renal cortex arterioles

The adenylate cyclase assay in a final volume of 100 µl, 30 mM Tris-HCl buffer (pH 7.5) contained, 1 mM 3-isobutyl-1-methylxanthine, 3 mM $MgCl_2$, 10 mM phosphocreatin, 30 µg creatin kinase, 0,1 % bovin serum albumine, 14-24 µg arteriolar protein, 0.2 mM [α^{32}P] ATP (20-30 cpm/pmol), 3-5.10^{4} cpm of [2,8 ^{3}H] cyclic AMP (recovery measurements) and test substance(s) (GTP and/or hormones). The assay components including bPTH-(3-34) with or without 10^{-4} M GTP, were preincubated at 37°C for 3 min after which bPTH-(1-34) and substrate were added. The reaction was allowed to proceed at 37°C for 10 min and was terminated by additing 100 µl of a solution containing 20 mg/ml ATP and 2 % SDS. After the addition of 800 µl H_2O, [α^{32}P] ATP was evaluated with the method of Salomon et al. (8). All assays were performed in duplicate and adenylate cyclase activity was expressed in pmol of cyclic AMP formed per mg of arteriolar protein and per min.

RESULTS

Effect of synthetic bPTH-(1-34)

The basal adenylate cyclase activity of the isolated rabbit renal arterioles was 32.1 $\pm$ 1.7 pMol cyclic AMP/min/mg protein (mean $\pm$ S.E. n=12). Synthetic bPTH-(1-34) caused a dose-related activation of adenylate cyclase whether 100 µM GTP was present or not (see Fig. 1).

Apparent km (ED50) and maximum stimulation rates in the absence or presence of exogenous GTP are shown in Table 1.

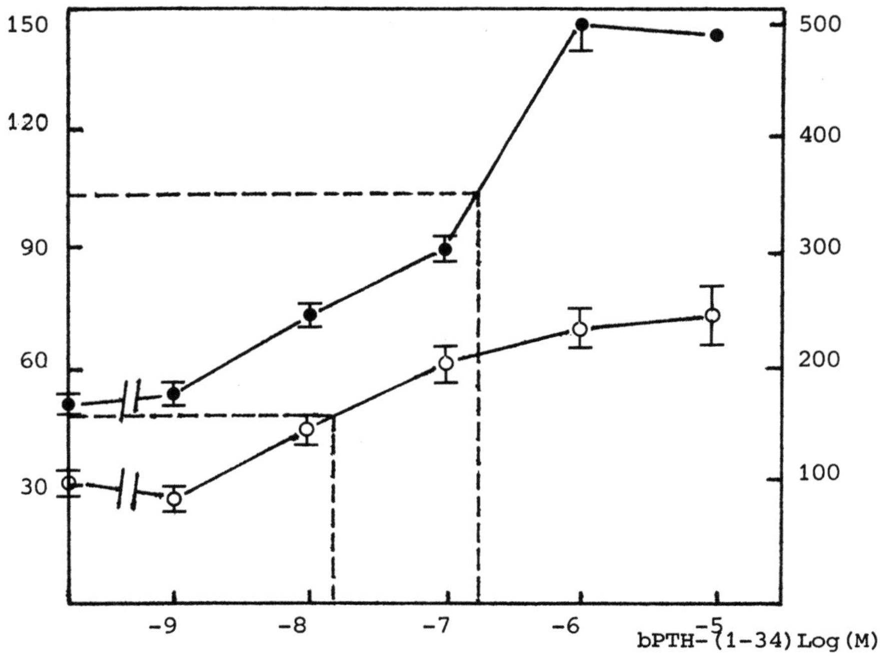

Fig. 1 : Stimulation of arteriolar adenylate cyclase by bPTH-(1-34)
Adenylate cyclase activity was measured in the basal state and with various concentrations of bPTH-(1-34) either in the absence (o-o) or presence of 100 μM GTP (●-●) Each plot is the mean of four experiments. Vertical lines indicate S.E.M. Dotted lines show half-maximal stimulation.

Table 1. Maximum stimulation rates and apparent km of bPTH-(1-34) on arteriolar adenylate cyclase.

Experimental conditions	Maximum stimulation rate (Δ %)	Apparent km (M)
bPTH-(1-34)	+ 135.9 ± 25.2	$4.5.10^{-8}$
GTP	+ 68.6 ± 24.9	-
bPTH-(1-34)+GTP	+ 377.6 ± 23.0	$5.2.10^{-7}$

Means are shown ± SE (n=4). Adenylate cyclase stimulation rates are given for 10^{-6}M bPTH-(1-34) and/or 10^{-4}M GTP.

The addition of 100 µM GTP to the incubation mixture enhanced the maximum stimulation rate of the enzyme and the apparent Km in the presence of GTP was about 12 time higher than in the absence of GTP.

Inhibition of bPTH-(1-34) action

At 5.10^{-6}M, the specific PTH inhibitor [$Nleu^{8,18}$, tyr^{34}]-bPTH-(3-34) amide reduced the action of 10^{-6}M bPTH-(1-34) by 60,4 % in the absence of GTP. However, this (3-34) substituted fragment only inhibited the action of bPTH-(1-34) by 40 % when tested in the presence of 100 µM GTP. bPTH-(3-34) alone was completely devoid of agonist activity even at 5 µM whether 100 µM GTP was present or not.

Table 2. Effect of PTH inhibitor on the action of bPTH-(1-34) on arteriolar adenylate cyclase.

Conditions	pM cAMP/min/mg	Δ %	% Inhibition
Control	32.8 ± 2.0	0	
bPTH-(3-34)amide	31.6 ± 2.6	- 3.7	
bPTH-(1-34)	63.9 ± 2.5	+ 94.8	
bPTH-(3-34)amide + bPTH-(1-34)	45.1 ± 2.6	+ 37.5	60.5
GTP	53.2 ± 3.1	0	
bPTH-(3-34)amide + GTP	47.8 ± 1.4	- 9.0	
bPTH-(1-34) + GTP	136.3 ± 0.7	+156.2	
bPTH-(1-34) bPTH-(3-34)amide + GTP	103.2 ± 7.2	+ 94.0	39.8

Mean are shown ± SE (n=8). Adenylate cyclase activity was measured with 10^{-6}M bPTH-(1-34) and/or 5.10^{-6}M [$Nleu^{8,18}$, tyr^{34}]-bPTH-(3-34) amide and/or 10^{-4}M GTP.

DISCUSSION

Almost simultaneously with the present communication, Huang et al. (5) reported that both bPTH-(1-84), and bPTH-(1-34) which contains the aminoacid sequence required for the known biological activity of the hormone, caused dose-related activation of brain microvascular adenylate cyclase in the presence of exogenous GTP. Synthetic bPTH-(1-34) was more potent than the native hormone with an apparent km of 6.3 x 10^{-9} M and 8-fold enzyme stimulation.

The present work demonstrates the presence of bPTH-(1-34) dependent adenylate cyclase in arterioles isolated from rabbit kidney cortex. Even without exogenous GTP, bPTH-(1-34) at 10^{-6} M stimulated renal arteriole adenylate cyclase. In brain vessels no stimulation has been seen in the absence of GTP (5). In the present work, the apparent km values when no GTP added, was about 12 times higher than in the presence of 100 μM GTP (Fig. 1 and Table 1). Exogenous GTP thus enhanced maximum stimulation rate of adenylate cyclase activity and reduced the apparent affinity of the hormone for its receptor. Guanyl nucleotide potentiation of PTH stimulated adenylate cyclase has been illustrated in canine renal cortical membranes (10-12) and in chicken renal plasma membranes (13). These studies showed that guanyl nucleotides enhanced the coupling of the occupied PTH receptor to the adenylate cyclase catalytic unit and the dissociation rate of receptor-bound PTH. Our results could be explained by the presence of high and low affinity bPTH-(1-34) action sites on the renal cortex arterioles. Low affinity action site would require higher GTP concentration for maximum activation of enzyme activity resulting from the partial "uncoupling" of the PTH-receptor and the adenylate cyclase catalytic unit and/or the low dissociation rate of the receptor-bound PTH. Stimulated activity when no GTP was added was probably due to the presence of trace amounts of endogeneous GTP. Further investigations are obviously necessary to assess these conclusions. Nevertheless, the apparent km values reported here are lower than those in canine renal cortical membranes (11) cultured bone tumor cells, skin fibroblasts (14) and brain microvessels (5). This difference may reflect intrinsic properties of tissue receptors or may be due to methodological factors. However, similar apparent km have been obtained in isolated rat glomeruli (1.1x10^{-7}M) and rabbit glomeruli (2.3x10^{-7}M) when no exogenous GTP was present (18,19).

Earlier studies have demonstrated that the substituted 3-34 fragment of bovine PTH competitively inhibited the stimulated bPTH (1-34) adenylate cyclase in canine cortical membranes (15,16) and cultured bone tumor cells (14). The data presented here show that this analogue is a powerful inhibitor of the bPTH-(1-34)-stimulated enzyme of renal cortical arterioles. The inhibition was less effective when GTP was added than in the absence of guanyl nucleotide. According to the above-mentioned hypothesis, low affinity PTH receptors might be less sensitive to bPTH-(3-34) amide.

Previous observation by other workers (1-34) showed that PTH dilates several vascular beds. The present results and those of Huang et al. (5) show that this effect is probably mediated by cAMP production. It is very likely that the PTH receptor are localized on the periarteriolar smooth muscle cells. In fact parathyroid extract acts on ^{45}Ca exchange in isolated rat aorta (4) and it is currently thought that cellular calcium physiology is pivotal in the regulation of these cells.

The renal microvessels and especially the afferent arteriole are characterized by high renin activity and by the absence of glomerular and tubular contaminations (6). In fact, the afferent arteriole has a thick coat of cells containing collections of cytoplasmic granules : the juxtaglomerular granular cells. These cells are currently thought to be a source of renin (9). Several drugs, such as the β agonists or certain prostaglandins, are potent vasodilatators and stimulators of renin release from the kidney (cf. 17). These results therefore raise the question of whether PTH plays a physiological role in regulating intracortical microcirculation by relaxing perivascular smooth muscle cell and stimulating renin release from the walls of these microvessels.

This work was supported by a "Contrat de Recherches libres INSERM, France, n° 815018. The authors gratefully acknowledge the continued encouragment and helpful suggestions of the followings Prof. C. BOLLACK (Director of the René Leriche Laboratory), Prof. R. ARDAILLOU, Prof. J. GEISERT, Prof. G. REBEL (Maître de Recherches, CNRS) and Prof. P. MANDEL. We also wish to thank Miss E. FRIEDMANN, Miss J. KRILL and Mrs. S. WENDLING for their skilled technical assistance.

REFERENCES

1. G. A. Charbon. An rapid and selective vasodilator effect of parathyroid hormone. European J. Pharmacol. 3:275 (1968).
2. G. A. Charbon and P. F. Hulstaert, Augmentation of arterial, hepatic and renal flow by extracted and synthetic parathyroid hormone. Endocrinology 95:621 (1974).
3. A. Berthelot and A. Gairard. Action of parathormone on arterial pressure and on contraction of isolated aorta in the Rat. Experientia 31:457 (1975).
4. R. Schleiffer, A. Berthelot and A. Gairard. Action of parathyroid extract on arterial blood pressure and on contraction and ^{45}Ca exchange in isolated aorta of the rat. European J. Pharmacol. 58:163 (1979).
5. M. Huang, D. A. Hanley and O. P. Rorstad. Parathyroid hormone stimulates adenylate cyclase in rat cerebral microvessels. Life Sciences, 32:1009 (1983).
6. J. J. Helwig, A. N. K. Yusufi, C. Judes, V. Varga, P. Mandel and C. Bollack. Isolation and some properties of a preglomerular arteriolar fraction from rabbit kidney, in : "Biochemistry of kidney Functions. INSERM Symposium n°21" F. Morel, ed., Elsevier Biomedical Press B.V. p.p.59-68.(1982).

7. O. H. Lowry, N. J. Rosebrough, A. L. Farr and R. S. Randall. Protein measurement with the folin phenol reagent. J. Biol. Chem., 128:1319 (1951).
8. Y. Salomon, C. Londos and M. Rodbell. A highly sensitive adenylate cyclase assay. Anal. Biochem. 58:401 (1974).
9. W. F. Cook, J. W. Fisher ed., Hormones and kidney, Academic Press., N. Y. pp. 117-128 (1974).
10. R. A. Nissenson, S. R. Abbott, A. P. Teitelbaum, O. H. Clark and C. D. Arnaud. Endogeneous biologically active human PTH : measurement by a guanyl nucleotide - amplified renal adenylate cyclase assay. J. Clin. Endocrin. Metab. 52:840 (1981).
11. D. Goltzmann, E. N. Callahan, G. W. Tregear and J. T. Potts. Influence of guanyl nucleotides on PTH-stimulated adenylate cyclase activity in renal cortical membranes. Endocrin. 103: 1352 (1978).
12. E. Bellorin-Font and K. J. Martin. Regulation of the PTH-receptor-cyclase system of canine kidney : effects of calcium, magnesium and guanine nucleotides. Am. J. Physiol. 241:F364 (1981).
13. R. A. Nissenson, K. O. Nyiredy and C. D. Arnaud. Guanyl nucleotide potentiation of PTH stimulated adenylate cyclase in chicken plasma membranes : a receptor-independent effect. Endocrin. 108:1949 (1981).
14. S. R. Goldring, J. M. Dayer and M. Rosenblatt, Factors regulating the response of cells cultured from human giant cell tumors of bone to PTH. J. Clin. Endocrin. Metab. 53:295 (1981).
15. M. Rosenblatt, E. N. Callahan, J. E. Mahaffey, A. Pont and J. D. Potts. PTH inhibitors. J. Biol. Chem. 252:5847 (1977).
16. A. P. Teitelbaum, R. A. Nissenson and C. D. Arnaud. Coupling of the canine renal PTH receptor to adenylate cyclase modulation by guanyl nucleotides and N-Ethylmaleimide. Endocrinol. 111:1524 (1982).
17. S. Suzuki, R. Franco-Saenz and P. S. Mulrow. The role of renal prostaglandins in the renin response to isoproterenol in the rat in vitro. Endocrinol. 108:1654 (1981).
18. J. Sraer, R. Ardaillou, N. Loreau and J. D. Sraer. Evidence for PTH sensitive adenylate cyclase in rat glomeruli. Mol. Cell. Endocrin. 1:285 (1974).
19. M. Imbert, D. Chabardes and F. Morel with the technical assistance of M. Montegut and A. Clique. Hormone sensitive adenylate cyclase in isolated rabbit glomeruli. Mol. Cell. Endocrin. 1:295 (1974).

THE EFFECTS OF CHANGES IN SERUM CALCIUM AND PARATHORMONE ON PLASMA RENIN ACTIVITY IN INTACT MONGREL DOGS

Edward T. Zawada, Jr. and Michael Johnson

McGuire VA Medical Center and
Medical College of Virginia
Richmond, Virginia

ABSTRACT

Studies were undertaken to extend previous observations of the interaction between calcium and parathormone on renin synthesis by the kidney. Intact normovolemic mongrel dogs between 15 and 25 kg were used for all studies. Plasma renin activity (PRA) was measured by radioimmunoassay. Hypocalcemia produced by thyro-parathyroidectomy or chelation with EDTA resulted in an elevated PRA of 3.76 $\pm$ .86 ng/ml/hr in 17 dogs compared to 1.5 $\pm$ .29 ng/ml/hr in 14 controls ($p < .05$). In 5 renovascular dogs calcium-channel blockade with nifedipine resulted in a higher PRA of 31.8 $\pm$ 0.5 compared to 11.9 $\pm$ 1.1 ng/ml/hr in 23 renovascular controls, $p < .001$.

The reactive hyperreninemia following angiotensin blockade was greater in 22 hypocalcemic (10.94 $\pm$ 2.03 ng/ml/hr) dogs compared to 14 controls (1.32 $\pm$ .34 ng/ml/hr), $p < .001$. Results with calcium antagonism on PRA levels in renovascular dogs were found similar to those described with angiotensin blockade.

We conclude from these studies that calcium-channel blockade or calcium reduction independent of a rise in parathormone was associated with an elevation of PRA in normal and renovascular hypertensive dogs. The rise in PRA could occur without changes in blood pressure or volume, consistent with an interruption of the short feedback loop control of renin synthesis by calcium antagonism. Finally, hypocalcemia and calcium-channel blockade resulted in reactive hyperreninemia greater than or equal to that seen after angiotensin blockade in both groups of dogs, again suggesting interference with the short feedback loop control of renin synthesis.

INTRODUCTION

There have been a number of clinical reports linking plasma renin activity with clinical disorders of calcium and/or parathormone.[1,2] In these reports elevated plasma renin activity (PRA) has been seen with hyperparathyroidism. Surgical therapy resulted in a return of PRA toward normal. However, it has never been clear whether the hypercalcemia or the increased parathormone is a stimulus to PRA. In isolated perfused kidneys contradictory results of the effects of calcium on renin have been reported.[3,4] Some studies have shown that calcium stimulates renin production[3]; others showed calcium suppresses renin synthesis.[4] In view of these controversies and contradictions, no clear idea emerges as to the interactions between serum calcium and parathormone versus renin, especially in whole-animal preparations. To further explore these relationships, studies were undertaken using normal and renovascular hypertensive mongrel dogs to determine the effect of changes in serum calcium and/or parathormone and calcium-channel blockade on plasma renin activity under conditions of normal activity of the renin-angiotensin axis and under conditions of a stimulated renin-angiotensin axis.

MATERIALS AND METHODS

Intact normovolemic mongrel dogs between 15 and 25 kg were used for all studies. All animals had silastic catheters surgically placed into a femoral artery for blood pressure measurements and a femoral vein for sampling. A peripheral intravenous catheter placed into a forelimb vein was used for drug administration. Blood pressure (BP) was measured by a Beckman (Schiller Park, Ill.) quartz transducer connected to a Beckman (Schiller Park, Ill.) physiological recorder that had been calibrated with a mercury manometer prior to each study. All measurements in non-hypertensive dogs were done with the animals unanesthetized, standing in a canvas sling. All measurements in renovascular hypertension were done in animals anesthetized with Nembutal.®

Plasma renin activity (PRA) was measured in blood drawn into tubes kept chilled on ice using the Clinical Assays® (Cambridge, Mass.) radioimmunoassay kit described by our laboratory previously.[5] Serum calcium was measured by autoanalyzer. Thyroparathyroidectomy (TPTX) was performed as described previously by our group[5]

Renovascular hypertension was created by a model of bilateral renal artery ischemia. A midline abdominal approach was used. The left kidney was isolated first, and an occluding cuff (In Vivo Metrics, Heraldsburg, Ca.) was placed around the vessel. A snug fit was desired, so several sizes ranging from 2-4 mm were kept on hand. Then the right renal artery was located. A suture tie was placed loosely around the vessel for later tieoff. After baseline measurements were made, the right renal artery was tied off. Then the occluding cuff on the left renal artery was inflated, and blood pressure monitoring was begun. After 30 minutes of renal ischemia, the mean arterial pressure rose and stabilized at a significantly higher lever.

Ten groups of studies were performed. Group I consisted of measurements of BP and PRA after 15 minutes of upright posture in 14 conscious normocalcemic dogs standing in a canvas sling. Group II studies were similar measurements of BP and PRA in 17 hypocalcemic conscious dogs. Twelve of these were dogs two days after surgical thyroparathyroidectomy. Five of these were animals receiving a one-hour intravenous infusion of ethylenediamine-tetraacetic acid (EDTA) in a dose of 2.5 mg/kg/min. Group III studies consisted of 23 BP and PRA measurements in anesthetized dogs 1 hour after renovascular hypertension was created. Group IV consisted of 5 anesthetized renovascular hypertensive dogs 30 minutes after a 10 Ug/kg/min infusion of the calcium-channel blocking drug nifedipine was begun. Group V consisted of 30 measurements of PRA in conscious normocalcemic dogs at the lowest blood pressure sustained for one minute within 30 minutes after angiotensin blockade with either .143 mg/kg of the competitive antagonist saralasin (15 studies) or .356 mg/kg of the non-competitive inhibitor captopril (15 studies). Group VI consisted of 22 measurements of PRA and BP as described for Group V in conscious hypocalcemic dogs (15 TPTX, 7EDTA) after angiotensin blockade. Group VII consisted of 5 measurements of PRA and BP as before in anesthetized renovascular dogs receiving angiotensin blockade 30 minutes after nifedipine infusion was begun. Group VIII consisted of 14 studies of PRA and BP as before in anesthetized renovascular dogs receiving angiotensin blockade and EDTA infusion as described. Group IX consisted of 22 studies of PRA and BP as before in anesthetized renovascular dogs after angiotensin blockade alone. Group X consisted of 9 measurements of BP and PRA in anesthetized renovascular hypertensive given EDTA alone.

The dose of EDTA employed in these studies was a dose which from our previous studies produced a significant reduction of serum calcium in normal conscious dogs.[5] The doses of angiotensin blockade were those which from other previous studies [6] by our group significantly reduced blood pressure in renovascular hypertensive dogs. All results are reported as mean values plus or minus the standard error of the mean. The student t-test for paired variables was used in all comparisons. The statistics were performed on a Hewlett-Packard programmable calculator and their Stat-Pac®.

RESULTS

In Figure 1 it can be seen that hypocalcemia in normal dogs resulted in a rise of PRA from 1.52 ± .29 to 3.76 ± .86 ng/ml/hr ($p < .05$) without a significant fall in blood pressure or apparent change in plasma volume.

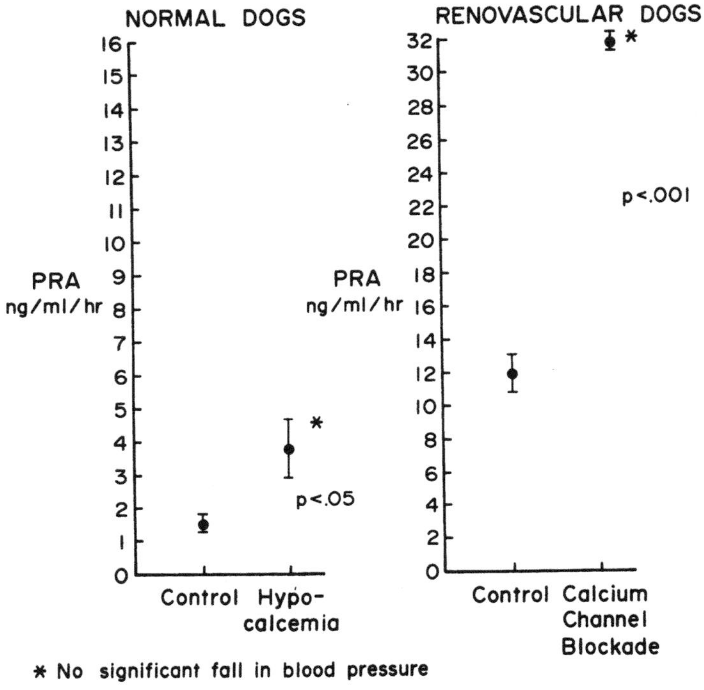

Figure 1.

In Figure 1 also it can be seen that another form of calcium antagonism, calcium-channel blockade with nifedipine, resulted in an even more significant increase in PRA levels to 31.8 ± .5 from 11.9 ± 1.1 ng/ml/hr ($p < .001$) in renovascular hypertensive dogs again without a significant fall in blood pressure or change in plasma volume.

In Figure 2, it can be seen that the reactive hyper-reninemia following angiotensin blockade was greater, $p < .001$, in hypocalcemic dogs (10.94 ± 2.03 ng/ml/hr) compared to normocalcemic dogs ($1.32 \pm .34$ ng/ml/hr). In both groups in the doses used of angiotensin blockers, both normocalcemic and hypocalcemic groups had significant reductions of blood pressure.

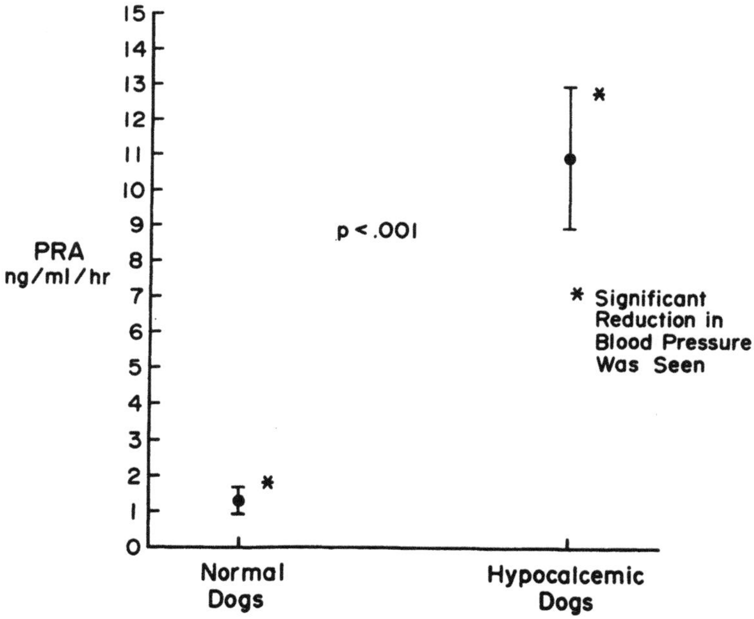

Figure 2.

Figure 3 summarizes all measurements of PRA in renovascular hypertensive dogs.

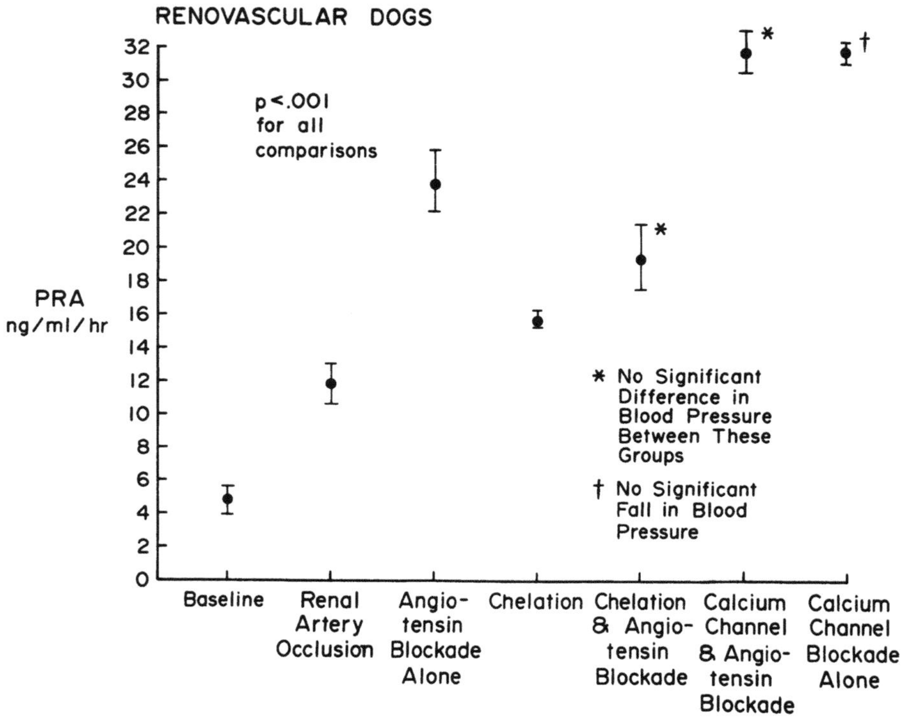

Figure 3.

Chelation with EDTA resulted in a significant rise in PRA from 11.9 ± 1.1 to 15.7 ± .5 ng/ml/hr, $p < .05$, which accompanied a significant fall in blood pressure. PRA after chelation and angiotensin blockade was significantly higher at 19.5 ± 1.9 ng/ml/hr. However, PRA after chelation and angiotensin blockade was not higher than PRA after angiotensin blockade alone. The highest PRA levels were seen after calcium channel blockade, 31.8 ± 0.5 ng/ml, and calcium channel blockade and angiotensin blockade 31.8 ± 1.1 ng/ml/hr. Importantly, in the studies with calcium channel blockade, there was no significant fall in blood pressure preceding the rise in PRA.

DISCUSSION

These studies showed that hypocalcemia due to TPTX or antagonism of calcium by either chelation or calcium-channel blockade was associated with a rise in PRA in normal dogs and an even more significant rise in renovascular hypertensive dogs. Since the rise in PRA was seen even in animals who had undergone TPTX, we conclude that the fall in calcium or its antagonism per se (independent of potential compensatory elevations of parathormone) is sufficient for the rise in PRA to occur. The greater changes seen with calcium-channel blockade would suggest that it is interference with intracellular entry of calcium that leads to the rise in PRA levels. The greater rise in PRA with calcium antagonism in a model of a stimulated renin-angiotensin axis suggested to us a dependency of renin synthesis on calcium antagonism. Conversely, calcium entry into cells seemed necessary to shut off renin synthesis. Antagonism of calcium interfered with such a negative feedback system to further stimulate renin synthesis.

To test this concept further we analyzed these studies in light of known determinants of PRA levels. In Group II & IV, the rise in PRA occurred without a significant fall in blood pressure or obvious change in volume status. In addition, the reactive rise in PRA after angiotensin blockade in hypocalcemic non-hypertensive dogs (Group VI) was greater than that in normocalcemic dogs (Group V) despite similar degrees of blood pressure reduction. The reactive rise in PRA after angiotensin blockade is another form of stimulation of the renin-angiotensin axis.[7,8] The greater increase in reactive PRA in hypocalcemic dogs is consistent with less restriction on renin synthesis during hypocalcemia. Finally, in renovascular dogs, calcium-channel blockade resulted in a greater reactive rise in PRA after angiotensin blockade than chelation pointing again to the need for intracellular entry of calcium to shut down renin synthesis. The greater rise in reactive PRA after calcium-channel blockade and angiotensin blockade occurred despite comparable reduction of blood pressure to chelation and angiotensin blockade.

More concisely, our studies led to the conclusion that reduction of serum calcium and more importantly reduction of intracellular entry of calcium uncouples a negative feedback loop controlling renin synthesis. This feedback loop is due to direct inhibition of renin synthesis by angiotensin II levels. Our previous studies [5,7] have demonstrated angiotensin antagonism by calcium antagonism. Such angiotensin antagonism could blunt the expression of angiotensin in the short feedback loop control of renin synthesis. In this way calcium antagonism, especially blockade of intracellular entry of calcium, may interrupt the short feedback loop control of renin synthesis. This conclusion fits best with our previous results of angiotensin antagonism by calcium antagonism.

REFERENCES

1. G. S. Brinton, W. Jubiz, and L. D. Lagerquist, Hypertension in primary hyperparathyroidism: The role of the renin-angiotensin system, J. Clin. Endocrinol. Metab. 41:1025 (1975).
2. E. T. Zawada, Jr., A. S. Brickman, M. H. Maxwell, and M. A. Tuck, Hypertension associated with hyperparathyroidism is not responsive to angiotensin blockade, J. Clin. Endocrinol. Metab. 50:912 (1980).
3. D. S. Chen, and A. M. Poisner, Direct stimulation of renin release by calcium, Proc. Soc. Exp. Biol. Med. 152:565 (1976).
4. J. S. Fray, Stimulation of renin release in the perfused kidney by low calcium and high magnesium, Am. J. Physiol. 237:F377 (1977).
5. E. T. Zawada, Jr., E. P. Bennett, M. Johnson, and D. Bennett, Effects of changes in serum calcium on blood pressure in conscious dogs, Nephron 33:260 (1983).
6. E. T. Zawada, Jr., M. Johnson, Does calcium mediate high renin renal hypertension?, Clin. Res. 30:467A (1982).
7. M. H. Maxwell, P. Varady, E. T. Zawada, Jr., J. F. Burkhalter, U. Waks, L. S. Marks, Maximal discrimination of renovascular from essential hypertension by the saralasin test, Clin. Sci. Mol. Med. 55:2975 (1978).
8. D. B. Case, and J. H. Laragh, Reactive hyperreninemia in renovascular hypertension after blockade with saralasin or converting enzyme inhibitor, Ann. Intern. Med. 91:153 (1979).

MODIFICATION OF THE RENAL EFFECTS OF OUABAIN BY CALCIUM CHANNEL BLOCKERS

Manuel A. Cruz-Soto and Manuel Martínez-Maldonado

Renal Metabolic Laboratory, Medical and Research Service Veterans Administration Center and the Department of Medicine and Physiology, University of Puerto Rico School of Medicine, San Juan, Puerto Rico

INTRODUCTION

Ouabain, a specific inhibitor of Na^+K^+ ATPase, has been shown to inhibit renin release and exert natriuretic and renal vasoconstrictive effects in the dog (1, 2, 3, 4).

The mechanism of the cardiac glycosides-induced natriuresis is inhibition of tubular Na^+K^+ ATPase (1, 2). On the other hand, the precise way in which cardiac glycosides cause vasoconstriction and renin inhibition have not been completely elucidated. Studies *in vitro* suggest that these effects may be mediated through increases in free cytosolic calcium in effector cells (5, 6, 7, 8).

Studies utilizing rat kidney slices (6, 7, 9) have suggested that ouabain exerts its effect on renin release by altering calcium content of granular cells. The present studies were undertaken to examine *in vivo* the role of calcium in the renal vasoconstriction and renin suppression induced by ouabain.

Materials and Methods

Mongrel dogs of either sex (10 to 15 kg body weight) were anestherized with sodium pentobarbital (30 mg/kg i.v.) after overnight food deprivation, small doses were administered as needed to maintain light anesthesia. An endotracheal tube was inserted and connected to a Harvard Respirator. A catheter in the femoral artery was used to sample blood and to monitor blood pressure (American Optical Blood Pressure Monitor). Through a femoral vein catheter solutions of inulin (5 g in 375 ml of 0.9% saline) paraaminohippurate (PAH, 5g in 100 ml of 0.9% saline) were infused at a rate of 0.5 ml/min. Their clearance was used as markers of glomerular filtration rate (GFR) and renal plasma flow (RPF). Renal blood flow (RBF) in the experimental kidney was also directly measured with a flowmeter (Gould Statham SP 2202, Oxnard, Ca). The ureters were exposed by a midline abdominal incision and cannulated for urine collection. The left kidney pedicle was then exposed and the artery and vein were visualized. Samples of renal venous blood for renin and PAH determination were obtained through a catheter advanced from the left spermatic or ovarian vein into the renal vein. A hooked 23 gauge needle was inserted into the renal artery and used for intra-arterial infusions.

All clearance periods were of 10 min. duration with blood sampling at midpoint for electrolytes and plasma renin activity (PRA). After surgical preparation and infusion of inulin and PAH an equilibrium period of at least 45 min. was allowed before starting collections. Blood and urine losses were replaced with Ringer's lactate. In all groups two control collection periods were obtained before any experimental maneuvers. The following groups of dogs were studied:

Group 1 (n=7) After control collections, ouabain (1 ug/kg/min) was infused into the renal artery for 70 to 80 minutes, while collection periods were obtained.

Group 2 (n=6) After the control phase, verapamil (100 ug/min) was infused into the renal artery and two collections were obtained. Ouabain was then superimposed as in Group 1. In this group clearance collections were started 30 min after commencing ouabain infusion.

Group 3 (n=6) These dogs were handled as those in Group 2, but another calcium channel blocker, nifedipine (10 ug/min) was used. Nifedipine is a calcium channel blocker which is structurally different from verapamil.

Sodium and potassium concentration in plasma and urine were determined with a Beckman Flame Photometer. Calculation of renal blood flow from PAH clearances and hematrocrit values correlated within 5% with flow meter measurements. PRA was measured by radioimmunoassay (New England Nuclear, Boston, Ma). The renin secretory rate (RSR) was calculated from the arteriovenous difference of renin and the renal plasma flow as previously described (10). Statistical analysis utilized Student's t test; analysis of variance was used whenever appropriate. Only values for the experimental kidney are presented; changes in the contralateral kidney have been previously shown to be slight and of little consequence (10).

Results

Effects of ouabain on renal function. The renal effects of ouabain are detailed in Table 1. As reported previously, ouabain infusion into the renal artery elicited progressive increases in urine flow rate and fractional excretion of sodium (4, 11). The GFR decreased steadily throughout the experiments. The fact that natriuresis occurred while the GFR was low illustrates the primary tubular effect of ouabain.

The renal blood flow fell and remained low for the first 50 to 60 min of ouabain infusion, but then returned spontaneously to baseline values. The renin secretory rate diminished and remained low while ouabain was infused. The blood pressure remained unchanged, while the heart rate fell progressively and there were no changes in hematocrit or in serum electrolytes (not shown).

TABLE 1 Renal and systemic effects of ouabain

	GLOMERUALR FILTRATION RATE ml/min	RENAL BLOOD FLOW ml/min	URINE FLOW RATE ml/min	FE_{Na} %	RENIN SECRETORY RATE ng/ml/hr. ml/min
CONTROL	18.2±3.2	109±20	0.99±0.13	3.7±0.7	387±75
20 min	15.5±3.2	79±7[a]	1.09±0.21	4.2±0.8	184±65[b]
40 min	14.1±2.7[c]	79±8[a]	1.85±0.44[a]	12.9±2.2[a]	193±29[b]
60 min	13.2±2.5[d]	91±12	1.98±0.40[b]	16.1±2.4[c]	197±29[b]
80 min	13.7±2.2[c]	95±16	2.73±0.66[c]	20.9±3.4[d]	124±28[c]

Results are means ± SE. The letters in superscript represent the degree of significance as compared to control values (<0.05=a, <0.02=b, <0.01=c, <0.001=d).

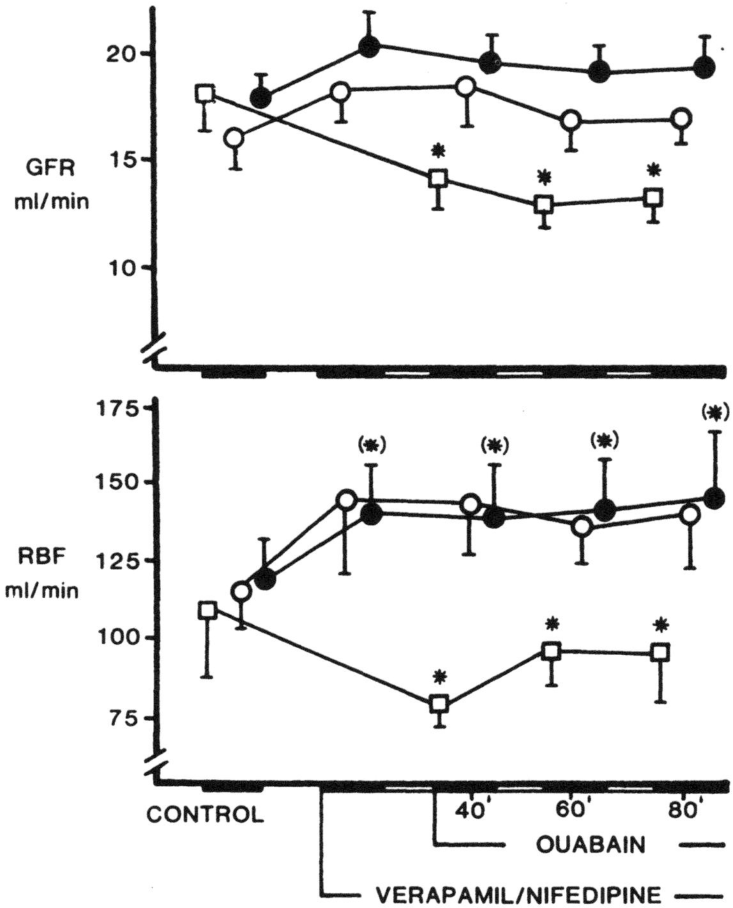

Figure 1 - <u>Effects of calcium channel blockers on the renal action of ouabain</u>: GFR and RBF

Results are means ±SE of the corresponding renal function parameter in the ordinate. The horizontal bars in the abcissa represent the experimental phases indicated at the bottom of the figure □, Group 1-ouabain alone; ○, Group 2-verapamil plus ouabain; ●, Group 3-nifedipine plus ouabain. GFR, glomerular filtration rate; RBF, renal blood flow. *, $p<0.05$ compared with Group 1. (*) $p<0.05$ compared with control values in Group 2 and 3.

<u>Effects of calcium channel blockers on renal function and on the renal action of ouabain</u>. Verapamil infusion into the renal artery

elicited a significant increase in renal blood flow (116±12 → 147±23 ml/min), whereas the GFR did not change (16±2 → 17±2 ml/min). As a consequence the filtration fraction fell. The urine flow rate (2±0.2 → 5±0.5 ml/min) and the fractional excretion of sodium (5±0.2 → 13±1%) rose significantly, whereas the mean arterial pressure (MAP) and the heart rate decreased. Nifedipine exerted identical effects, although the FENa increase (6±1 → 9±3%) did not achieve statistical significance.

The effects of verapamil and nifedipine upon the action of ouabain are depicted in Figure 1. In the presence of a calcium channel blocker ouabain did not decrease GFR or RBF, as compared to ouabain alone. There was a massive increase in urine flow rate and FE_{Na} when ouabain was added. The natriuretic effect of nifedipine, in combination with ouabain, was less pronounced than that with verapamil despite identical increase in urine flow rate and similar hemodynamic effect.

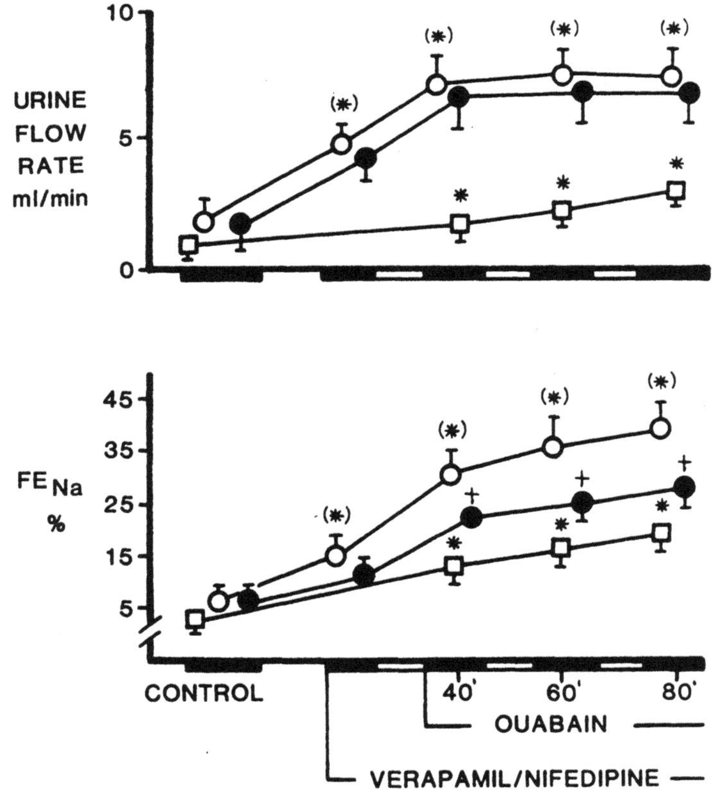

Figure 2 - Effects of calcium channel blockers on the renal action of ouabain: urine flow rate and sodium excretion (FE_{Na}). Legend as in Figure 1. †, $p<0.05$ when Groups 2 and 3 were compared.

The MAP did not change further when ouabain was superimposed, whereas the heart rate decreased (not shown). The hematocrit and serum electrolytes remained unchanged throughout the experiments (not shown). The changes in renin secretion in response to calcium channel blockers or in combination with ouabain are depicted in Figure 3. The renin secretory rate after calcium channel blockers rose in most experiments, but these changes did not achieve statistical significance. These values were even greater when ouabain infusion was superimposed during calcium channel blockers administration. The increases in renin secretion under these circumstances were statistically significant. Verapamil increased renin secretion significantly as compared to the control and to when it was infused alone. The change after combined nifedipine and ouabain was significantly different only from control.

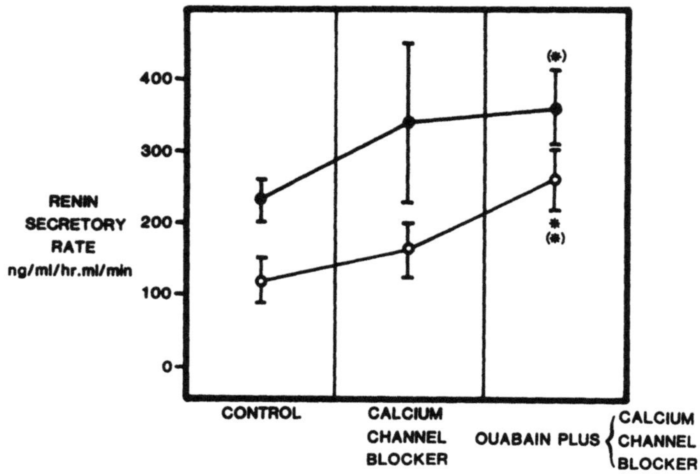

Figure 3 - Modification of the effects of ouabain on renin secretion by calcium channel blockers

Results are mean ± SE ○, Group 2-verapamil plus ouabain ●, Group 3-nifedipine plus ouabain *, $p<0.05$ compared with previous value. (*), $p<0.05$ compared with control values.

Discusssion

These data strongly suggest that the renal vasoconstrictive and renin inhibitory effects of ouabain are calcium dependent. The results of the studies with calcium channel blockers give credence to the possibility that entry of calcium from the extracellular fluid into smooth muscle and granular cells is essential for the actions of cardiac glycosides. Moreover, it is evident that the natriuresis of ouabain is not affected by drugs which reduce calcium entry into cells.

We have previously shown that ouabain reduced renal blood flow due to a direct vasoconstrictive action and inhibits renin secretion in the dog in vivo (4). Studies in kidney slices have shown that the renin inhibitory effect of ouabain is dependent upon changes in cell calcium (6, 7, 9). In the present studies, verapamil and nifedipine prevent the decrease in renal blood flow and in renin secretion induced by ouabain. Thus, these data provide compelling evidence supporting the dependence of the effects of ouabain upon the increase of calcium in the cytosol.

Inhibition of $Na^{+}K^{+}$ ATPase promotes cell membrane depolarization. Consequently, the decrease in membrane potential allows the opening of voltage-dependent calcium channels and facilitates entry of calcium into the cytosol. Accumulation of sodium inside the cell will also decrease Na-Ca exchange in the cell membrane. The diminished calcium efflux would accentuate the increase in cysotolic calcium (12). In support of this, we have also shown that nifedipine and verapamil blunt the renal effects of vanadate, suggesting a similar mechanism of action of the element to that of ouabain (10, 13).

The spontaneous reversal of ouabain vasoconstriction cannot be easily explained. Several possibilities can be considered. It is well known that increases in free cytosolic calcium call into play several homeostatic mechanisms to keep its concentration within a narrow range. For example, calcium-ATPase translocates calcium away from the cytosol into organelles (14, 15). Thus, it is possible that ouabain increases cytosolic calcium leading to the initial vasoconstriction, activation of Ca-ATPase would restore calcium to normal, allowing vasodilatation (16). Other intracellular homeostatic mechanisms for calcium may also participate in reversing ouabain induced vasoconstriction (15).

Enhancement of the natriuresis of ouabain by calcium channel blockers suggest that these agents have direct tubular effects on sodium reabsorption. This suggestion is strengthened by the fact that there were no changes in filtered load of sodium and that the reduction in filtration fraction induced by the calcium channel blockers remained constant. Moreover, mean arterial pressure fell, a circumstance that should enhance proximal reabsorption under conditions of renal vasodilation or vasodilatation. Evidence that calcium channel blockers may have direct tubular actions in the dog has also been advanced by Mc. Crorey et al (17).

Acknowledgement

We are indebted to Mr. José L. Gotay, Mr. Eliseo Rivera, Mr. George Crespo and Ms. Joyce Bou-Vierno for technical assistance, and to Mrs. Victoria D. de Pérez for secretarial assistance.

This work was supported by funds from the Veterans Administration Central Office (Merit Review Program), 2-S06-RR-08102-10

Support for University Biomedical Education (SUBE) and by grant 1R01 AM 30201-01 from the NIH.

References

1. M. Martínez-Maldonado, M. J. C. Allen, G. Eknoyan, W. Suki and A. Schwartz, Renal concentrating mechanism: Possible role for sodium potassium activated adenosive triphosphatase. Science 165:807 (1969).

2. M. Martínez-Maldonado, M. J. C. Allen, C. Inagaki, N. Tsaparas and A. Schwartz, Renal sodium-potassium-activated adenosine triphosphatase and sodium reabsorption. J. Clin. Invest. 51: 2544 (1972).

3. P. C. Churchill and F. McDonald, Effect of ouabain on renin secretion in anesthetized dogs, J. Physiol. 242:635 (1974).

4. M. A. Cruz-Soto, J. E. Benabe, J. M. López-Novoa and M. Martínez-Maldonado, Renal Na^+-K^+-ATPase in renin release. Am. J. Physiol. 243 (Renal Fluid Electrolyte Physiol. 12):F598 (1982).

5. L. Belardinelli, D. Harder, N. Sperelakis, R. Rubio and R. M. Berne, Cardiac glycoside stimulation of inward Ca^{++} current in vascular smooth muscle of canine coronary artery. J. Pharmacol. Exp. Ther. 209:62 (1979).

6. P. C. Churchill, Possible mechanism of the inhibitory effect of ouabain on renin secretion from rat renal cortical slices. J. Physiol. London 294:123 (1979).

7. C. S. Park, and R. L. Malvin, Calcium in the control of renin release. Am. J. Physiol. 235 (Renal Fluid Electrolyte Physiol.): F22 (1978).

8. C. S. Park, D. S. Han and J. C. S. Fray, Calcium in the control of renin secretion: Ca^{2+} influx as an inhibitory signal. Am. J. Physiol. 240 (Renal Fluid Electrolytes Physiol. 9):F70 (1981).

9. H. J. Lyons, and P. C. Churchill, The influence of ouabain on *in vitro* renin secretion. Proc. Soc. Exp. Biol. Med. 145:1148 (1973).

10. J. M. López-Novoa, J. C. García, M. A. Cruz-Soto, J. E. Benabe, and M. Martínez-Maldonado, Effect of sodium orthovanadate on renal renin secretion in vivo. J. Pharmacol. Exp. Ther. 222: 447 (1982).

11. M. Martínez-Maldonado, G. Eknoyan, J. C. Allen, W. N. Suki and A. Schwartz, Urine dilution and concentration after digoxin infusion into the renal artery of dogs. Proc. Soc. Exp. Biol. Med. 134:855 (1970).

12. M. P. Blaustein, Sodium ions, calcium ions blood pressure regulation, and hypertension: a reassessment and a hypothesis Am. J. Physiol. 232:C165 (1977).

13. J. E. Benabe, M. A. Cruz-Soto, and M. Martínez-Maldonado, Critical role of extracellular calcium in vanadate-induced renal vasoconstriction in the dog. Clin. Res. 30(5):881A (1982).

14. W. Hasselback and M. Makinose, ATP and active transport. Biochem. Biophys. Res. Comm. 7:132 (1982).

15. A. Schwartz, Calcium and sarcomplasmic reticulum. In: Calcium and the Heart, P. Harris, and L. H. Opie, eds., Academic Press London and New York, (1971).

16. H. G. Ferreira and V. L. Lew, Use of ionophore A23187 to measure cytoplasmic Ca buffering and activation of the Ca pump by internal Ca. Nature 259:47 (1976).

17. H. L. McCrorey, T. Berl, T. J. Burke, A. de Torrente and R. Schrier, Effect of calcium transport inhibitors on renal hemodynamics and electrolytes excretion in the dog. In: Hormonal Regulation of Sodium Excretion. B. Licardus, R. W. Schrier, and J. Ponel, eds. Elsevier/North Holland Biomedical Press, Amsterdam, (1980).

IMPORTANCE OF CALCIUM IN THE RENAL HEMODYNAMIC CHANGES INDUCED BY VANADATE

Julio E. Benabe and Manuel Martínez-Maldonado

Renal Metabolic Laboratory, Medical and Research Service
Veterans Administration Center and the Department of
Medicine and Physiology, University of Puerto Rico School
of Medicine, San Juan, Puerto Rico

INTRODUCTION

Vanadate has been recognized as an inhibitor of (Na^+, K^+)-ATPase (1, 5). Several groups have emphasized it's potential role as a regulator of the enzyme in the kidney (6), an organ where vanadium tends to accumulate (7). In the dog, intraarterial infusion of vanadate produces a marked vasoconstriction, a decrease in renal blood flow and glomerular filtration rate as well as a decrease in urine flow and sodium excretion (8, 9). In addition to the hemodynamic changes there is also a decrease in renin secretion (10, 11), suggesting that the vasoconstriction is a direct result of the inhibition of the vascular ATPase system. Inhibition by vanadate of sodium or calcium pumps may increase the influx of Ca++ or reduce its efflux from the cytoplasm of muscle cell. This increase in cytoplasmic Ca++ may serve as a stimulus for vasoconstriction.

The following experiments were performed to examine the role of calcium in the renal effects of vanadate in the dog.

Methods

Mongrel dogs weighing 12 to 20 kg. were studied. The animals were deprived of food but not water overnight. Anesthesia was induced with sodium pentobarbital (30 mg/kg I.V.). Animals were ventilated with room air through an endotracheal tube connected to a Harvard respirator. Inulin (12.5 gm/l) and PAH (5 mg/l) diluted in Ringer's solution were given through a femoral vein at a rate of 0.5 ml/min. Both ureters were cannulated with polyethylene catheters (PE 100) through a midline incision. The left kidney was exposed and a hooked 23 gauge needle was inserted into the renal artery.

When more than one drug was to be infused a second needle was inserted. To maintain patency of the lines an infusion of isotonic saline was given through each line at a rate of 0.5 ml/min. All compounds (vanadate, verapamil and calcium) were infused through the lines in the renal artery. The renal vein was catheterized for blood sampling for serum calcium when necessary. An electromagnetic flowmeter (Gould Statham Sp-202, Oxnard, California) cuff probe was placed around the renal artery and renal blood flow (RBF) was measured continously throughout the experiment. The value for each clearance period was obtained by recording mean flow only during the mid-point of blood collection. Blood pressure was measured through a femoral artery catheter using a pressure transducer (Statham Instruments Hato Rey, Puerto Rico). Throughout the experiments the animals received an infusion of saline sufficient to replace the losses of urine and blood. In addition the animals received 100 ml of saline to replace surgical losses so that modest volume expansion existed when the experiment began.

An equilibrium period of at least 45 minutes was allowed before collections. All clearance periods were of 10 minutes duration with arterial and renal vein blood samples collected at midpoint for electrolytes, inulin and PAH determinations.

Three groups of animals were studied. Group I, verapamil (VER) group (n=7). Following three control periods in which Ringer's solution was infused into the left renal artery at a rate of 0.5 ml/min, verapamil diluted in Ringer's solution, (200 μg/ml), was infused at 0.5 ml/min through a second needle into the renal artery and three clearance periods of 10 min each were obtained. This was followed by the simultaneous infusion of VER and Na_3VO_4. The orthovanadate (Na_3VO_4) was disolved in Ringer's solution and infused at a rate of 0.5 μmol/min (0.5 ml/min). Three clearance periods were obtained during its infusion. Three final clearance periods were obtained infusing Na_3VO_4 alone after stopping the VER.

Group II-Thyroparathyroidectomy (TPTX) and vanadate (n=8). TPTX was performed 24 hrs. before the experiments. After control clearance collections, VO_4 was infused as in the previous group (0.5 μmols/min).

Group III-TPTX and vanadate (n=6). After control clearance were obtained vanadate was infused alone for two periods. This was followed by two clearance periods in which during VO_4 infusion a calcium chloride solution calculated to restore normal serum calcium was also given through a second needle in the renal artery. Blood calcium was measured in samples of renal venous blood.

Verapamil was a generous gift from Knoll Pharmaceutical Co. (Whippany, N.J.). Sodium orthovanadate was purchased from Alfa Products (Danvers, MA).

Na^+ and K^+ were measured by flame photometry, Ca^{++} by a spectrophotometric micromethod. Results are presented as mean ± standard errors. Analysis of variance and paired t-test were used for statistical analysis.

Results

Group I (Verapamil and vanadate). The results in this group are shown in Table 1. Verapamil infusion had no effect on RBF. There were also no significant changes in GFR, V and FE_{Na^+}. Simultaneous infusion of vanadate decreased RBF to 82% of control without significantly changing GFR, which decreased to only 89% of control. Urine flow and FE_{Na^+} decreased only to 80% of control, a change which was not significant, but it decreased to 52% of the values obtained with verapamil plus vanadate.

TABLE 1 Renal effects of verapamil and vanadate (Group I)*

	RBF ml/min	GFR ml/min	V ml/min	FE_{Na^+} %
CONTROL	126.7 ±7.1	18.4 ±1.7	0.98 ±0.15	5.4 ±1.5
VERAPAMIL	144.1 ±11.1	19.5 ±2.1	1.88 ±0.40	7.7 +1.9
VERAPAMIL + VANADATE	104.0 ±11.5	16.3 ±2.4	1.95 ±0.39	8.5 ±2.0
VANADATE	† 55.6** ±7.1	† 9.1** ±2.9	† 0.60** ±0.12	4.3 ±1.0

*Means ± SE; significant values ($p<0.05$) are indicated by † (different from control) and by ** (different from previous values). RBF=renal blood flow; GFR-glomerular filtration rate; V=urine flow; FE_{Na}=fractional sodium excretion.

Group II (TPTX and vanadate). The results of these experiments are shown in Table 2. TPTX resulted in a significant reduction in serum calcium from 8.78±0.29mg% to 4.98±0.25mg% ($p<0.0001$). When vanadate was infused under this conditions it decreased RBF to 80% of control ($p<0.025$). There were no significant changes in GFR, V or FE_{Na^+} throughout the experiment.

TABLE 2 Effect of TPTX on renal response to vanadate (Group II)*

	RBF ml/min	GFR ml/min	V ml/min	FE_{Na^+} %
CONTROL	167.0 $\pm$28.5	23.0 $\pm$2.8	1.10 $\pm$0.37	4.02 $\pm$1.03
VANADATE	132.0† $\pm$19.3	20.4 $\pm$2.7	1.21 $\pm$0.44	4.15 $\pm$1.19

*Symbols as in Table 1

Group III (TPTX, vanadate and calcium infusion). The results are shown in Table 3. Vanadate decreased RBF to only 84% control ($p<0.05$) in TPTX dogs (serum calcium 5.41$\pm$0.40 mg%) but upon restoring calcium to normal (9.74$\pm$0.74mg%), RBF fell to 49% of control ($p<0.001$) The changes in GFR induced by vanadate in TPTX were not significant, but restoration of serum calcium was associated with a sharp fall in GFR to 42% control ($p<0.02$) and to 53% of the value when vanadate was infused while serum calcium was low ($p<0.02$). Urine flow and FE_{Na^+} did not change significantly when vanadate was infused in the TPTX dogs. Restoration of serum calcium to normal did not change V (92% control) but led to a significant rise in FE_{Na^+} ($p<0.02$).

TABLE 3 Effects of TPTX on renal response to vanadate and calcium infusion*

	RBF ml/min	GFR ml/min	V ml/min	FE_{Na^+} %
CONTROL	156.4 $\pm$29.9	19.1 $\pm$4.1	1.3 $\pm$0.4	7.7 $\pm$2.1
VANADATE	131.8† $\pm$30.7	15.2 $\pm$3.1	1.6 $\pm$0.8	9.3 $\pm$3.7
CALCIUM + VANADATE	76.8**† $\pm$18.9	8.1**† $\pm$1.6	1.2 $\pm$0.3	13.3**† $\pm$3.2

*All symbols as in Table 1.

Discussion

The renal vasoconstrictive effect of VO_4 in intact rats, isolated perfused rat kidney, the cat, and intact dogs have been recently discribed (9, 12, 13).

We have postulated that the vasoconstrictive effects of vanadate might be related to increased intracellular calcium (9, 11) possibly secondary to inhibition of (Na^{+}, K^{+})-ATPase. A similar suggestion was considered by Rapp (14). This investigator used aortic rings from Dahl salt-sensitive and salt-resistant rats in an attempt to assess if the contractile effects of vanadate were the results of inhibition of (Na^{+}, K^{+})-ATPase, which in turn would cause intracellular calcium to rise (14). Using indirect methods (The activity of the enzyme was not measured), this investigator concluded that vanadate (up to 10^{-3} M) does not inhibit (Na^{+}, K^{+})-ATPase in intact smooth muscle cells. Similar conclusions were reached by Ozaki and Urakawa (15) who also employed indirect methods to assess enzyme activity in guinea pigs aortic strips.

From the present experiments we can not ascertain whether (Na^{+}, K^{+})-ATPase inhibition mediated in part or completely the renal vascular effects of vanadate. However, in view of our results it seems certain that the extracellular calcium concentration is critical. Since vasoconstriction is dependent on intracellular calcium concentration it is clear that vanadate must have increased the influx of extracellular calcium into the cell. Although changes in calcium efflux could have been taking place, this is an unlikely explanation in view of the result with verapamil and TPTX.

Equally unlikely is the possibility that increased intracellular calcium could have also resulted from intracellular calcium redistribution as a result of inhibition of Ca-ATPase activity in plasma membranes or in endoplasmic reticulum (16, 17, 18, 19). It should be pointed out that Ca-ATPase activity has not been shown to be altered by diminished extracellular calcium nor by a slow calcium channel blocker.

Verapamil blocked the effects of vanadate almost completely. These findings strengthens the previous suggestion from this laboratory that voltage-dependent channels are required for calcium entry into the cytosol in vanadate induced vasoconstriction (9, 11) the alternative, that verapamil blocks the entry of vanadate into cells is unlikely since vanadate enters cells by the same system that transports phosphate (20, 21) or through an anion exchange system (22) and these systems are not known to be affected by calcium-channel blockers.

Finally, we feel that the experiments in TPTX dogs from Group III conclusively indicate the critical role of extracellular calcium concentration in the hemodynamic changes induced by VO_4. The infusion of VO_4 reduced RBF and GFR by 20% or less (not statistically significant). By contrast, restoration of pre-TPTX plasma calcium levels led to a 51% decrease in RBF and a 58% decrease in GFR. Despite this, during hypocalcemia, vanadate increased V by 23% while normocalcemia abolished the rise.

An important aspect of this study resides in the demonstration that vanadate is clearly natriuretic in the dog during the hypocalcemia of TPTX. Once natriuresis was established when hypocalcemia was present, restoration of serum calcium did not prevent natriuresis despite falls in RBF and GFR. This strongly suggest that VO_4 had reached its intracellular sites of action in the tubular epithelium and strenghtens our previous suggestion that intense vasoconstriction is responsible for most, if not all, the antidiuresis and antinatriuresis of VO_4 in the dog.

Granting that the evidence put forth is indirect, in the aggregate, they strongly suggest that extracellular calcium concentration is critical in mediating the renal vasoconstrictive effects of vanadat

Acknowledgements

We are indebted to Mr. José L. Gotay, Mr. George Crespo and Ms. Joyce Bou-Vierno for technical assistance, and to Mrs. Victoria D. de Pérez for secretarial assistance.

This work was supported by funds from the Veterans Administration Central Office (merit Review Program) and by NIH grants RR-08102 (SUBE for Support for University Biomedical Education) and AM-30201.

REFERENCES

1. L. A. Beaugé and I. M. Glynn, Commercial ATP containing traces of vanadate alters the responce of (Na^+-K^+)-ATPase to external potassium. Nature London 272:551 (1978).

2. M. D. Blaustein, Sodium ions, calcium ions blood pressure regulation, and hypertension: a reassessment and a hypothesis. Am. J. Physiol. 232:C165 (1977).

3. U. Borchard, K. Greeff, D. Hafner, E. Noack, and K. Rojsathaporn, Effects of vanadate on heart and circulation. J. Cardiovasc. Pharmacol. 3:510 (1981).

4. L. C. Cantley, Jr., and P. Aisen, The fate of cytoplasmic vanadium: implications on (Na, K)-ATPase inhibition. J. Biol. Chem. 254: 1781 (1979).

5. L. C. Cantley, Jr., L. Josephson, R. Warner, M. Yanagisawa, C. Lechene, an G. Guidotti. Vanadate is a potent (Na^+, K^+)-ATPase inhibitor found in ATP derived from muscle. J. Biol. Chem 252: 7421 (1977).

6. J. J. Grantham, The renal sodium pump and vanadate. Am. J. Physiol 239:F97 (1980).

7. P. L. Jorgensen, Sodium and potassium ion pump in kidney tubules. Physiol. Rev. 60:864 (1980).

8. D. J. Inciarte, R. P. Steffen, D. E. Dobbins, B. T. Swindall, J.Johnston, and F. J. Haddy, Cardiovascular effects of vanadate in the dog. Am. J. Physiol. 239:H47 (1980).

9. J. M. López-Novoa, V. Mayol and M. Martínez-Maldonado, Renal actions of orthovanadate in the dog. Proc. Soc. Exp. Biol. Med. 170:418 (1982).

10. P. C. Churchill and M. C. Churchill, Vanadate inhibits renin secretion from rat kidney slices. J. Pharmacol. Exp. Ther. 213: 114 (1980).

11. J. M. López-Novoa, J. C. García, M. A. Cruz-Soto, J. E. Benabe, and M. Martínez-Maldonado, Effect of sodium orthovanadate on renal renin secretion in vivo. J. Pharmacol. Exp. Ther. 222: 447 (1982).

12. A. Kamur and C. N. Corder, Diuretic and vasoconstrictor effects of sodium orthovanadate on the isolated perfused rat kidney. J. Pharmacol.. Exp. Ther. 213:85 (1980).

13. J. A. Larsen, O. Thomsen, and O. Hansen, Vanadate induced oliguria in the anesthetized cat. Acta Physiol. Scan. 106:495 (1979).

14. J. P. Rapp, Aortic responses to vanadate: independence from (Na^+ and K^+)-ATPase and comparison of Dahl salt-sensitive and salt-resistant rats. Hypertension 3:1168 (1980).

15. H. Ozaki, and N. Urakawa, Effects of vanadate on mechanismal responses and Na+ - K+ pump in vascular smooth muscle. Eur. J. Pharmacol. 68:339 (1980).

16. S. G. O'Neal, D. B. Rhoads and E. Racker, Vanadate inhibition of sarcoplasmic reticulum Ca++ - ATPase and other ATPases. Biochem. Biophys. Res. Comm. 89:845 (1979).

17. L. Varecka and E. Caratoli, Vanadate-induced movements of Ca++ and K+ in human red blood cells. J. Biol. Chem. 257:7414 (1982).

18. R. L. Smith, K. Zinn, and L. C. Cantley, A study of the (Na+, K+) ATPase, evidence against interacting nucleotide site models. J. Biol. Chem. 255:9852 (1980).

19. T. Wang, L. I. Tsai, R. J. Solaro, A. O. Grassi de Gende and A. Schwarts, Effects of potassium on vanadate inhibition of sarcoplasmic reticulum Ca^{++}-ATPase from dog cardiac and rabbit skeletal muscle. Biochem. Biophys. Res. Comm. 91:356 (1979)

20. L. C. Cantley, Jr., M. D. Resh and G. Guidotti, Vanadate inhibits the red cell (Na^+, K^+)-ATPase from the cytoplasmic side. Nature London 272:552 (1978).

21. I. G. Macara, K. Kustin, and L.C. Cantley, Jr., Glutathione reduces cytoplasmic vanadate: mechanism and physiological implications. Biochim. Biophys. Acta 629:95 (1980).

22. A. Heinz, K. A. Rubinson, and J. J. Grantham, The transport and accumulation of oxyvanadium compounds in human erythrocytes in vitro. J. Lab. Clinc. Med. 100:593 (1982).

MINERALS AND MYOPATHIES

NORMAL MUSCLE ENERGY METABOLISM

Martin J. Kushmerick

Department of Physiology & Biophysics
Harvard Medical School
Boston, Massachusetts 02115

INTRODUCTION

In all cells, ATP plays a central role in providing a chemical form of potential energy which is enzymatically converted through specific coupling mechanisms into useful work of the cell, e.g. macromolecular synthesis, osmotic, electrical and mechanical work. Striated muscle cells, and skeletal muscle cells in particular, are excellent preparations for studies of the regulation of this energy production and utilization. The reason is that, in contrast with other cells which operate under steady physiological states, the metabolic rate of muscle cells can be increased ten- to fifty-fold above the basal rate by stimulating the muscle to mechanical activity. This large increase in metabolic rate allows exploration of non-steady state energy perturbations, which gives important insight into general aspects of metabolic regulation.

BASIC SCHEME

The basic paradigm with which experimentors who are interested in muscle energetics work incorporates concepts developed from studies of isolated muscles and exercising animals (Kushmerick, 1982). The paradigm has two aspects: (1) there is a net decrease in chemical potential energy content during muscle activity--for brief contractions the major reaction is the utilization of phosphoryl-creatine (PCr); and (2) there exists a recovery period after mechanical relaxation in which oxidative metabolism utilizes substrate to regenerate the initial precontraction steady state of high-energy content. At least under certain experimental conditions, it is thought possible to separate completely the processes occurring in the contraction phase (e.g. PCr splitting) from those occurring in the recovery phase (e.g. oxygen consumption). The basis for the separability into two phases lies in the greatly differing time constants of the relevant chemical processes. For mammalian skeletal and cardiac muscles which differ in mitochondrial content, there is a wide variation in the relative rates of high-energy phosphate resynthesis as compared to high-energy phosphate utilization.

This energetic paradigm is schematically illustrated in Fig. 1. The contractile phase is on the left; progression from left to right indicates a contraction-recovery cycle. Figure 1A shows the development of isometric force upon stimulation. During the recovery period (on the right) there is no mechanical activity. In Fig. 1B, the ATPase rate is the most direct and explicit measure of energy utilization. Before stimulation, there is a small positive value equivalent to the basal rate of energy metabolism (dashed line). With the onset of stimulation, the ATPase rate rises rapidly. Current evidence suggests it passes through a maximum, and during the maintained tetanus settles on a steady rate very much higher than the basal rate. As a consequence of the increased rate of ATP

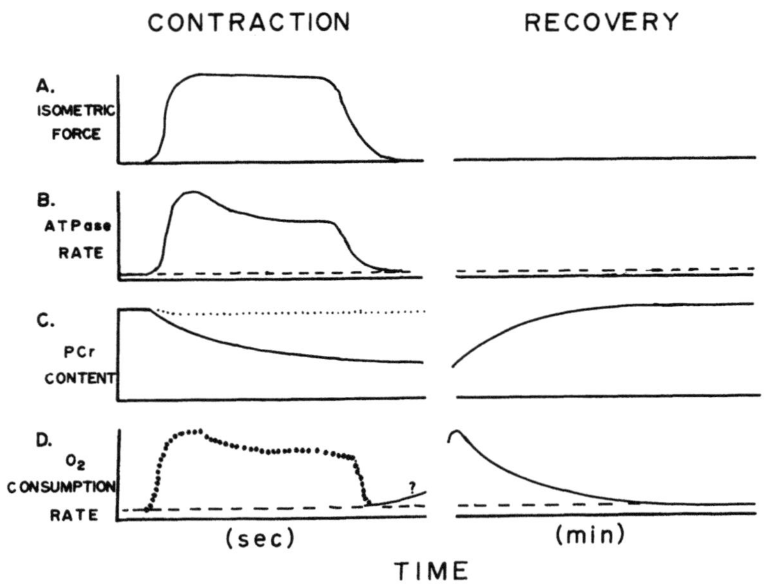

Fig. 1. Schematic diagram of chemical and mechanical events during contraction and recovery phases of a complete cycle of muscular activity is shown. For details, see text. Figure reproduced from Kushmerick, 1982.

utilization and on the condition that PCr and ATP are maintained near equilibrium, the PCr levels follow the time course indicated in Fig. 1C: the rate of decrease is proportional to the ATP turnover rate. Figure 1D shows the condition in which oxygen consumption remains at basal levels during brief contractions (dashed line).

Obviously, a feature of the model is that the contractile events are so rapid that the appropriate metabolic signals have not reached the mitochondria to increase the rate of oxidative metabolism during contraction. At some time during a long contraction or at some time after a brief contraction, the oxygen consumption declines exponentially from this elevated value to basal values as PCr levels are restored. Note that this elevated rate of oxygen consumption is considerably less than the maximal rate of which the muscle is capable. The return of oxygen consumption to basal values marks the end of the recovery period. The increased rate of oxygen consumption above basal during recovery, and the low basal ATPase rate during the recovery period (Fig. 1B on the right), allow the PCr levels to be returned to precontractile levels (Fig. 1C on the right). The rate of PCr synthesis is directly proportional to the oxygen consumption rate in this simple model.

To emphasize alternatives, I have diagrammed an extreme form of another energetic model. Consider the possibility that the rates of ATP utilization and the rates of ATP synthesis by oxidative metabolism might always be equivalent at rest and during the contraction; i.e., oxidative phosphorylation is always able to maintain ATP and PCr levels nearly constant. Such a possibility appears to be the case for smooth muscle. In this situation there would be an ATPase rate associated with the contractile processes, but the net decrease in PCr would be minimal because of a simultaneous increase in oxygen consumption (dotted line, Fig. 1D on the left) proportional to the ATPase rate. Thus, the PCr levels would fall only slightly during a transition from basal steady state to contractile steady state (dotted line, Fig. 1C on the left). Obviously the division between a contractile phase and recovery energetic phase is meaningless in this second type of energetic model.

Time Course of High Energy Phosphate Utilization During Contraction

Thus, the two features that distinguish the non-steady state of muscle contraction from the more common steady state behavior of other cells are (1) the rate of ATP utilization by actomyosin and other ATPases following activation usually exceeds by an order of magnitude the rate of its resynthesis by glycolysis and oxidative phosphorylation; and (2) striated muscle cells have a large content of creatine phosphate (three to five times the content of ATP) which serves as a back-up supply by equilibration between ATP and creatine phosphate via the enzyme creatine phosphokinase (CPK). There is evidence that the reaction:

$H^+ + PCr + ATP = ATP + Cr$

is near equilibrium in cells (see below). Figure 2 shows the results obtained from isolated in vitro mouse hind limb muscles at 20°C when quantitative data of the extent of energy consumption is plotted against the duration of a continuous tetanus (Crow and Kushmerick, 1982a). In the slow-twitch soleus mucle, the rate of coupled hydrolysis of PCr and ATP (Δ~P) is averaged over 3 sec intervals of a continuous 15 sec tetanus. Quantitatively, the results are identical

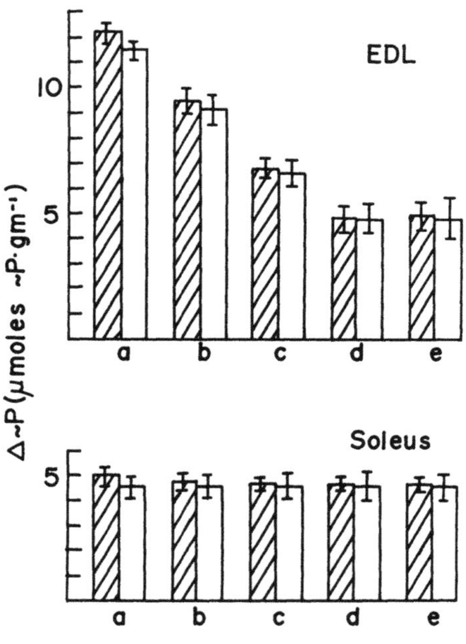

Fig. 2. Utilization of chemical potential energy during a continuous isometric tetanus of in vitro mouse soleus and extensor digitorum longus (EDL) is graphed in units of high energy phosphate change during serial 3 sec intervals (a to e) of a 15 sec tetanus. Open bars indicate directly measured depletion of PCr and ATP; hatched bars indicate total recovery oxygen consumption X 6.3. Data repeated from Crow and Kushmerick, 1982a.

whether the energy utilization was measured directly as changes in PCr content or by total oxygen consumption. This equivalence shows a biochemical energy balance between ~P and oxidative metabolism in whole cells as observed in isolated mitochondria. In the fast-twitch EDL muscle, during a maintained tetanic contraction in which there is nearly a steady isometric force (force typically decreases to not less than 80% of its initial value at 15 sec), there is a more than two-fold decrease in the rate of coupled ~P hydrolysis. The initial more rapid rate in the fast-twitch muscle is three times the rate of energy consumption in the slow-twitch muscle for the same force per cross sectional area.

One conclusion of this type of study is that it is not safe to assume that during a steady physiological process, here isometric muscle contraction, that the rate of energy consumption is also constant. Thus, it is always necessary to ask whether the coupling coefficient in any physiological process is quantitatively constant in time.

A mechanism which may explain the increase in isometric economy in fast-twitch muscle, but not in the slow-twitch muscle, involves a covalent modification of a component of the myosin molecule, the 18,000 dalton light chain. We and others have observed that during stimulation, phosphorylation of a myosin light chain occurs concurrently with the decrease in rate of high energy utilization during an isometric tetanus (Crow and Kushmerick, 1982b); reduction in myofibrilar ATPase rate has also been observed under conditions of myosin phosphorylation (Cooke et al., 1982).

A similar pattern of chemical changes is observed during a period of steady-state activity consisting of intermittent stimulation (trains of isometric twitches), an experimental manipulation analogous to a brief period of steady-state exercise. An example of such an experiment in an isolated cat soleus muscle studied by ^{31}P-NMR is shown in Fig. 3. Spectrum a is characteristic of an unstimulated muscle, in which the PCr/ATP ratio is typically 3 and the Pi constant is nearly equal to ATP in these slow-twitch muscles. Spectra b, c and d show the changes in content of these compounds that result from a 15 min period of twitches at 1 per sec; the isometric force (not shown) was steady from the onset of the stimulation. The stimulus was stopped commencing with the onset of spectrum e, and the recovery period from this "exercise" is shown in spectra e-h. There is no detectable change in the ATP level, nor is there any detectable ADP present. However, there is a clear decrease in PCr levels, and a concomitant and stoichiometric equivalent increase in Pi. Within a 15 min period at 25°C, these intracellular chemical changes, as well as oxygen consumption rate (data not shown) become steady. Thus, although there is an increased rate of ATP splitting during the stimulation period, the metabolic system adjusts to a lower PCr/Cr ratio, and a higher Pi level. This means that the

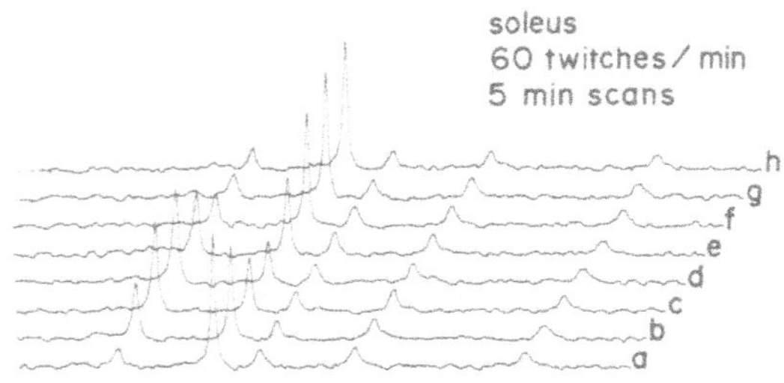

Fig. 3. Series of ^{31}P-NMR spectra were obtained from an arterially-perfused cat soleus muscle in vitro. Each spectrum was obtained at 109.3 MHz and is the average of twenty free induction decays repeated every 15 sec with 90° pulses. Peaks are left-to-right: Pi, PCr, γ, α and β of ATP. a: unstimulated muscle; b-d: continuous 15 min stimulation at one isometric twitch per sec; e-h: recovery after stimulation stopped. Spectra are sequentially offset to the right.

ATP/ADP ratio is also lower as a consequence of the near equilibrium position of the CPK reaction. These chemical changes serve to stimulate mitochondrial respiration. Upon cessation of the stimulus, oxygen consumption rate gradually returns to the resting level, while the original PCr and Pi levels are restored. It should be emphasized that the steady-state oxygen consumption rate during the "exercise period" is much less than the maximum the muscle can achieve. In this experiment, the muscle was given supra-maximal electrical stimulation directly, so that all of the constituent muscle cells were activated with each stimulus. With this experimental protocol, various levels of decrease in creatine phosphate, increase in Pi and increase in oxygen consumption rate could be reproducibly achieved by varying the stimulation rate during the "exercise period". This example serves to indicate that the general energetic scheme outlined earlier appears valid for steady-state exercise periods as well as for steady-state maximal contractions of much shorter duration described earlier.

Intracellular pH Changes During Contractile Activity

An important prediction of the basic energetic model and of the creatine phosphokinase reaction already described is that the cytoplasm should become alkaline during muscle activation if net PCr splitting is the only quantitatively significant reaction occurring. A convenient way to measure intracellular pH is by the chemical shift of inorganic phosphate by ^{31}P-NMR (Moon and Richards, 1973). The bases of this method and its applications to physiological problems are presented in Dr. Ross' paper, and have been reviewed elsewhere (e.g. Gadian, 1982). We developed arterially-perfused muscles for ^{31}P-NMR study (Meyer et al., 1982): the cat soleus muscle, a pure slow-twitch muscle; the cat biceps, a pure fast-twitch muscle. Our

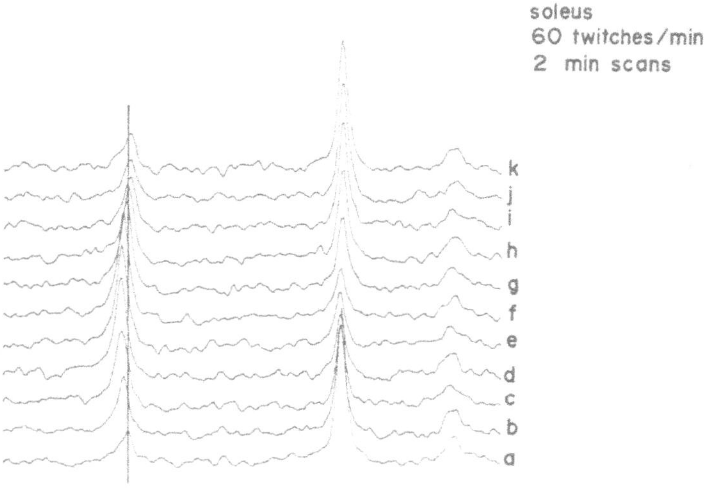

Fig. 4. Series of ^{31}P-NMR spectra was obtained from a cat soleus muscle as described in Fig. 3, except that only eight free induction decays were averaged to give a 2 min time resolution. a: unstimulated muscle; b-f: continuous 10 min stimulation; g-k: recovery. Spectra are aligned so that the PCr peaks coincide. The vertical line indicates the chemical shift corresponding to an intracellular pH of 7.1. Deviations to the left indicate more alkaline pHs; those to the right, more acidic.

experiment was to stimulate the muscles with a train of stimuli at a rate sufficient to decrease PCr to one third the initial level. The records for soleus (Fig. 4) show the expected alkalinization of the cytoplasm as PCr falls. As recovery metabolism commences and restores creatine phosphate to its original level, the expected acidification occurs. An important feature of this recovery metabolism, revealed by NMR, is that the rate of recovery of intracellular pH always is slower than that of creatine phosphate and of Pi. The rate of increase of PCr is quantitatively equivalent to the rate of decrease in Pi during recovery. From the magnitude of the decrease in PCr and from the increase in pH, the calculated buffer capacity ($\Delta H^+/\Delta pH$) is 49 mM, in good agreement with values reported for mammalian muscle by other techniques.

In contrast, the intracellular pH change in the fast-twitch biceps has a different pattern for the same relative change in creatine phosphate; because of a higher ATP and creatine phosphate level, there is a greater absolute decrease in creatine phosphate per gram of muscle. First, the degree of alkalinization is very attenuated,

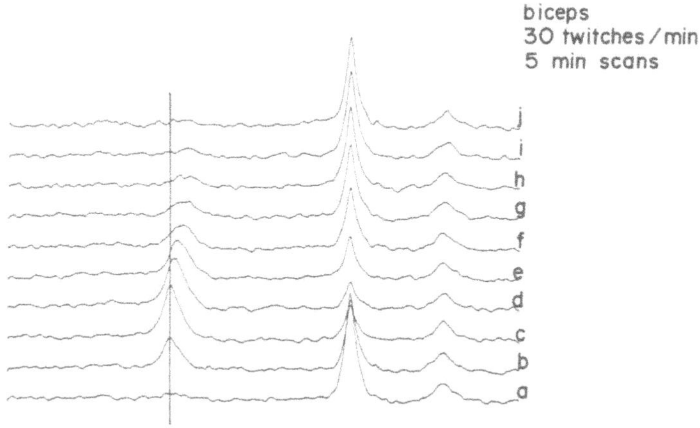

Fig. 5. Series of ^{31}P-NMR spectra was obtained from a cat biceps muscle by methods similar to those described in Fig. 3. a: unstimulated muscle; b-d: continuous 15 min stimulation at 30 twitches/min; e-j: recovery. Spectral alignment and pH calibration by the vertical line is the same as in Fig. 4.

and usually not seen, as the example in Fig. 5 shows. Secondly, the degree of acidification during the recovery period is much more marked. Lastly, in contrast to the spectra obtained in the soleus muscle, there is considerable broadening of Pi peaks in the biceps, which indicates heterogeneity of pH, probably among different cells types because the cat biceps is known to be composed of both glycolytic and oxidative-glycolytic fibers. Most likely, the greater glycolytic capacity of the fast-twitch fibers and the consequent production of lactate overshadow the H^+ uptake associated with net PCr decrease, and enhances the degree of acidification during the recovery period. Also note the very much lower Pi levels in unstimulated biceps muscles compared to the slow-twitch soleus.

The conclusion from these studies is that even though the pattern of changes in high energy phosphate utilization is similar in skeletal muscles during a stimulation-recovery cycle (i.e., the non-steady state pattern of energy utilization and resynthesis described in the first section), it does not follow that other chemical events occur or occur to the same extent. Certainly changes in intracellular pH are not the same either in magnitude or direction when observed by ^{31}P-NMR.

Is the CPK Reaction Near Equilibrium?

The unique feature of ^{31}P-NMR is its ability to measure unidirectional chemical reaction fluxes by spin transfer techniques (Meyer et al., 1982). Without going into the details of the measurements, some of which are given by Dr. Ross, I can summarize our results as follows: the forward and backward fluxes catalyzed by CPK in the cat biceps are equal to each other, and equal to 5 μmol ~P/g/sec. This exchange rate is about 10^3 times the net rate of ATPase in resting muscle as determined from oxygen consumption measurements. The maximal rate of high energy phosphate utilization during contraction has not been measured in the biceps, but is expected to be on the order of 1 μmol/g/sec based on measurements of the energy consumption in other fast-twitch muscles. Thus, even if the chemical exchange fluxes through the CPK reaction do not increase in stimulated muscle, it is clear that this reaction can remain near equilibrium in resting muscle, and is likely not to deviate far from equilibrium in contracting muscle. Supporting this conclusion is the fact that the same total enzymatic activity of CPK, whether in the cytosolic composition and ionic strength, gives the same measured chemical flux by NMR methods. Our experiments on this subject are still underway, but so far it is clear that we do not need to invoke separate pools of ATP, creatine phosphate, or CPK to explain these results in the fast-twitch biceps muscle.

Mg^{++} Levels in the Cytosol

Since the chemical shift of the β phosphate of ATP is altered according to the degree of saturation of the nucleotide with Mg^{++} or other divalent cations (Cohn and Hughes, 1962), unbound cytosolic inorganic Mg^{++} levels can be calculated. As with the measurements in intracellular pH by ^{31}P-NMR, the accuracy of the measure depends on knowledge of the appropriate binding constants under the conditions in the cytosol. Confirming the ^{31}P-NMR published work of others, we find the free Mg^{++} in biceps and soleus muscle is about 2 mM, somewhat less than what is measured by Mg^{++}-sensitive dyes (Baylor et al., 1982), and microelectrodes (Hess et al., 1982). However, we always found in perfused rabbit uterus and urinary bladder that the β peak of ATP was shifted with respect to that observed in all striated muscles; one example is shown in Fig. 6. This chemical shift indicates a free Mg^{++} concentration of 0.4 mM, or nearly an order of magnitude lower than reported for other types of muscle cells so far studied by ^{31}P-NMR or by other methods measuring the cytosolic Mg levels. We have been unable to alter the chemical shift of the β ATP by making the perfusate Mg^{++} free, or by adding 20 mM Mg^{++} to the perfusate, confirming the low permeability of cell

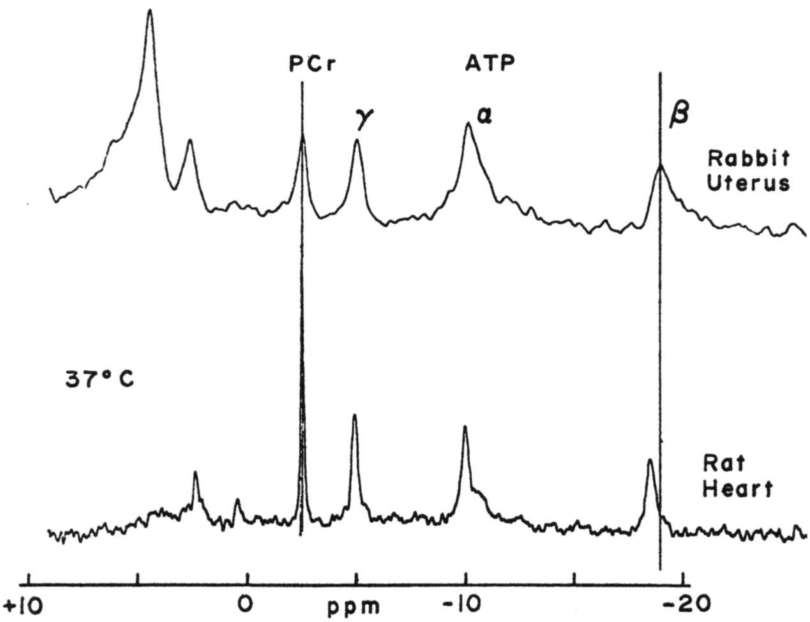

Fig. 6. ^{31}P-NMR spectrum of a perfused rabbit uterus in vitro is compared with one obtained from a rat heart. Chemical shifts of the PCr peak are aligned with each other at -2.52 ppm. The β peak of ATP is shifted -0.4 ppm in the uterus compared to that of the heart, indicating a smaller fraction of ATP is bound to divalent cation in the uterus than in the heart.

membranes to Mg^{++}. Also, the cytosolic Mg^{++} does not change during carbachol stimulation of the bladder. Thus, these smooth muscle cells appear to buffer effectively the cytosolic Mg^{++}, but at a level lower than other muscle cells. The physiological significance of this finding is not clear, but it may have important bearing on our understanding of the regulation of actomyosin ATPase and of phosphorylation of smooth muscle actomyosin, and on the formation of myosin thick filaments, all of which are studied _in vitro_ at millimolar concentrations of Mg^{++}.

CONCLUSION

Skeletal muscle cells have a pattern of energy metabolism that distinguishes them from the steady state patterns found in smooth muscle and non-muscle cells: during normal physiological activity high energy phosphate stores, PCr (and ATP in the extreme) are depleted. Clearly, this is a non-steady state condition of limited duration, which must be followed by a phase of contractile inactivity and a phase of metabolic recovery in which ~P stores are replenished. Spin transfer NMR experiments indicate in the fast-twitch muscle (the biceps, the only one we have studied in some detail so far) that the CPK reaction is at equilibrium under resting conditions, and therefore can function as a store of chemical potential energy which will maintain ATP levels at the expense of PCr during contraction. A marked difference in the intracellular pH changes during contractile activity was observed between fast-twitch and slow-twitch muscles. This result highlights the necessity for measuring properties of the constituent cell types when averaging NMR or other information over an entire organ when more than one cell type is present.

REFERENCES

Baylor, S.M., Chandler, W.K., and Marshall, M.W., 1982, Optical measurements of intracellular pH and magnesium in frog skeletal muscle fibres, _J. Physiol. (London)_, 331:105.

Cohn, M., and Hughes, T.R., Jr., 1962, Nuclear magnetic resonance spectra of adenosine di- and triphosphate. II. Effect of complexing with divalent metal ions, _J. Biol. Chem._, 237:176.

Cooke, R., Franks, K., and Stull, J.T., 1982, Myosin phosphorylation regulates the ATPase activity of permeable skeletal muscle fibers, _FEBS Lett._, 144:33.

Crow, M.T., and Kushmerick, M.J., 1982a, Chemical energetics of slow- and fast-twitch muscles of the mouse, _J. Gen. Physiol._, 79:147.

Crow, M.T., and Kushmerick, M.J., 1982b, Phosphorylation of myosin light chains in mouse fast-twitch muscle associated with reduced actomyosin turnover rate, _Science_, 217:835.

Gadian, D.G., 1982, "Nuclear Magnetic Resonance and its Applications to Living Systems," Oxford University Press, Oxford (England).

Hess, P., Metzger, P., and Weingart, R., 1982, Free magnesium in sheep, ferret and frog striated muscles at rest measured with ion-selective micro-electrodes, J. Physiol. (London), 333:173.

Kushmerick, M.J., 1982, Chemical energy balance in amphibian and mammalian skeletal muscles. Introduction, Fed. Proc., 41:147.

Manning, D.R., and Stull, J.T., 1979, Myosin light chain phosphorylation and phosphorylase A activity in rat extensor digitorum longus muscle, Biochem. Biophys. Res. Comm., 90:164.

Meyer, R.A., Kushmerick, M.J., and Brown, T.R., 1982, Application of ^{31}P-NMR spectroscopy to the study of striated muscle metabolism, Am. J. Physiol., 242:CI.

Moon, R.B., and Richards, J.H., 1973, Determination of intracellular pH by ^{31}P magnetic resonance, J. Biol. Chem., 248:7276.

THE MYOPATHY OF EXPERIMENTAL MAGNESIUM DEFICIENCY

James P. Knochel and Robert E. Cronin

Dallas VA Medical Center and
University of Texas Southwestern Medical School
Dallas, Tx

Selective deficiency of magnesium has not been considered to be a cause of structural disorganization of skeletal muscle cells in man. In contrast, the well-known functional consequences of magnesium depletion and hypomagnesemia appear to affect conduction in perpheral nerves rather than dysfunction at the neuromuscular junction. At the latter location and on the skeletal muscle cell, changes in concentration of magnesium ions required to induce functional alterations are beyond the range of disturbances seen in clinical magnesium deficiency or excess. In humans, experimental magnesium deficiency leads to symptoms of neuromuscular irritability, but these appear to be marked or persistent only when they occur in the presence of hypokalemia and hypocalcemia (1).

EXPERIMENTAL MAGNESIUM DEFICIENCY IN LABORATORY ANIMALS

Structural alterations of skeletal muscle in animals fed magnesium deficient diets otherwise replete in minerals and nutrients have been described in rats (2-5), calves (6), and dogs (7). Common to most other element deficiencies, there exists distinctive species intervariations. In 1969, Heggtveit (2), studying 70 gram Sprague-Dawley rats, examined the effects of feeding a magnesium deficient diet for a period of 60 days. His studies were limited to histologic examination of muscles from the anterior thigh. As described by many observers, after only one week the animals displayed hyperemia of the skin, edema, hyperexcitability and a propensity toward convulsive seizures. This was followed by patchy loss of hair and ulcerations of the skin. Of importance, and common to many studies examining the effect of diets selectively deficient in one element, the animals apparently did not eat and grew at only 50% of the normal rate.

The first lesions in skeletal muscle were noted at seven days. Scattered muscle fibers showed Zenker's hyaline degeneration, swelling and loss of cross striation. The sarcoplasm of the fibers appeared homogeneous and became intensely acidophilic. Progression of the lesion lead to vacuolization of degenerating fibers, granularity and clumping of sarcoplasm. The latter changes appeared to be focal within individual muscle fibers. By 14 days, floccular necrosis was a major finding. At this point, neutrophils and macrophages invaded the necrotic zones and of some interest, a generous accumulation of eosinophils was also noted. Muscle necrosis peaked at 21 days at which time some of the lesions evolved into focal granulomonous nodules with proliferation of fibroblasts. As noted in every tissue ever examined in magnesium deficiency, calcium accumulated in skeletal muscle and in this study became apparent as distinctive calcifications in degenerating myofibers.

Accumulations of eosinophils has been an interesting finding that at least in experimental models, has been observed only in rats. Lowenhaupt (3) also examined the effect of magnesium deficiency in rats and described a widespread perivascular inflammatory process with necrotic foci localized within muscle fibers. Many of the cells in the perivascular inflammatory exudate were eosinophils. It is of interest that myocardial lesions in alcoholic patients who have expired of acute cardiomyopathy are often associated with accumulations of eosinophils in the inflammatory areas of the myocardium. At least two authors showed that eosinophilic glucocyte accumulation and degenerating muscle were not perivascular in location (2,4).

Robeson and her associates (5) examined the ultrastructural effects of magnesium deficiency on skeletal muscle. Mitochondrial swelling appeared on day 14. Total disorganization of the sarcoplasmic reticulum was apparent by day 26.

Moore and his coworkers (6) examined the effect of a magnesium deficient diet for five months in calves. The earliest changes, as described in rats, appeared to be swelling and loss of cross striations of the muscle fiber which stained more deeply with eosin than normal. At a later time, fragmentation of the degenerated fibers could be seen followed in some instances by liquefaction necrosis. Eventually, calcification appeared.

Skeletal Muscle Structure in the Magnesium Deficient Dog

Cronin and his associates (7) studied skeletal muscle samples from the lateral thigh in dogs fed a magnesium deficient diet in constant quantities for a period of ten to eleven weeks. Tissue samples were obtained upon completion of the study. By light microscopy, four of the ten animals examined had normal muscle.

Three others showed focal necrosis of individual muscle cell fibers and the remaining three frank rhabdomyolysis. As will be discussed subsequently, animals with extensive muscle necrosis tended to have much lower total phosphorus content of skeletal muscle than normal. Specimens examined by transmission electron microscopy revealed a wide range of abnormalities while some myofibrils appeared quite normal, others exhibited minimal changes including swelling of the mitochondria and elements of the sarcoplasmic reticulum. Some myofibrils also show disruption of sarcomere (Z-Z) banding together with focal fragmentation of the A band with an apparent loss of the normal A-I banding pattern. The primary mitochondrial abnormality was swelling, especially in mitochondria in the areas of banding disarrangement. Focal areas of sarcomere banding disruption resulting from a disarrangement of the myosin-actin filament interaction (A-band degradation) were apparent as was a loss of glycogen deposits. In addition to focal necrosis, some myofibrils exhibited gross necrosis with myofibrillar degeneration and pockets of swollen mitochondria and other residual myofibrillar elements. Mitochondria in areas of severe necrosis exhibited large dense flocculent matrix granules. The latter apparently represent calcium deposits.

Muscle Cell Composition in Experimental Magnesium Deficiency

Before considering alterations of univalent and divalent ion composition of skeletal muscle in experimental animals produced by magnesium deficiency, one should be aware of two important facts. First, white and red fibers have different element composition. Second, depending upon the species of animal, muscles may be composed of all red, all white or mixtures of such fibers. Sreter and Woo (8) and independently Chutkow (9) have shown that in the rat, concentrations of potassium, magnesium and calcium are greater and the concentration of sodium is considerably less in muscle composed predominantly of white fibers as compared to that composed predominantly of red fibers. Such changes also correspond to resting electrical membrane potential difference of muscle cells. In the laboratory rat, certain muscles are composed of either red or white fibers. Thus it becomes immediately apparent that if one were to base any conclusion on analysis of a muscle, for example the soleus, which is composed predominantly of red fibers, that the results may be entirely different than if a muscle sample were collected from the medial head of the gastrocnemius which is predominantly a white muscle. On the other hand, in dogs and humans, almost all muscles contain essentially equal numbers of red and white fibers, except that extensive physical conditioning or training might convert white fibers to red. Some of the foregoing variations might account for the information to be presented concerning the observation that magnesium deficiency in some experiments causes a loss of potassium ions from skeletal muscle where as in others it does not.

One of the most interesting and as yet unexplained findings in skeletal muscle collected from magnesium deficient animals is the observation that muscle magnesium content often remains within normal limits. This has been true for laboratory rats (4,5,10,12,14), newly hatched chickens (11) and dogs (7). For example, skeletal muscle magnesium content in chicks fed a magnesium deficient diet for a period of 7-21 days showed a control value of 11.1 mEq/100 g FFDW compared to 11.3 mEq/100 g FFDW after feeding the deficient diet (11). On the other hand, MacIntyre and Davidson (13) studied magnesium deficient rats for a period of 11-70 days and showed that magnesium content of muscle fell from a value of 10.1 to 8.7 mEq/100 g FFDW. In the study reported by Whang and Welt (14) rats fed a magnesium deficient diet for 31 days showed a value of 10.1 before and 10.0 mEq/100 g FFDW after magnesium deficiency had occurred, despite a drop in serum magnesium from 1.85 to 0.64 mEq/L. Table I shows data from Chutkow's studies (15) on element composition in white vs. red muscle of the normal rat. Each of these values is significantly different. It is readily apparent that if a study were performed in which a white muscle sample was biopsied as a control specimen and a red sample collected as an experimental specimen, one would observe a statistically significant difference in muscle cell element composition without any experimental intervention whatsoever. Table II compares data on white and red muscle before and after 12 days of feeding a diet deficient in magnesium. This shows that a modest magnesium deficiency occurred in both groups. Calcium rose in white muscle but not in red, potassium deficiency did not occur and finally, the tissue gained sodium.

A review of the aforementioned literature on magnesium deficient rats shows that tissue deficiencies of magnesium and phosphorus are variable, elevated tissue calcium content is usual, and all studies uniformally show elevations of sodium and chloride. In the study by Reddy and his associates (11) on chickens, muscle content of magnesium, calcium, sodium and potassium remained within normal limits. Grace and O'Dell (16) examined the effects of a magnesium deficient diet on weanling guinea pigs. After 36 days of a magnesium deficient diet, muscle magnesium and potassium contents remained within normal limits. Muscle sodium and chloride contents both rose.

When the tissue content of both sodium and chloride become elevated as a result of dietary manipulation, there is uncertainty whether this is explained by an increase in the extracellular space of the tissue sample as a result of edema or a result of decreased resting electrical membrane potential difference which in turn would permit entry of chloride ions into the interior of the cell. As a means to avoid this dilemma, Cronin and his associates (7) induced magnesium deficiency in dogs and measured membrane

TABLE I COMPOSITION OF WHITE VS. RED MUSCLE OF THE NORMAL RAT

	Mg	Ca	K	Na
WHITE (GASTROC)	5.46	5.65	50.6	8.4
RED (SOLEUS)	4.27	4.24	44.4	13.7

CHUTKOW PROC. SOC. EXP. BIOL. MED. 1973

VALUES EXPRESSED AS MOLS/dg FFDW.

TABLE II COMPOSITION OF WHITE VS. RED MUSCLE IN MG DEFICIENCY OF 12 DAYS DURATION

		Mg	Ca	K	Na
WHITE	CONTROL	5.42	5.27	49.9	7.48
	DEFICIENT	4.95*	7.87*	48.3	9.88*
RED	CONTROL	41.6	4.60	40.9	12.2
	DEFICIENT	38.0*	4.72	40.3	13.5*

* STATISTICALLY DIFFERENT FROM CONTROL

CHUTKOW MAYO CLIN. PROC. 1974

potential along with tissue element composition. Table III shows the concentration of minerals and electrolytes in plasma from these dogs before, at seven weeks and again at ten weeks of depletion.

Serum magnesium fell appreciably. Serum sodium rose from 147 to 153 mEq/L, a finding that has been reported previously in magnesium deficiency. Serum potassium and phosphorus did not change. Although hypocalcemia was anticipated (11) the average value fell but this was not a statistically significant change. In Table IV lists values for membrane potential and muscle element content. This indicates that in dogs with severe hypomagnesemia, although muscle magnesium content fell modestly in early magnesium depletion, the value later rose to normal. Values for muscle calcium, sodium and chloride contents became elevated. Muscle potassium remained normal. Table V illustrates the value of measuring membrane potential as a tool to calculate intracellular ion concentrations. This showed an unexpected finding, namely, the muscle cells became hyperpolarized. This occurred in early magnesium depletion and was associated with an elevation of intracellular sodium and a decline of intracellular potassium. Both of these values became normal with continued magnesium depletion. Of interest, muscle intracellular chloride concentration remained within normal limits. These findings suggest two interesting possibilities. First, an ongoing sodium leak might have increased ATPase activity in muscle sufficiently so that the increased rate of sodium efflux resulted in electrical hyperpolarization as an expression of the electrogenic effects of the sodium pump. This would maintain intracellular chloride concentration within a normal or even less than normal value. This would also tend to readjust intracellular potassium concentrations back toward normal, as was observed. Of interest, Mazzocco and his associates observed an increase in renal cortical Na, K-ATPase activity in magnesium deficient rats (17).

Phosphorus Deficiency Induced by Magnesium Deficient Diets.

Studying rats, Whang and Welt (14) showed that magnesium deficient rats tended to become hyperphosphatemic and showed a net rate of phosphorus excretion into the urine that far exceeded their simultaneous intake. They also showed that this occurred in potassium deficiency. They did not measure muscle phosphorus content. Cronin and his associates (7) measured muscle phosphorus content and showed that its values fell appreciably, indeed to the same levels seen when dogs are fed a phosphorus deficient diet. It is of interest that this occurred despite feeding the animals a generous phosphorus intake. At the present time, there is no good explanation for mobilization of muscle phosphorus, the tendency toward hyperphosphatemia and phosphaturia to produce a net negative phosphorus balance as a result of magnesium deficiency.

TABLE III PLASMA MINERALS AND ELECTROLYTES IN MAGNESIUM-DEPLETED DOGS

	Wk	Mg^{2+}, meq/liter	Na^{+} meq/liter	K^{+} meq/liter	PO_4 mg/dl	Ca^{2+}, mg/dl
CONTROL (n=11)	0	1.5 ± 0.2	147 ± 1	4.2 ± 0.6	5.6 ± 1.4	10.2 ± 0.6
MAGNESIUM DEPLETION (n=9)	7	0.5† ± 0.1	151 ± 3	3.8 ± 0.3	6.2 ± 2.6	9.4 ± 0.9
MAGNESIUM DEPLETION (n=9)	10	0.5† ± 0.2	153* ± 3	4.1 ± 0.7	5.0 ± 2.2	9.3 ± 1.5

VALUES ARE MEANS $\pm$ SD. * $P < 0.05$. † $P < 0.001$.

TABLE IV Em AND SKELETAL MUSCLE COMPOSITION IN MAGNESIUM-DEPLETED DOGS

	Wk	MEASURED Em, MV	Mg^{2+}, mM/100 g FFDS	PO_4, mM/100 g FFDS	Ca^{2+}, mM/100 g FFDS	Na^+ meq/100 g FFDS	K^+, meq/ 100 g FFDS	Cl^- meq/100 g FFDS
CONTROL (n=11)	0	94.8 ±2.4	3.8 ±0.2	29.5 ±1.8	0.64 ±0.11	13.2 ±2.6	35.9 ±1.9	5.8 ±0.8
SEVEN DAYS	7	94.8 ±7.3	3.1 † ±0.4	22.0 ‡ ±1.6	0.93* ±0.17	22.9 ‡ ±4.7	33.0 ±4.1	8.2‡ ±1.6
NINE DAYS	10	103.9 † ±8.3	3.5 ±0.4	24.8 ‡ ±2.8	0.85* ±0.26	17.8 † ±2.0	36.3 ±2.0	6.8* ±0.6

TABLE V DERIVED DATA FROM Em AND MUSCLE COMPOSITION

	WK	MEASURED Em, mV	WATER		INTRACELLULAR		
			EC, ml/100 g FFDW	IC, ml/100 g FFDW	Na^+, meq/liter	K^+ meq/liter	Cl^- meq/liter
CONTROL (n=10)	0	94.8	38.9	265.5	27.0	136.3	3.6
MAGNESIUM DEPLETION (n=7)	7	94.8	55.3	279.0	56.6*	120.0	3.7
MAGNESIUM DEPLETION (n=8)	10	103.9†	45.6	275.0	37.3	135.0	2.7

VALUES ARE MEANS ± SD. EC, EXTRACELLULAR; IC, INTRACELLULAR. * $P < 0.05$. † $P < 0.005$.

DISCUSSION

A specific myopathy consequent to isolated magnesium deficiency has not been described in man. Nevertheless, based upon studies performed in this laboratory on other selective ion deficiencies and the information available on experimental magnesium deficiency, it is likely that such an entity exists. The foregoing data indicate that it is impossible to produce isolated magnesium deficiency in skeletal muscle tissue without affecting the balance of other components. Especially striking among these is the fact that magnesium deficiency causes severe phosphorus deficiency. Indeed, phosphorus levels in the skeletal muscle in magnesium deficient dogs was more severe than that produced by feeding an animal a diet selectively deficient in phosphorus and replete in all other elements (18). Although magnesium deficiency may play a role in alcoholic myopathy, the issue is certainly not a clear one. Animals fed alcohol chronically develop deficiencies of phosphorus, magnesium and potassium and show appreciable gain of sodium chloride in calcium in their muscle tissue (19,20). These changes resemble those measured in patients with severe alcoholism and clinical evidence of myopathy. Nevertheless, the fact that magnesium deficiency in an experimental animal usually does not reduce muscle magnesium content while alcohol administration does, suggest that a fundamental difference exists between the two myopathies (21,22).

In conclusion, it seems obvious that dietary magnesium deficiency can induce abnormalities of skeletal muscle in rats, dogs and cattle. Based upon studies in the dog, frank rhabdomyolysis may occur in those animals displaying hyperexcitability and a propensity toward convulsive seizures. Other experiments on several animal models such as hypokalemia (23) and hypophosphatemia (24) suggest that violent muscle contractions such as those experienced during convulsive seizures are sufficient to induce acute rhabdomyolysis in a variety of situations provided cellular injury preexists. Thus, we propose that magnesium deficiency in dogs may induce a sufficient subclinical muscle cell injury so that the violent muscle contractions imposed by convulsive seizures result in frank rhabdomyolysis. The muscle cell hyperpolarization is probably explainable on the basis of a sodium leak, the consequent increased active transport of sodium from the cell and in the process, generation of a higher potential difference due to the electrogenicity of the sodium pump. The calculated normal value for chloride in muscle cell water corresponds to the ultrastructural finding that sarcoplasmic reticulum and transverse tubules are dilated, suggesting an expansion of the extracellular space in magnesium deficiency. Except for abnormally low muscle magnesium content in chronic alcoholic dogs, the remainder of the findings in isolated magnesium deficiency resemble findings in alcoholic patients very closely.

It would seem very likely that much more pronounced changes would be observed in dogs if magnesium deficiency were continued for a much longer period of time. One might predict that overt calcification of skeletal muscle would occur similar to that noted in rats and cattle.

REFERENCES

1. Shils, M.E.: Medicine 48: 61-82, 1969.
2. Heggtveit, H.A.: Ann. N.Y. Acad. Sci. 162:758-765, 1969.
3. Lowenhaupt, E., Schulman, M.P., and Greenberg, D.M.: Arch. Path. 49:427-433, 1950.
4. Ko, K.W., Fellers, F.X., and Craig, J.M.: Lab. Invest. 11:294-305, 1962.
5. Robeson, B.L., Martin, W.G., and Friedman, M.H.: J. Nutr. 110:2078-2084, 1980.
6. Moore, L.A., Hallman, E.T., and Sholl, L.B.: Arch. Path. 26:820-838, 1938.
7. Cronin, R.E., Ferguson, E.R., Shannon, W.A., Jr., and Knochel, J.P.: Am. J. Physiol. 243:F113-120, 1982.
8. Sreter, F.A., and Woo, G.: Am. J. Physiol. 205:1290-1294, 1963.
9. Chutkow, J.G.: Proc. Soc. Exp. Biol. Med. 143:430-432, 1973.
10. Heggtveit, H.A., Herman, L., and Mishra, R.K.: Am. J. Path. 45:757-782, 1964.
11. Reddy, C.R., Coburn, J.W., Hartenbower, D.L., Friedler, R.M., Brickman, A.S., Massry, S.G., and Jowsey, J.: J. Clin. Invest. 52:3000-3010, 1973.
12. Elin, R.J., Armstrong, W.D., and Singer, L.: Am. J. Physiol. 220:543-548, 1971.
13. MacIntyre, I. and Davidsson, D.: Biochem. J. 70:456-462, 1958.
14. Whang, R., and Welt, L.G: J. Clin. Invest. 42:305-313, 1963.
15. Chutkow, J.G.: Mayo Clin. Proc. 49:448-454, 1974.
16. Grace, N.D., and O'Dell, B.L.: J. Nutr. 100:45-50, 1970.
17. Ryan, M.P., and Hingerty, D.: I. J. Med. Sci. 2:137-140, 1969.
18. Fuller, T.J., Carter, N.W., Barcenas, C., and Knochel, J.P.: J. Clin. Invest. 57:1019-1024, 1976.
19. Ferguson, E.R., Blachley, J.D., and Knochel, J.P.: Trans. Assoc. Am. Phys. 95:61-72, 1981.
20. Blachley, J.D., Ferguson, E.R., Carter, N.W., and Knochel, J.P.: Trans. Assoc. Am. Phys. 93:110-122, 1980.
21. Anderson, R., Haller, R., Elms, J., Carter, N.W., and Knochel, J.P.: Miner. Electrolyte Metab. 4:106-112, 1980.
22. Knochel, J.P., Bilbrey, G.L., Fuller, T.J., and Carter, N.W.: Ann. NY Acad. Sci. 252:274-286, 1975.
23. Knochel, J.P., and Schlein, E.M.: J. Clin. Invest. 51:1750-1758, 1972.
24. Knochel, J.P.: Trans. Assoc. Am. Phys. 91:156-168, 1978.

THE MYOPATHY OF PHOSPHATE DEPLETION

Nachman Brautbar and Shaul G. Massry

Division of Nephrology, University of Southern

California, School of Medicine, Los Angeles, California

Phosphate depletion is commonly associated with proximal muscle weakness, muscle pain, impaired resting membrane potential (1) and mild elevation of creatine phosphokinase and aldolase (1). Phosphorus depletion in experimental animals has been shown to cause severe muscle weakness and creatinuria (2). Fuller and associates (1) examined the effect of phosphate depletion and repletion on skeletal muscle in the dog; they found that resting muscle membrane potential and muscle content of potassium and total phosphorus fell, while muscle sodium, chloride and water content rose with phosphate depletion. All these abnormalities returned to, or towards, normal with phosphate repletion. Further studies by the same group of investigators demonstrated that overt rhabdomyolysis may be precipitated by the superimposition of severe hypophosphatemia on pre-existing subclinical myopathy (3). In addition, a rise in creatine phosphokinase occurs in patients who develop acute fall in the serum levels of phosphorus (4). The observation that myopathic symptoms develop only in severe hypophosphatemia (4), and that acute hypophosphatemia may be associated with acute rhabdomyolysis suggest that both serum and cellular inorganic phosphorus levels play an important role in the myopathy.

These clinical and experimental observations suggest that skeletal myopathy of phosphate depletion may be at least in part the result of abnormalities in cellular inorganic phosphorus turnover and impaired functional integrity of cell membrane. This study was designed to examine the effects of experimental phosphate depletion on skeletal muscle cellular aerobic and anaerobic energy metabolism and membrane biochemical integrity.

METHODS

150-200 g Sprague-Dawley rats were studied after short term, (4 weeks) moderate (8 weeks) and long term (12 weeks) of selective dietary phosphorus restriction. The animals were fed rat chow containing 0.025% phosphorus. Another group of weight and age matched, pair-fed rats received diets containing 0.35% phosphorus and served as control. At the day of sacrifice, skeletal muscle samples were obtained from the gastrocnemius muscle for the analysis of phosphorylated intermediates and mitochondrial energy production as described previously (5). Energy utilization was examined in isolated myofibrils as described by Solaro et al (6). Samples were also processed for acid extractable phospholipid precursors, glycerol and glycogen, (7) as well as butanol extractable tissue phospholipids. Blood was collected for the measurement of serum inorganic phosphorus.

Phospholipids were extracted as described by Bligh and Dyer (8) and were separated utilizing high pressure liquid chromatography (9) and thin layer chromatography (10). Inorganic phosphorus was then determined with the methods of Bartlett (11).

RESULTS

I. Cellular Energy Metabolism

a. Anaerobic energy production

Skeletal muscle glycogen and glucose 6-phosphate concentration fell significantly at 8 and 12 weeks of phosphate depletion (Table I). There were significant correlations between the muscle content in glucose 6 phosphate ($p<0.01$) and glycogen ($p<0.01$) and those of inorganic phoshorus.

b. Aerobic energy production and utilization

The changes in cellular inorganic phosphorus, ATP, ADP, and creatinine phosphate are shown in Figures (1-3). There was a marked fall in cellular inorganic phosphorus in early phosphate depletion, and levels remained low at 8 and 12 weeks but the content of adenine nucleotides and creatine phosphate levels did not change. The cells maintained energy charge, but phosphorylation potential calculated from the ratios of $\frac{ATP}{ADP \times P}$ (12), was significantly elevated in (Table I).

Mitochondrial oxygen consumption (energy production) and transport were significantly impaired already at 4 weeks of phosphate depletion, (Figure 4 and 5), and myofibrillar energy utilization (myofibrillar creatine phosphokinase activity) was also reduced (Figure 6), as well as total extractable cellular creatine phosphokinase activity (Figure 7), and these changes were correlated with the changes in cellular inorganic phosphorus, ($p < 0.01$).

II. Biochemical integrity of cellular membrane

The concentration of glycerol phosphate was markedly reduced at 4 weeks of phosphate depletion and remained low throughout the study (Table II). The fall in glycerol phosphate was correlated with the fall in cellular inorganic phosphorus, ($p<0.01$).

There was a marked fall in the concentration of major cellular phospholipids including phosphatidylcholine, phosphatidylethalamine and 1,2 diglyceride, Table II.

TABLE I. Skeletal Muscle Glycogen, Glucose 6 Phosphate, and Phosphorylation Potential at 4,8, and 12 weeks of Phosphate Depletion

	Glycogen/mg Protein	Glucose 6 Phosphate μmol/g Protein	Phosphorylation Potential
4 weeks			
Control	61.0±8.4	4.0±0.3	2020±120
PD	-	3.8±1.2	4160±102*
8 weeks			
Control	71.0±7.0	4.65±0.17	2000±330
PD	35.8±2.1*	2.40±0.20*	2830±140
12 weeks			
Control			
PD			

Data are presented as mean ±SE, * $p<0.01$, ** $p<0.05$.

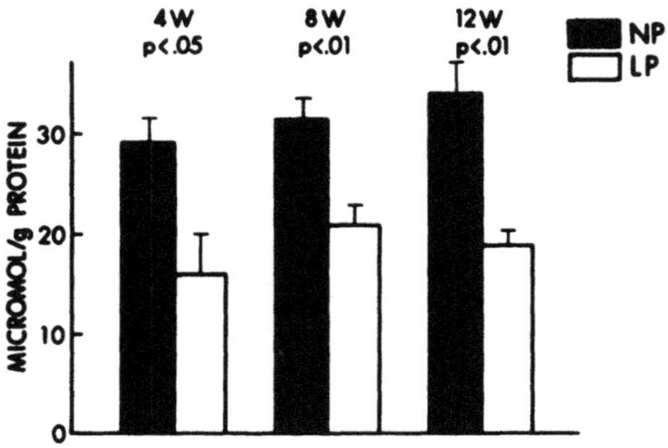

Figure 1: The changes in inorganic phosphorus content of skeletal muscle of rats induced by various periods of phosphate depletion.

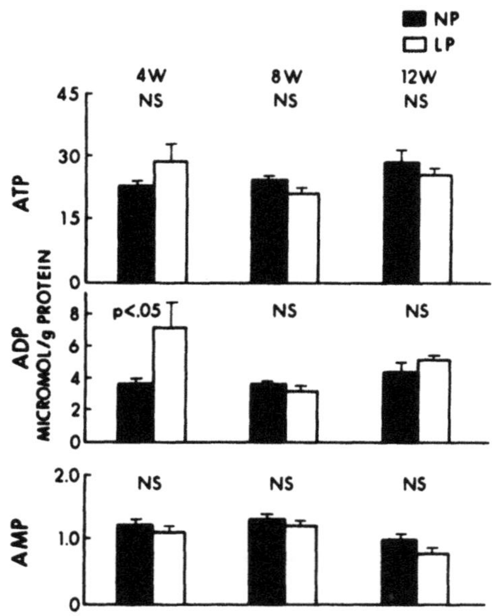

Figure 2: The changes in adenine nucleotide content of skeleton muscle of rat induced by various periods of phosphate depletion.

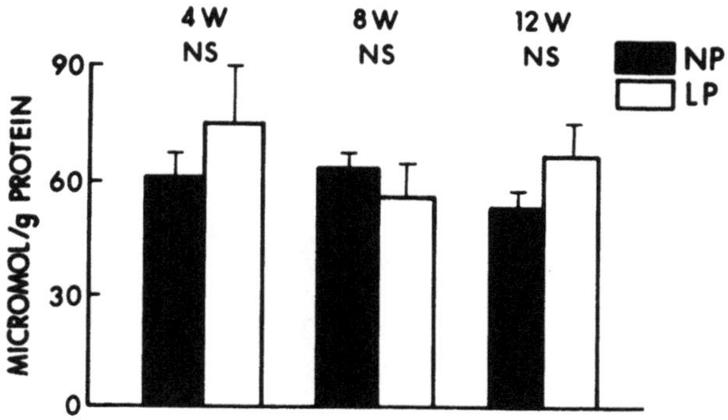

Figure 3: The changes in creatine phosphate content of skeletal muscle of rat induced by various periods of phosphate depletion.

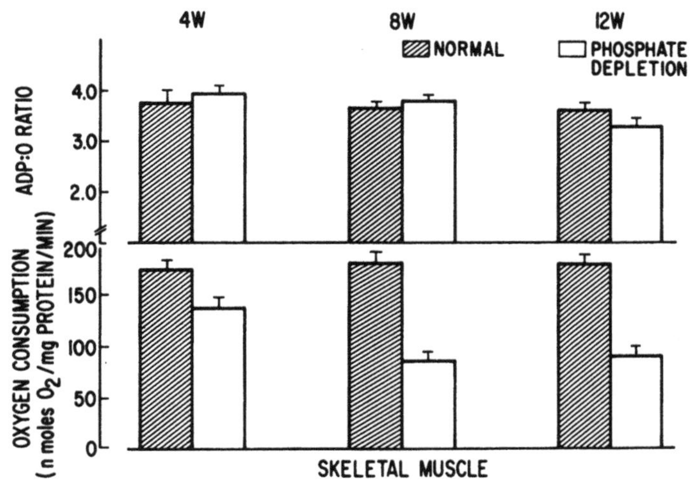

Figure 4: Effect of various durations of phosphate depletion on mitochondrial oxygen consumption and on ADP:O ratio.

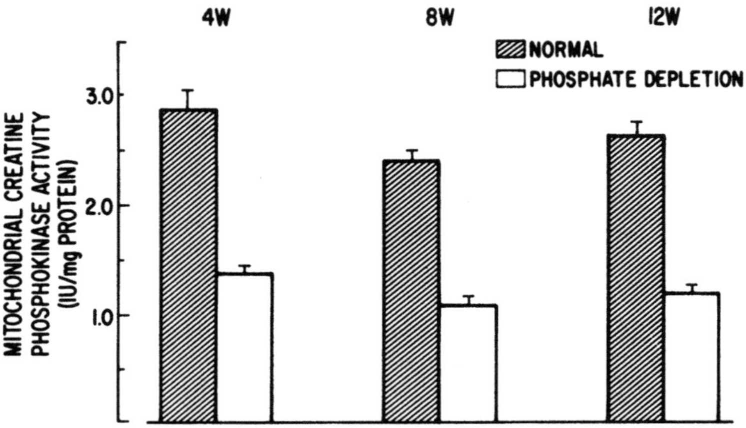

Figure 5: Effect of various durations of phosphate depletion in the activity of mitochondrial creatine phosphokinase.

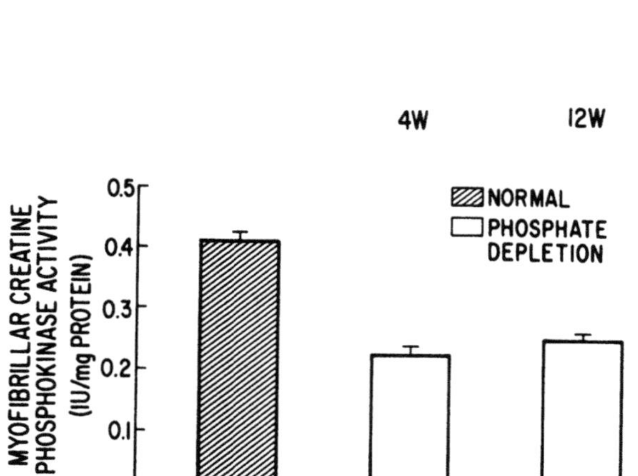

Figure 6: Effect of various durations of phosphate depletion on the activity of myofibrillar creatine phosphokinase.

TABLE II. SKELETAL MUSCLE PHOSPHOLIPID PRECURSORS AND MAJOR PHOSPHOLIPIDS

	Glycerol Phosphate nmol/gram protein	Cytidine Triphosphate n/mol gram protein	Phosphatidyl-choline % Inorganic Pi	Phosphatidyl-ethanolamine % Inorganic Pi	Phosphatidyl-choline Phosphatidyl-ethanolamine
4 weeks					
Control	670±60	430±40	-	-	-
PD	380±40*	530±30			
8 weeks					
Control	680±70	-	-	-	-
PD	320±10*	-	-	-	-
12 weeks					
Control	740±40	380±30	45.0±6.0	13.4±1.4	3.3±0.08
PD	330±30*	190±40*	23.0±3.8*	4.8±0.8*	2.8±0.01**

Data are presented mean±SE, * = $p<0.01$, ** $p<0.05$

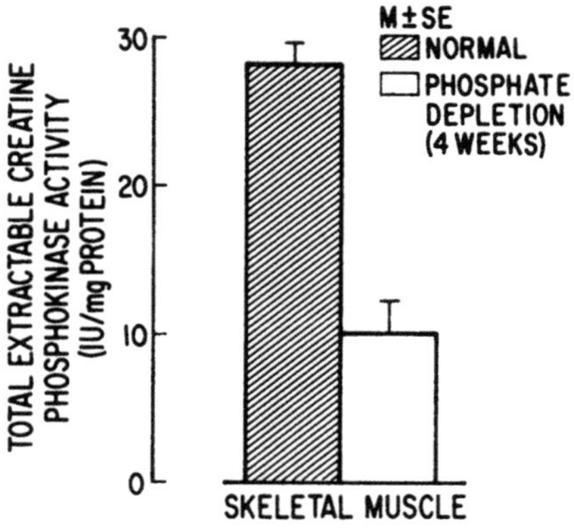

Figure 7: Effect of 4 weeks of phosphate depletion on the activity of total extractable creatine phosphokinase.

DISCUSSION

The results of our studies show that phosphate depletion is associated with alterations in anaerobic and aerobic energy production, energy transport and utilization and an impaired phospholipid metabolism indicating impaired biochemical integrity of cell membrane.

The current concept of skeletal muscle energy metabolism is shown in Figure (8) and is based on the principal of microcompartmentation of the energy (13), and control of energy produced via respiration, by cytosolic inorganic phosphorus (14) and the availability of ADP. Thus, three steps are recognized:

Step I: Energy is produced in the mitochondria in the form of ATP which cannot permeate the mitochondrial membrane; and therefore, there is a need to initiate steps for energy transport.

Step II: Energy from ATP is converted to diffusible energy in the form of creatine phosphate. This step is mediated via the mitochondrial adenine nucleotide translocase, creatine phosphokinase isoenzyme, cytosolic ADP and creatine. The creatine phosphate diffuses through the cytosol to the myofibrils for use in the contraction process.

Step III: The utilization of the energy from creatine phosphate at the myofibrillar site is accomplished via the myofibrillar isoenzyme of creatine phosphokinase and CA ATPase. The ADP released during muscle contraction is phosphorylated to ATP, and free creatine and the latter diffuses back to the mitochondrial site for rephosphorylation. Thus, creatine phosphate, creatine and creatine phosphokinase isoenzyme form a shuttle which is called the creatine phosphate energy shuttle (13).

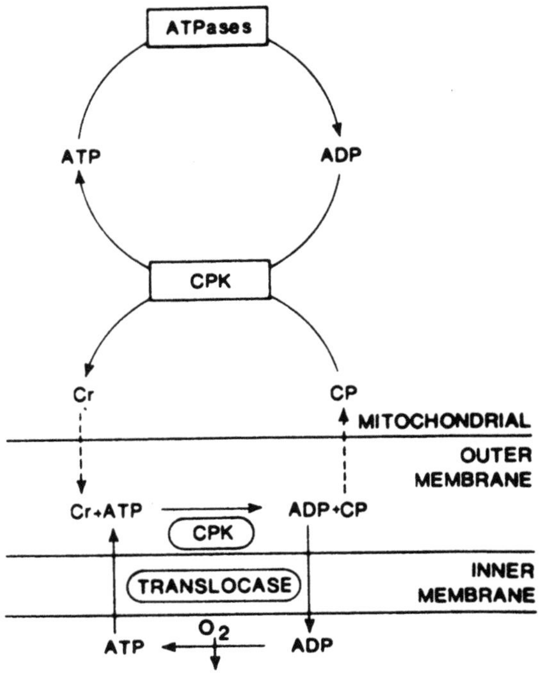

Figure 8: Schematic presentation of the current concept of skeletal muscle energy metabolism.

The first changes to occur with short term hypophosphatemia are 1) reduction in cellular inorganic phosphorus content, 2) reduced activity of mitochondrial and myofibrillar creatine phosphokinase activity, 3) elevation of phosphorylation potential and reduction in mitochondrial respiration. It is of interest that despite the reduction in mitochondrial and cytosolic ATP production, there was no fall in absolute ATP and creatine phosphate values, even at 8 and 12 weeks of phosphate depletion. The reason for this could be that the biopsy values of ATP and creatine phosphate represent static levels in a non exercised muscle, and do not discriminate between mitochondrial and myofibrillar ATP. Since energy utilization by the myofibrils is reduced as well, is it possible that the total ATP and creatine phosphate may not change. Indeed, recent studies by Hettelman et al (15) have shown that ATP levels after muscle stimulation are reduced in phosphate depleted mice.

The fall in creatine phosphokinase isoenzyme activity occurred early in the course of phosphate depletion and was associated and correlated with the fall in cellular inorganic phosphorus. Whether creatine phosphokinase has any relationship with inorganic phosphorus concentration is not known, but it is possible that like other enzymes (such as phosphofructokinase), creatine phosphokinase activity might be in part determined by the cellular concentration of inorganic phosphorus.

The fall in glucose 6 phosphate concentration and the

reduced levels of glycogen are compatible with reduced glycolysis, glucose phosphorylation, and reduced glycogen synthesis. Indeed, decreased glucose uptake as well as insulin resistance have been reported in hypophosphatemic patients (16) and rats (17). Increased glucose-6-phosphate utilization could also be present and contribute to its reduced cellular content. Our data do not support or refute this possibility. However, the metabolic pathway of glucose-6-phosphate is facilitated by phosphofructokinase. This enzyme is sensitive to the cellular concentration of inorganic phosphorus and is inhibited when the latter is low. It is reasonable to suggest that in phosphate depletion, the activity of this enzyme is reduced, and therefore, increased utilization of glucose-6-phosphate does not occur.

The reduced cellular levels of glycogen are consistent with impaired glucose phosphorylation and glycogen synthesis, but the possibility of increased glycogen breakdown cannot be ruled out. Indeed, Horl et al (18) have reported both decreased glycogen synthesis and increased glycogen breakdown in the myocardium of PD rabbits.

Several lines of evidence suggest an abnormality of cell membrane integrity in phosphate depletion. Insulin resistance and impaired cellular glucose uptake have been described in phosphate depleted dogs (19), rats (17), and patients (16). Fuller et al (1) reported reduced resting membrane potential in skeletal muscle of phosphate depleted dogs and Saglikes et al (20) reported recently an end organ resistance to vasopressor agonists. The derangement in cell membrane integrity may be due to abnormalities in phospholipid biosynthesis. Indeed, the findings of reduced phosphatidylcholine (PC) phosphatidylethanolamine (PE) and total phospholipid phosphorus in the skeletal muscle of phosphate depleted rats demonstrate impaired biochemical integrity of cell membrane. Furthermore, the observation of altered ratios of PC/PE is compatible with membrane phospholipid abnormality and possibly function.

These changes in phospholipids may have occurred in the membrane of the intact cell, sarcoplasmic reticulum, or mitochondria. We have measured total phospholipids, and our data do not allow to differentiate between changes in these various cellular sites. However, certain information may shed light on this issue. The observation of a reduced resting rate of mitochondria respiration in phosphate depleted rats is against an impairment of mitochondrial membrane, since the latter is associated with increased resting mitochondrial oxygen consumption. Kreusser et al (21) reported a reduction in phospholipid content in the sarcoplasmic reticulum from phosphate depleted rabbits indicating an effect on the membrane of this cellular membrane.

The reduced cellular levels of cytidine (CTP) triphosphate and glycerol phosphate in phosphate depletion suggest a defect in the synthesis of phospholipids rather than increased breakdown since CTP is a major coenzyme in the biosynthesis of phospholipids.

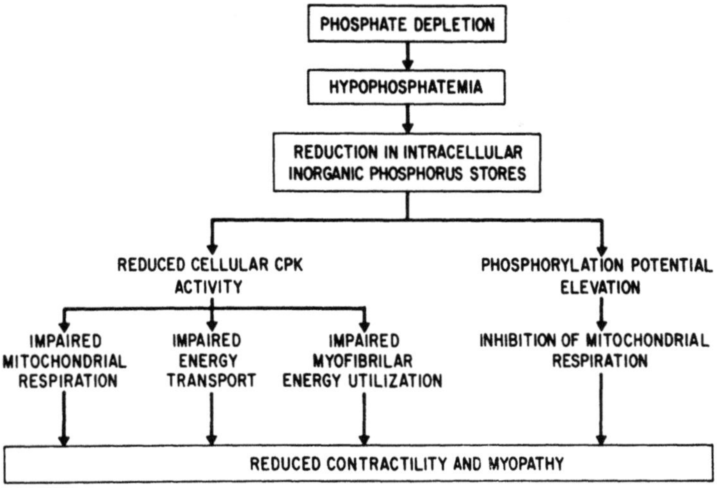

Figure 9: Schematic presentation of the possible mechanisms underlying the myopathy of phosphate depletion.

Recent studies by Carpenter et al (22) have shown that inhibition of creatine phosphokinase activity was associated with reduced protein and lipid synthesis. Since all of the abnormalities described in our study were preceded by a fall in cellular inorganic phosphorus and creatine phosphokinase isoenzymes, we propose the following cellular mechanism to mediate the skeletal myopathy of phosphate depletion, (Figure 9).

Prolonged hypophosphatemia causes a reduction in intracellular inorganic phosphorus stores and, this in turn reduces the activity of the creatine phosphokinase isoenzymes. Since these enzymes are of major regulatory role in mitochondrial respiration (23,24) energy transport (13), and myofibrillar energy utilization (13,24), phosphate depletion would result in impairment in all these steps. The reduction in creatine phosphokinase activity also impairs phospholipid synthesis, and in turn cellular membrane functional integrity will be impaired.

Since phosphate depletion is not an isolated metabolic abnormality and is associated with hypomagnesemia and hypercalcemia, it is not possible to rule out some effects of intracellular magnesium depletion or calcium overload in addition to the reduction intracellular inorganic phosphorus stores.

References

1. T.J. Fuller, N.W. Carter, C. Barcenas, J.P. Knochel, Reversible changes of the muscle cell in experimental phosphorus deficiency, J. Clin. Invest. 57:1019 (1976).
2. H. Schneider and H. Steenbock, A low phosphate diet and the response of rats to vitamin D, J. Biol. Chem. 128:159 (1939).

3. J.P. Knochel, C. Barcenas, J.R. Cotton, Hypophosphatemia and rhabdomyolysis, J. Clin. Invest. 62:1240 (1978).
4. J.P. Knochel, Hypophosphatemia, West. J. Med. 134:15 (1981).
5. N. Brautbar, R. Baczynski, C. Carpenter, S. Moser, P. Geiger, P. Finander, S.G. Massry, Impaired energy metabolism in rat myocardium during phosphate depletion, Amer. J. Physio. 242:F699 (1982).
6. R.J. Solaro, D.C. Panyg, F.N. Briggs, The purification of cardiac myofibrils with triton X-100. Biochem. Biophys. Acta 245:259 (1971).
7. Methods of Enzymatic Analysis. Editor: H.W. Bergmeyer, Volume I, pp. 473-474, Academic Press, Inc., New York, 1974.
8. E.G. Bligh and E.G. Dyer, A rapid method of total lipid extraction and purification, Can. J. Physiol. 37:911 (1959).
9. N. Brautbar, J. Tabernero-Romo, J. Coats, S.G. Massry, Impaired myocardial lipid metabolism in phosphate depletion, Kidney Int. (In Press).
10. J.K. Kaitaranta and S.P. Bessman, Determination of phospholipids by a combined liquid chromatography-automated phosphorus analyzer, Anal. Chem. 53:1232 (1981).
11. G.R. Barlett; Phosphorus assay in column chromatography, J. Biol. Chem. 234:466 (1959).
12. R.L. Veech, W.R. Lawson, N.W. Cornell, Cytosolic phosphorylation potential, J. Biol. Chem. 254:6538 (1979).
13. S.P. Bessman and P.J. Geiger: Transport of energy in muscle: The phosphorylcreatine shuttle, Science. 211:448 (1981).
14. M. Erecinska, M. Stubbs, Y. Miyaa, Regulation of cellular metabolism by intracellular phosphate, Biochem. Biophys. Acta. 462:20 (1977).
15. B.D. Hettleman, R.L. Sabina, M.K. Drezner, E.W. Holmes, J.L. Swain, Defective adenosine triphosphate synthesis. An explanation for skeletal muscle dysfunction in phosphate deficient mice, J. Clin. Invest. 72:582, 1983.
16. R.A. DeFronzo and R. Lang, Hypophosphatemia and glucose intolerance: Evidence for tissue insensitivity to insulin, New Engl. J. Med. 303:1259 (1980).
17. J.L. Davis, S.B. Lewis, T.A. Schultz, R.A. Kaplan, J.D. Wallin, Acute and chronic phosphate depletion as a modulator of glucose uptake in rat skeletal muscle, Life Science, 24: 629 (1979).
18. W.H. Horl, W. Kreusser, A. Heidland, E. Ritz, Abnormalities of glycogen metabolism in cardiomyopathy of phosphorus depletion. In: Phosphate and Minerals in Health and Disease. Editors: S.G. Massry, E. Ritz, and H. Jahn, pp. 343-350, Plenum Press, New York, 1980.

19. L.N. Gold, S.G. Massry, R.M. Friedler, Effects of phosphate depletion on renal tubular reabsorption of glucose, J. Lab. Clin. Med 89:554 (1977).
20. V.M. Campese, Y. Saglikes, N. Brautbar, R. Brandt, S.G. Massry, Effect of phosphate depletion on blood pressure, Proceedings of the Amer. Soc. Nephrol, p 4A (1982).
21. W. Kreusser, H. Scholz, W. Rascher, A. Schomig, R. Dietz, D. Klormann, E. Ritz, Circulatory response to pressor agents in phosphorus depletion. In: Regulation of Phosphate and Mineral Metabolism. Ed. S.G. Massry, J. Letteri, E. Ritz, Plenum Press, New York, 1982, pp. 259-266.
22. C.L. Carpenter, C. Mohan, P.S. Bessman, Inhibition of protein and lipid synthesis in muscle by 2,4 dinitroflurobenzene, an inhibitor of creatine phosphokinase, Biochem. Biophys. Res. Com. 111:884 (1983).
23. Seraydarian, M.W. and L. Artaza, Regulation of energy metabolism by creatine in cardiac and skeletal muscle cells in culture, J. Mol. Cell. Cardiol. 8:669 (1976).
24. V.A. Saks, V.V. Kupriyanov, G. Elizarova, Studies of energy transport in heart cells, J. Biol. Chem. 255:755 (1980).

MYOPATHY OF UREMIA

Eberhard Ritz, Wilhelm Kreusser
Michael Rambausek, Otto Mehls

Dept. of Internal Medicine and Pediatrics
University of Heidelberg (Germany)

1. The clinical spectrum of myopathy in uremia

Myopathy of uremia has to some extent been a Cinderella of clinical nephrology. It is widely overlooked because signs and symptoms are usually discrete: easy fatiguability and asthenia, difficulty in performing acts involving tonic contractions of shoulder or pelvic girdles, e.g. climbing or descending stairs, arising from a squatting or kneeling position etc. On physical examination, the patients exhibit muscle weakness, particularly of the proximal muscles of the lower extremities and muscles appear flaccid on palpation.

Table 1
Causes of myopathy in renal failure

- Secondary to associated disease
  SLE, polyarteritis, systemic sclerosis, diabetes mellitus ...
- Drug toxicity
  glucocorticoid, clofibrate
  P_i depletion
  Al-intoxication?
  Fe-intoxication (hemosiderosis)?
- Catabolism, disturbed vitamin D metabolism, PTH excess

It deserves mentioning that overzealous use of oral phosphate binders not uncommonly causes phosphate depletion with its associated myopathic features. There is also some suspicion that aluminium may not only cause osteomalacia and encephalopathy but also myopathy (2). As early as 1974, Floyd et al. (3) reported on 11 patients with metabolic bone disease and myopathy who improved dramatically after dialysis with deionized water. Recent work of our laboratory in chronically aluminium (Al) intoxicated rats (140 mg Al ip) shows unchanged basal muscle ATP (CO: 2.63 ± 0.14; Al: 2.46 ± 0.12 mmol/g ww; $\bar{x} \pm$ SEM) and diminished basal cAMP (CO: 5.59 ± 0.42; Al 4.6 ± 0.98 pmol/mg protein; p 0.05) with a trend for diminished cAMP after a isoproterenol bolus (100 ng/kg). Electrolyte and water composition was unchanged.

One report claims that hemodialysed polytransfused patients, particularly those with hemochromatosis alleles HLA-A3, B7 or B14, show iron deposition in periseptal macrophages and within myofibers, associated with muscle weakness and normal electromyograms (4). Dr. Bommer (5) was recently able to demonstrate coprecipitation of Fe and Al in lysosomes of dialysed patients - obviously the possibility of mutual enhancement of Al and Fe toxicity with respect to myopathy deserves further study.

After all such extrinsic causes of myopathy have been excluded, one still encounters "idiopathic" myopathy in uremic patients and this has been related - amongst others - to catabolism, disturbed vitamin D metabolism and PTH excess (1).

2. Ultrastructural evidence for myopathy

Evidence for the existence of some specific myopathy of uremia, unrelated to polyneuropathy, has come from histochemical and ultrastructural studies (6). Apart from preferential type II fiber atrophy secondary to neural damage, the following features of abnormal cytoarchitecture point to coexisting non-neuronal damage: focal dysorganisation of myofibrillar pattern, moth-eaten appearance of type I fibers, decay of mitochondria, lysosomal aggregation at cell periphery, fragments of myofilaments, and dispersion of Z-line material. However, frank myopathic features, e.g. necrosis and phagocytosis of fibers are usually absent.

3. Potential etiological factors

Muscle is a target organ for catabolism and also a target organ for abnormal hormonal metabolism (e.g. vitamin D metabolites, PTH, insulin, catecholamines). This review will selectively focus on some recent work relating to the roles of catabolism and $1,25(OH)_2D_3$ in myopathy of uremia.

4. Muscle as a target organ for catabolism in uremia

It has long been recognized that uremic patients or uremic animals are hypercatabolic (7, 8). This is illustrated by table 2 which demonstrates that subtotally nephrectomized rats gain less total body nitrogen (Kjeldahl-technique) in the carcass than do sham operated pairfed rats despite identical intake of energy and protein.

Table 2

	Whole body N (g)	m.soleus (mg dw)
CO (14)	2.62 ± 0.34	166 ± 13
NX (14)	2.24 ± 0.29	139 ± 24

after Mehls O. et al., Int. J. Ped. Nephrol. 1, 34, 1980 (ref. 5).

This is associated with diminished muscle weight indicated by m. soleus as a reference muscle. It is of note that despite generalized wasting of skeletal muscle, consistent myocardial hypertrophy is observed in uremic rats. Such hypertrophy can be dissociated experimentally from hypertension, sympathetic overactivity, anemia, parathyroid oversecretion etc. (9). A true gain of myocardial fiber mass was verified by micromorphometric measurements and this was associated with a change of isomyosin patterns. These findings illustrate that catabolism is selective for skeletal muscle.

Several hypothesis have been advanced to explain muscle wasting.

Hörl et al. (10) observed altered subcomponent composition of the troponin system in acutely uremic rats, presumably resulting from proteolysis, with diminution of the inhibitory I-component. They suggested that this should lead to uncontrolled actomyosin ATP'ase activity and wasteful expenditure of energy. The particular susceptibility of troponin to proteolysis, possibly by Ca activated neutral proteases, is well known (11), but normal ATP and CP levels in muscle of uremic rats (12, 13) argue against uncontrolled ATP'ase activity.

In a series of brilliant experiments, Harter et al. (12, 13) examined the dependence of in vitro amino acid release (as an index of catabolism) on dietary protein, insulin etc. in uremic rats. Of particular note was the finding that $25(OH)D_3$, but not $1,25(OH)_2D_3$, given in vitro reduced AA-release with no change of P nucleotides, cAMP or protein synthesis. These experiments suggest that 25(OH)D is one mediator of muscle wasting; reduced uptake of ^{3}H-labelled $25(OH)D_3$ by muscles of uremic rats (13) could indicate a state of 25(OH)D resistance in uremia.

Recent experiments on the genesis of catabolism may have some bearing on catabolism of uremia (14, 15). In patients with septicemia or trauma, the presence of a short chain neuraminic acid containing peptide of approx. 4 kDal was demonstrated (14) which markedly increased protein degradation in both human and rat muscle in vitro. The substance has been related to, although it is not identical with, the macrophage secretory product interleukin I. Indeed, human leucocytic pyrogen, presumably interleukin I, was shown to stimulate lyosomal thiol proteases in muscle via increased prostaglandin E_2 synthesis (15). Elevated acute phase proteins and abnormal trace element metabolism in acute uremia are compatible with the notion of excess interleukin action. Furthermore, on the basis of their molecular weight, the above substances may accumulate as "middle molecules". This hypothesis should be tested experimentally.

5. Muscle as a target organ for disturbed vitamin D metabolism

Myopathy of vitamin D deficieny has been recognized for centuries. Some findings point to the involvement of vitamin D (metabolites) in the myopathy of uremia (16), primarily as a consequence of diminished circulating $1,25(OH)_2D_3$ levels.

Impaired force generation and muscle metabolism has been directly demonstrated in experimental rickets and is not equally well documented in uremia. The following factors have been implicated in the genesis of these abnormalities:

- impaired excitation contraction coupling
- impaired function of actinomyosin-troponin-system and
- impaired provision of energy for contraction, e.g. by impaired mitochondrial metabolism.

Impaired transport of calcium, the key ion in mediating excitation contraction coupling, has been demonstrated for sarcolemma, sarcoplasmic reticulum and mitochondria of vitamin D deficient or uremic animals. Ross et al. (17) reported on impaired sarcolemmal Ca^{++} binding and transport in vitamin D deficiency. Curry et al. (18) observed diminished Ca^{++} transport in the sarcoplasmic reticulum (SR) of skeletal muscle in vitamin D deficiency. Pointon (19) found no impairment after administration of EHDP and concluded on such indirect evidence that the abnormality was unrelated to

$1,25(OH)_2D_3$. This conclusion is not supported by our recent experiments (20) which demonstrate impaired Ca^{++} transport in the SR of strontium-fed chicks. Sr has been shown to inhibit 1-alpha-hydroxylase so that a state of selective $1,25(OH)_2D_3$ deficiency should occur. This would be in agreement with our previous findings (21) of impaired SR Ca^{++} transport in skeletal muscle of uremic rabbits. This abnormality was reversible with in vivo administration of $1,25(OH)_2D_3$. More recently (22) the kinetics of this have been worked out in some detail. Vectorial translocation of Ca^{++} from the incubation medium into the interior of right side out SR vesicles requires interaction of Ca^{++} with a phosphorylated acyl-intermediate of the Ca^{++} ATP'ase (EP). Covalent modification occurs by transfer of gamma-phosphate of ATP to an aspartate residue. Ca^{++} translocation is mediated by cyclical phosphorylation and dephosphorylation with the attendant changes in Ca^{++} affinity. As shown in table 3, steady state concentrations of EP were diminished in NX rabbits and retured to normal after 4 days administration of $1,25(OH)_2D_3$ in vivo.

Table 3

Effect of $1,25(OH)_2D_3$ on steady state EP levels in experimental uremia

	Phosphoprotein level nmol ^{32}P. mg^{-1}protein	
	0.1 mM Ca^{++}	5 mM Ca^{++}
NX (7)	1.57 ± 0.23	1.55 ± 0.24
CO (7)	2.05 ± 0.25	2.17 ± 0.18
NX + 1,25 (7) (3x54 ng/kg p. o.)	2.01 ± 0.29	1.98 ± 0.22

R. Boland et al., Calc. Tiss.Int. 35, 195, 1983 (ref. 19)

The disturbance seems to be more complex than simple diminution of transport sites, since the rate of phosphoprotein (EP) formation under conditions of slow phosphorylation (ITP as substrate, 0°C) was clearly diminished.

Finally, abnormal mitochondrial Ca^{++} transport in the SR of vitamin D deficient chicks was demonstrated by Pleasure et al. (23) and this may be related to vitamin D dependent abnormalities of mitochondrial innermembrane proteins (24).

The above mentioned abnormalities of abnormal actinomyosin-troponin system and abnormal energy provision as a function of vitamin D status have not been explored in experimental uremia. In view of previous (25) and recent (26) demonstration of vitamin D dependent changes of skeletal muscle actomyosin content, this possibility should clearly be examined experimentally. Although basal ATP and CP levels are unchanged in experimental uremia (13), this does not exclude abnormal provision of energy during increased demand from activated contractile apparatus.

The above demonstration of direct actions of $1,25(OH)_2D_3$ on skeletal muscle is of particular note in view of previous observations of Birge (26) of in vitro effects of $25(OH)D_3$ on protein synthesis and energy charge of skeletal muscle in vitro which could not be imitated by $1,25(OH)_2D_3$ (table 4).

Table 4
Effect of vitamin D metabolites on muscle (m. epitrochlearis) in vitro

		Control	Treated	
		^{3}H leucine / mg protein		
$25(OH)D_3$ (20ng/ml)	1h	115 ± 8	105 ± 5	
	2.5h	240 ± 9	253 ± 9	
	5h	476 ± 4	522 ± 5	0.01
$1,25(OH)_2D_3$ (0.5ng/ml)	5h	490 ± 12	465 ± 15	
		nmol ATP/mg protein		
$25(OH)D_3$ (20 ng/ml)	2.5h	25.9 ± 1.7	53.2 ± 1.7	0.001

After Birge and Haddad, J.Clin.Invest. 56, 1100, 1975 (ref. 23).

The action of $1,25(OH)_2D_3$ on skeletal muscle in vivo is the more puzzling since we and others have been unable to demonstrate $1,25(OH)_2D_3$ receptors in skeletal muscle depite exhaustive search with adequate methodology. This may indicate that $1,25(OH)_2D_3$ actions on muscle are mediated by non-genomic pathways. Non-genomic actions of $1,25(OH)_2D_3$ have recently been described in several systems.

6. Potential implications of diminished skeletal muscle function in uremia

Abnormal skeletal muscle function may provide concepts for the understanding of disturbances in the uremic syndrome in organs other than skeletal muscle.

As one example, abnormal subcellular Ca^{++} transport

demonstrated by us in the myocardium (27) similar to skeletal muscle (21). Cardiomyopathy is of even greater clinical importance than myopathy of skeletal muscle.

Abnormal phagocyte function is a well known feature of vitamin D deficiency (28). The potential implications of abnormal vitamin D metabolism for defective phagocytosis in uremia remain to be explored.

Finally, vitamin D is known to affect structure and function of aortic smooth muscle (29), the key cellular element for proliferation in aortic plaques. Vitamin D intoxication strikingly aggravates atherogenesis in various feeding models and 1-alpha-hydroxy-vitamin D has been shown to accelerate atherogenesis and accentuate plaque formation in uremic animals (30).

7. Conclusions

The pathogenesis of uremic myopathy is poorly understood. Major causes include catabolism and disturbed vitamin D metabolism. Understanding of the mechanisms of myopathy may have implications for other facets of the uremic syndrome.

References

1. Ritz,E., Bundschu, H.D., Massry, S.G, Uremic myopathy, in: "Textbook of Nephrology",S.G. Massry, R.J. Glassock, eds., Williams and Wilkins, Baltimore,1983
2. Ackrill, P., Day, J.P., Garstang, F.M. et al., 1982, Treatment of fracturing renal osteodystrophy by desferrioxamin, Proc. EDTA, 19: 203.
3. Floyd, M., Ayyar, D.R., Barwick, D.D., Hudgson, P., Weightman, D., 1974, Myopathy in chronic renal failure, Quart. J. Med. 63: 509.
4. Knepshield, J.H., Bregman, H., Gelfand, M.C., Manz, H.J., Winchester, J.F., Iron overload and proximal myopathy: a new hazard for the hemodialysis patient, in: "Controversies in Nephrology", G.E. Schreiner, ed., Georgetown University, 2: 366,
5. Bommer, J., Waldherr, R., Wieser, P.H., Ritz, E., 1983 Concomitant lysosomal storage of iron and aluminium in dialysis patients, Lancet 1: 1390.
6. Bundschu, H.D., Schlote, W., 1974, Elektronenmikroskopische Untersuchungen der Skelettmuskulatur bei terminaler Niereninsuffizienz, J. Neurol. Sci., 23: 243.

7. Mehls, O., Ritz, E., Gilli, G., Bartholome, K., Beisbarth, H., 1980, Nitrogen metabolism and growth in experimental uremia, Int. J. Ped. Nephrol. 1: 34

8. Mehls, O., Ritz, E., Gilli,G., Kreusser, S., 1978, Growth in renal failure, Nephron 21: 237

9. Rambausek, M., Mehls, O., Kreusser, W., Bommer, J., Ritz, E., 1982, Increased heart weight in experimental uremia, Int. J. Ped. Nephrol., 3: 140A

10. Hörl, W.H., Sperling, J., Heidland, A., 1978, Enhanced glycogen turnover in skeletal muscle of uremic rats - cause of uncontrolled actomyosin ATP'ase, Am. J. Clin. Nutr. 31: 1861

11. Ebashi, S., Sugita, H., 1979, The role of calcium in physiological and pathological processes of skeletal muscle, in: Current topics in nerve and muscle research, Excerpta Medica, Amsterdam, p 73

12. Harter, H.R., Karl, I.E., Klahr, S., Kipnis, D.M., 1979, Effects of reduced renal mass and dietary protein intake on amino acid release and glucose uptake by rat muscle in vitro, J.Clin.Invest. 64: 513.

13. Harter, H.R., Birge, St.J., Martin, K.J., Klahr, S., Karl, I.E., 1983, Effects of vitamin D metabolites on protein catabolism of muscle from uremic rats, Kidney Int. 23: 465.

14. Clowes, G.H.A., George, B.C., Villee, C.A., Saravis, C.A., Muscle proteolysis induced by a circulating peptide in patients with sepsis or trauma, New Engl. J.Med., 308: 546.

15. Baracos, V., Rodemann, H.P., Dinarello, Ch.A., Goldberg, A.L., 1983, Stimulation of muscle protein degradation and prostaglandin E_2 release by leukocytic pyrogen (interleukin-1), New Engl.J.Med. 308: 553.

16. Ritz, E., Boland, R., Kreusser, W., 1980, Effects of vitamin D and parathyroid hormone on muscle: potential role in uremic myopathy, Am. J. Clin. Nutr. 33: 1522.

17. Ross, F.P., Palxas, G., Pittifor, J.M., 1982, Changes in sarcolemmal calcium binding and uptake in skeletal muscle of vitamin D deficiency rats, 5th Workshop Vitamin D, Williamsburgh, Va, Abstract, p 214

18. Curry, O.B., Bastein, J.G., Francis, M.J.O., Smith, R., 1974, Calcium uptake by the sarcoplasmic reticulum of muscle from vitamin D deficient rabbits, Nature, 249: 83.

19. Pointon, J.J., Francis, J.J.O., Smith, R., 1979, Effect of vitamin D deficiency on sarcoplasmic reticulum function and troponin C concentration of rabbit skeletal muscle, Clin. Sci. 57: 257.

20. Boland, R., de Boland, A.R., Ritz, E., Hasselbach, W., 1983, Effect of 1,25-dihydroxycholecalciferol on sarcoplasmic reticulum calcium transport in strontium-fed chicks, Calc. Tiss.Int. 35: 190.

21. Matthews, C., Heimberg, K.W., Ritz, E., Agostini, B., Fritsche, J., Hasselbach, W., Effect of 1,25-dihydroxycholecalciferol on impaired calcium transport by the sarcoplasmic reticulum in experimental uremia, Kidney Int. 11: 227, 1977

22. Boland, R., Matthews, C., de Boland, A.R., Ritz, E., Hasselbach, W., 1983, Reversal of decreased phosphorylation of sarcoplasmic reticulum calcium transport ATP'ase by 1,25-dihydroxycholecalciferol in experimental uremia, Calc.Tiss.Int. 35: 195.

23. Pleasure, D., Wyszynski, R., Summer, A., Schotland, D., Feldmann, B., Ungent, N., Hitz, K., 1979, Skeletal muscle calcium metabolism and contractile force in vitamin D deficient chicks, J. Clin. Invest. 64: 1157.

24. de Boland, A., Albornoz, L.E., Boland, R., The effect of cholecalciferol in vivo on proteins and lipids of skeletal muscle from rachitic chicks, Calc. Tissue Int. (in press)

25. Ströder, J., Arensmeyer, E., 1965, Der Aktomyosingehalt der Skelettmuskulatur bei experimenteller Rachitis, Klin. Wschr. 43: 1201.

26. Birge, S.J., Haddad, J.G., 1975, 25-hydroxycholecalciferol stimulation of muscle metabolism, J.Clin. Invest. 56: 1100.

27. Zebe, E., Rauch, B., Ritz, E., Hasselbach, W., Goy, W., 1976, Myocardial metabolism in experimental uremia, in: "Renal Insufficiency", A. Heidland, ed., Thieme, Stuttgart, p 268.

28. Ströder, J., Kasal, P., 1970, Phagocytosis in vitamin D deficient rickets, Klin. Wschr. 48: 383.

29. Kamio, A., Kummerow, F.A., Degeneration of aortic smooth muscle cells in swine fed excess vitamin D_3, Arch.Pathol.Lab.Med. 101: 378, 1977

30. Tvedegaard, E., Ladefoged, O., Nielsen, M., Kamstrup, O., Effect of 1-alpha-hydroxyvitamin D_3 and dietary calcium and phosphate on the aortic mineral content in rabbits with chronic renal failure, Nephron (in press)

CLINICAL TOPICS

ABNORMALITIES IN PARATHYROID HORMONE SECRETION IN PRIMARY AND SECONDARY HYPERPARATHYROIDISM

Jeremiah Morrissey, Kevin Martin, Keith Hruska, and Eduardo Slatopolsky

Renal Division, Department of Medicine, Washington University School of Medicine, St. Louis, MO

High levels of serum parathyroid hormone are present in patients with primary and secondary hyperparathyroidism. In primary hyperparathyroidism, approximately 90% of the patients have an adenoma of the parathyroid glands and hypercalcemia is usually seen in this disorder. On the other hand, patients with secondary hyperparathyroidism have hyperplasia of all four parathyroid glands and hypocalcemia. Although in the two above-described abnormalities the amount of parathyroid tissue is enlarged and the secretion of PTH increased, it will seem that other mechanisms also are involved in the abnormal secretion of PTH observed in these patients.

The concentration of calcium ion in the extracellular space is the primary factor which controls the secretion of PTH (1-4). However, the secretion of PTH is not completely suppressed during hypercalcemia and a basal rate of secretion of hormone persists (5,6). In addition to a decrease in hormone secretion, an increase in calcium decreases parathyroid cell cyclic AMP levels (7,8) or adenylate cyclase activity of isolated parathyroid membranes (9-13). A complicating issue of parathyroid research is whether the increase in extracellular calcium primarily affects cellular cyclic AMP levels, which subsequently affects hormone secretion, or whether this calcium-mediated parathyroid function is an epiphenomenon to hormone secretion.

There is increasing evidence that a variety of agents other than calcium may secondarily modify PTH secretion by affecting the cyclic AMP level of parathyroid cells (for reviews see 7,14-16). The majority of this information is derived from in vitro experiments using bovine parathyroid cells while a few in vitro experiments used hyperplastic human parathyroid cells. While there is a consistent increase in hormone secretion obtained from bovine parathyroid cells using agents which raise the cyclic AMP level of the cells (7), there is considerable variation in the results obtained from studies in human parathyroid tissue (17,18). The infusion of epinephrine into cows at physiologic doses which affect heart rate, blood glucose and fatty acid levels was shown to increase parathyroid hormone secretion (19). Insulin-induced hypoglycemia is a potent stimulus for endogenous epinephrine secretion in man (20). This maneuver or the actual infusion of epinephrine in humans to raise plasma epinephrine to an elevated physiologic range, produced the expected changes in heart rate but no changes in serum parathyroid hormone levels which could not be accounted for by changes in serum calcium levels (21). Thus, while the bovine parathyroid may respond to a variety of agents to increase hormone secretion, the human parathyroid generally does not. In addition, results may vary from patient to patient with the majority of patients not responding. It was suggested in the past that PTH secretion was mediated by calcium through cyclic AMP (22, for reviews see 7,14-16,23). This was based upon the observed parallel changes in cellular cyclic AMP levels and hormone secretion as a function of extracellular calcium ion concentrations. Recent studies, however, suggest that there is no causal linkage between calcium-mediated cellular cyclic AMP levels and the bulk of calcium-mediated hormone secretion (8,18,24,25). Calcium may regulate a small portion of steady state hormone secretion through cyclic AMP (24). Agonist-stimulated hormone secretion from bovine parathyroid glands or from human parathyroid cells, when it occurs, has been linked to changes in cell cyclic AMP levels (7,25).

A number of studies have suggested that the majority of calcium-regulated parathyroid hormone that is secreted is obtained from a recently synthesized pool of protein which is not in rapid equilibrium with the bulk of the hormone stored in the cell (8,24,26,27). Beta-agonist stimulated hormone secretion, which is cyclic AMP mediated, will take place in the presence of a protein synthesis inhibitor suggesting that this occurs from a pool of previously synthesized older protein (28). Phenomenologically, stimulation of hormone secretion by hypocalcemia as opposed to stimulation by agents which operate through cyclic AMP appear to occur through different mechanisms (8,18,19). The sum of the data describing the manner in which calcium and cyclic AMP-mediated secretagogues affect parathyroid hormone secretion suggest that there are two cellular pools of hormone available for secretion (Figure 1). Ionized calcium affects the secretion from a newly synthesized and an older pool of hormone (24). Agents which influence cellular cyclic AMP levels, on the other hand, seem to affect secretion from an older pool of stored hormone (24). The net amount of hormone that is secreted from each pool is not precisely

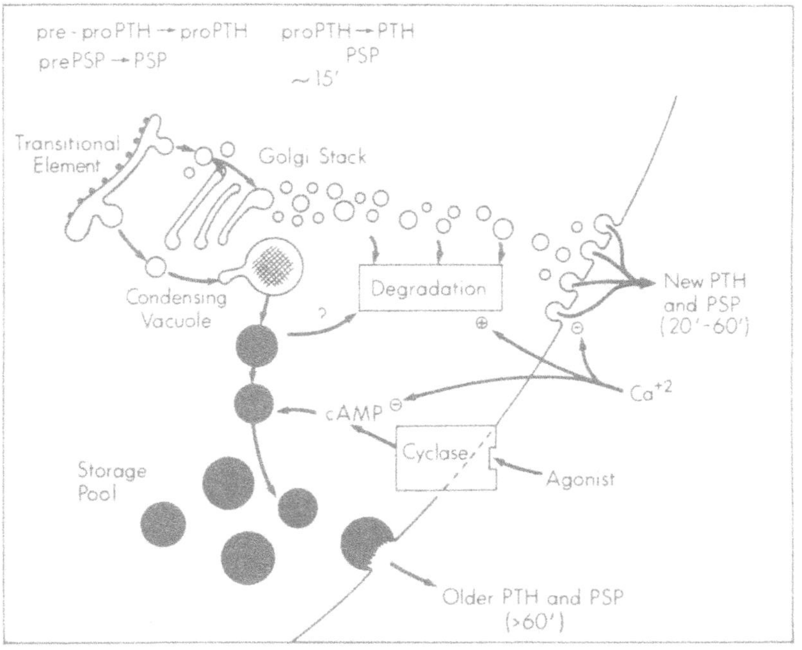

Fig. 1. Cellular pathways in the parathyroid cell for the secretion of parathyroid hormone. Calcium primarily effects the secretion of newly synthesized PTH (made within the last 20-60 minutes). Agents which influence cellular cyclic AMP levels effect the secretion of stored (older) hormone. This diagram summarizes aspects of hormone secretion described in references 8,24,26,27.

known. With at least two cellular mechanisms available for hormone secretion, agents may differentially effect hormone secretion depending on whether the agent affects calcium or cyclic AMP levels of parathyroid cells. The number of secretory granules, as visualized by electron microscopy, in human cells is highly variable (29). The secretory granule is the presumed storage form of hormone and the secretory granule content will in all probability determine the cyclic AMP-mediated responsiveness of the parathyroid cell. Variation in the secretory granule content of human parathyroid cells may account for the variable response of these cells to agents which are parathyroid secretagogues to bovine parathyroid cells.

Calcium is an inhibitor of the adenylate cyclase activity of isolated parathyroid membranes (9-13). Magnesium ion also influences adenylate cyclase activity. The cyclase of membranes prepared from 10 hyperfunctioning human parathyroid glands was shown to have an increased affinity for magnesium ion compared to the membranes of normal human or bovine parathyroid glands (12). As mentioned above, calcium inhibits the adenylate cyclase activity of membranes prepared from parathyroid glands. Membranes prepared from hyperplastic glands were less susceptible to the inhibition by calcium than membranes prepared from normal human parathyroid

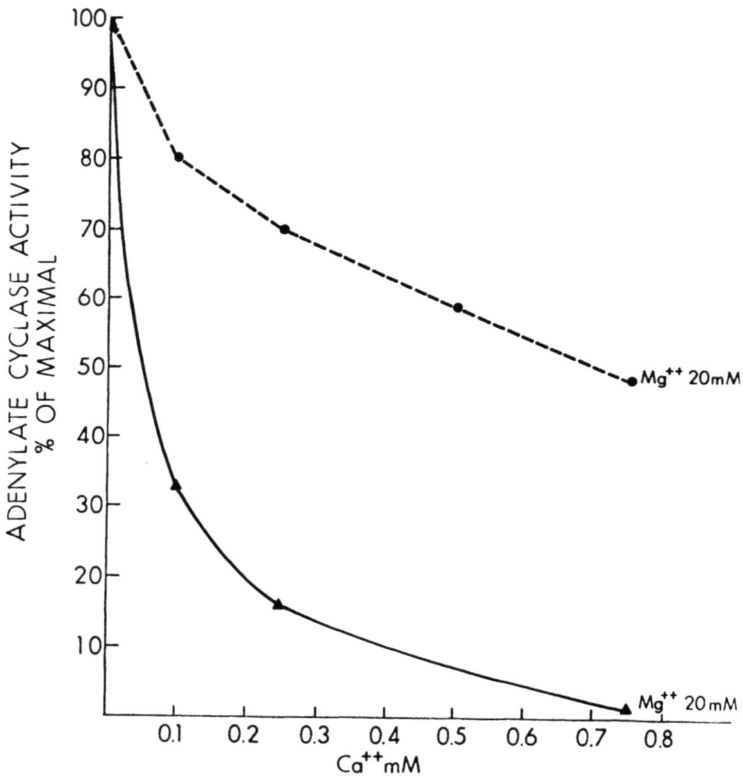

Fig. 2. Comparison of the effects of ionized calcium on adeny late cyclase activity in adenomatous human parathyroid gland (●---●) to activity in normal human parathyroid tissue (▲---▲) at 20 mM magnesium (see reference 12).

tissue (Figure 2). This suggests that the set point for calcium to inhibit parathyroid adenylate cyclase is elevated from normal in hyperfunctioning human parathyroid glands. In addition, the magnesium ion concentration influences the ability of calcium to inhibit the adenylate cyclase of membranes derived from both normal and hyperplastic parathyroid glands (12). An increase in the magnesium concentration led to an increase in the set point for calcium to inhibit the generation of cyclic AMP. These results have been qualitatively confirmed in another laboratory (13). Since calcium-mediated changes in cellular cyclic AMP cannot account for all the calcium-induced changes in hormone secretion, it is suggested that the elevated calcium set point for cyclase inhibition is a general manifestation of the hyperplastic state.

In addition to the altered set point for the inhibition by calcium of parathyroid adenylate cyclase in membranes obtained from hyperfunctioning human glands, there is an altered set point for calcium in the inhibition of hormone secretion (30-34). The accumulated data obtained for collagenase-dispersed human parathyroid cells indicates a set point in normal cells of 0.97 ± 0.04 mM calcium ion while in adenoma, primary and secondary hyperplasia the set point was found to be increased to 1.26 ± 0.13, 1.09 ± 0.15 and 1.17 ± 0.19 mM calcium ion respectively (34). Not only is the set point for calcium with respect to hormone secretion elevated in cells obtained from hyperplastic parathyroid tissue, but also the degree of responsiveness across the calcium sensitive range is altered. The degree of suppression of hormone secretion with increasing calcium is apparently less so for cells obtained from all types of hyperplastic glands than from normal glands (34). Thus, several factors can lead to elevated serum parathyroid hormone levels in man. These include: 1) an increase in tissue mass through cell hypertrophy and/or hyperplasia, 2) an increase in the set point for calcium to inhibit hormone secretion, and 3) a change in the degree of suppression by calcium throughout the calcium sensitive range, i.e. slope of the suppression line. These factors are diagrammatically illustrated in Figure 3. In this figure, the set point is defined as the calcium ion concentration causing a 50% decrease in overall hormone secretion. In Figure 3A is depicted the relative secretion rate of parathyroid hormone from a normal gland and gland which has doubled in size but the individual cells of the enlarged gland have retained a normal set point for calcium and their normal sharp responsiveness to calcium to suppress secretion. In this case, serum hormone levels will always be increased by an amount proportional to the increase in tissue mass at any calcium ion concentration provided there are no changes in the peripheral metabolism of the hormone. While each cell is operating in an essentially normal manner, the increase in the number of cells causes the hyperparathyroidism. Since there is a non-suppressible component to hormone secretion, there will be increased circulating hormone even in severe hypercalcemia. In

Figure 3B, in addition to an increase in tissue mass, there is also depicted the relative secretion rate when the set point for suppression is increased from the normal of 1.0 to 1.25 mM calcium.

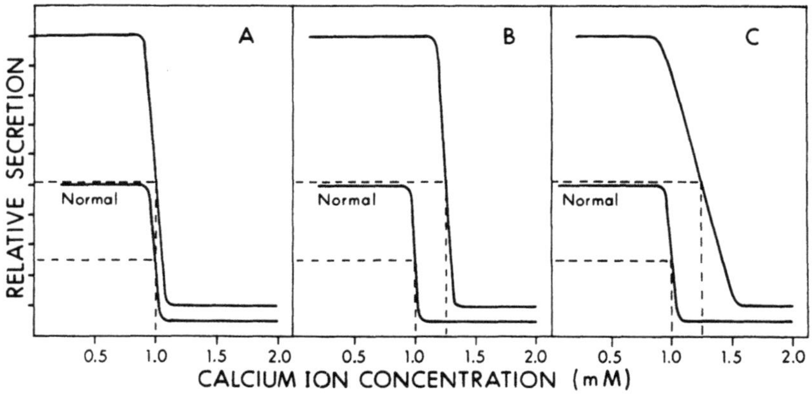

Fig. 3. Diagrammatic representation of factors contributing to abnormal parathyroid hormone secretion. A) Increase in tissue mass, B) Increase in tissue mass with an increase in set point, and C) Increase in tissue mass and set point with a decreased sensitivity to calcium. In each case, normal secretion is depicted. The dashed line indicates the set point for calcium.

The slope of the calcium suppression remains normal. In this situation, the hyperparathyroidism is a product of the increase in tissue mass and the lack of suppression by calcium in the normocalcemic range. The serum parathyroid hormone levels are then greater than the proportionate increase in tissue mass in normocalcemia and proportionate to the tissue mass in hypocalcemia and severe hypercalcemia. In Figure 3C, there is depicted not only an increase in tissue mass and an increase in the calcium set point but also there is less responsiveness of individual cells to calcium. Alternately, the change in slope to calcium sensitivity could be the result of autonomous drifting of the calcium set point of individual cells in the tissue mass with the majority of the cells adopting a set point higher than normal. From a summation of the available data obtained in vitro (34), the secretion of parathyroid hormone from hyperplastic human parathyroid cells approximates the diagrammatic representation in Figure 3C.

In our own experience with dialysis patients, we have observed changes in hormone secretion which are consistent with a change in calcium set point (35). Treatment of dialysis patients with a 1,25-dihydroxy vitamin D preparation given intravenously was found to decrease radioimmunoassayable serum parathyroid hormone levels at a time prior to decreases in hormone levels which could be attributed to an increase in serum ionized calcium. This suggests that 1,25-dihydroxyvitamin D may affect the sensitivity of human parathyroid cells to effects of calcium on secretion. If the 1,25-dihydroxyvitamin D caused a shift in the calcium set point toward normal, this could lead to a significant decrease in the secretion of hormone without a change in serum ionized calcium.

In summary, an increase in the calcium ion concentration surrounding parathyroid cells leads to a decrease in hormone secretion and cellular cyclic AMP levels. The changes in cellular cyclic AMP parallel the changes in hormone secretion but may be an epiphenomenon to secretion. During the process of cell hypertrophy and/or hyperplasia in human parathyroids there are changes in the set point for calcium with respect to hormone secretion and membrane adenylate cyclase activity. These changes in set point may reflect a pleiotropic effect on cellular function that is a reflection of the hyperplastic state of the parathyroid tissue. The set point for calcium on hormone secretion may be normalized by 1,25-dihydroxyvitamin D in uremic patients. Whether the vitamin D treatment does, indeed, affect the set point for calcium on hormone secretion and membrane adenylate cyclase activity remain to be determined.

REFERENCES

1. H.M. Patt and A.B. Luckhardt, Relationship of a low blood calcium to parathyroid secretion, Endocrinology 31:384 (1942).
2. D.H. Copp and G.F. Davidson, Direct humoral control of parathyroid function in the dog, Proc. Soc. Exp. Biol. Med. 107:1342 (1961).

3. L.M. Sherwood, G.P. Mayer, C.F. Ramberg, D.S. Kornfeld, G.D. Aurbach, and J.T. Potts, Jr., Regulation of parathyroid hormone secretion: proportional control by calcium, lack of effect of phosphate, Endocrinology 83:1043 (1968).
4. L.M. Sherwood, I. Herrman, and C.A. Bassett, Parathyroid hormone secretion in vitro: regulation by calcium and magnesium ions, Nature 225:1056 (1970).
5. R.F. Gittes, and I.C. Radde, Experimental hyperparathyroidism from multiple isologous parathyroid transplants: homeostatic effect of simultaneous thyroid transplants, Endocrinology 78:1015 (1966).
6. G.P. Mayer, J.F. Habener, and J.T. Potts, Jr., Parathyroid hormone secretion in vivo. Demonstration of a calcium-independent non-suppressible component of secretion, J. Clin. Invest. 57:678 (1976).
7. E.M. Brown, D.G. Gardner, R.A. Windeck, and G.D. Aurbach, Relationship of intracellular 3',5'-adenosine monophosphate accumulation to parathyroid hormone release from dispersed bovine parathyroid cells, Endocrinology 103:2323 (1978).
8. J.J. Morrissey, and D.V. Cohn, Regulation of secretion of parathormone and secretory protein-I from separate intracellular pools by calcium, dibutyryl cyclic AMP, and (l)-isoproterenol, J. Cell Biol. 82:93 (1979).
9. L.R. Dufresne, and H.J. Gitelman, A possible role of adenyl cyclase in the regulation of parathyroid activity by calcium, in: "Calcium, Parathyroid Hormone and the Calcitonins," R.V. Talmage and P.L. Munson, eds., Excerpta Medica Foundation, Amsterdam (1972).
10. S. Matsuzaki, and J.E. Dumont, Effect of calcium ion on horse parathyroid gland gland adenyl cyclase, Biochim. Biophys. Acta 284:227 (1972).
11. H.J. Rodriguez, A. Morrison, E. Slatopolsky, and S. Klahr, Adenyl cyclase of human parathyroid glands, J. Clin. Endocrinol. Metab. 47:319 (1978).
12. E. Bellorin-Font, K.J. Martin, J.J. Freitag, C. Anderson, G. Sicard, E. Slatopolsky, and S. Klahr, Altered adenylate cyclase kinetics in hyperfunctioning human parathyroid glands, J. Clin. Endocrinol. Metab. 52:499 (1981).
13. D.A. Ontjes, D.D. Mahaffee, and S.A. Wells, Adenylate cyclase activity in human parathyroid tissues: reduced sensitivity to suppression by calcium in parathyroid adenomas as compared with normal glands from normocalcemic subjects or noninvolved glands from hyperparathyroid subjects, Metabolism 30:406 (1981).
14. H. Heath, Biogenic amines and the secretion of parathyroid hormone and calcitonin, Endocrine Rev. 1:319 (1980).
15. J.A. Fisher, and J.W. Blum, Non-calcemic control of parathyroid hormone secretion, Min. Electr. Metab. 3:158 (1980).

16. E.M. Brown, PTH secretion in vivo and in vitro: Regulation by calcium and other secretagogues, Min. Electr. Metab. 8:130 (1982).
17. E.M. Brown, D.G. Gardner, R.A. Windeck, S. Hurwitz, M.F. Brennan, and G.D. Aurbach, β-adrenergically stimulated adenosine 3',5'-monophosphate accumulation in and parathyroid hormone release from dispersed human parathyroid cells, J. Clin. Endocrinol. Metab. 48:618 (1979).
18. E.M. Brown, Relationship of 3',5'-adenosine monophosphate accumulation to parathyroid hormone release in dispersed cells from pathological human parathyroid tissue, J. Clin. Endocrinol. Metab. 52:961 (1981).
19. J.W. Blum, J.A. Fisher, W.H. Hunziker, U. Binswanger, G.B. Picotti, M. DaPrada, and A. Guillebeau, Parathyroid hormone response to catecholamines and to changes of extracellular calcium in cows, J. Clin. Invest. 61:1113 (1978).
20. P.E. Cryer, Physiology and pathophysiology of human sympathoadrenal neuroendocrine system, N. Engl. J. Med. 303:436 (1980).
21. J. Body, P.E., Cryer, K.P. Offord, and H. Heath, Epinephrine is a hypophosphatemic hormone in man, J. Clin. Invest. 71:572 (1983).
22. M. Abe, and L.M. Sherwood, Regulation of parathyroid hormone secretion by adenyl cyclase, Biochem. Biophys. Res. Commun. 48:396 (1972).
23. D.V. Cohn, and R.R. MacGregor, The biosynthesis, intracellular processing and secretion of parathormone, Endocrine Rev. 2:1 (1981).
24. J.J. Morrissey, and D.V. Cohn, Secretion and degradation of parathormone as a function of intracellular maturation of hormone pools, J. Cell Biol. 83:521 (1979).
25. E.M. Brown, and J.C. Thatcher, Adenosine 3',5'-monophosphate (cAMP)-dependent protein kinase and the regulation of parathyroid hormone release by divalent cations and agents elevating cellular cAMP in dispersed bovine parathyroid cells, Endocrinology 110:1374 (1982).
26. R.R. MacGregor, L.L.H. Chu, J.W. Hamilton, and D.V. Cohn, Studies on the subcellular localization of parathyroid hormone in the bovine parathyroid gland: separation of newly synthesized from mature forms, Endocrinology 93:1387 (1973).
27. R.R. MacGregor, J.W. Hamilton, and D.V. Cohn, The by-pass of tissue hormone stores during the secretion of newly synthesized parathyroid hormone, Endocrinology 97:178 (1975).
28. D.A. Hanley, K. Takatsuki, M.E. Birnbaumer, A.B. Schneider, and L.M. Sherwood, In vitro perfusion for the study of parathyroid hormone secretion: effects of extracellular calcium concentration and beta-adrenergic regulation on bovine parathyroid hormone secretion in vitro, Calcif. Tiss. Internat. 32:19 (1980).

29. S.I. Roth and C.C. Capen, Ultrastructural and functional correlations of the parathyroid gland, in: "International Review of Experimental Pathology", Vol. 13, G.W. Richter and M.A. Epstine, eds., Academic Press, New York (1974).
30. J.F. Habener, Responsiveness of neoplastic and hyperplastic parathyroid tissue to calcium in vitro, J. Clin. Invest. 62:436 (1978).
31. E.M. Brown, M.F. Brennan, S. Hurwitz, R. Windeck, S.J. Marx, A.M. Spiegel, J.O. Koehler, D.G. Gardner, and G.D. Aurbach, Dispersed cells prepared from human parathyroid glands: distinct calcium sensitivity of adenomas vs. primary hyperplasia, J. Clin. Endocrinol. Metab. 46:267 (1978).
32. E.M. Brown, Set-point for calcium: Its role in normal and abnormal parathyroid secretion, in: "Hormonal Control of Calcium Metabolism," D.V. Cohn, R.V. Talmage, and J.L. Matthews, eds., Excerpta Medica, Amsterdam (1981).
33. E.M. Brown, R.E. Wilson, R.C. Eastman, J. Pallotta, and S.P. Marynick, Abnormal regulation of parathyroid hormone release by calcium in secondary hyperparathyroidism due to chronic renal failure, J. Clin. Endocrinol. Metab. 54:172 (1982).
34. E.M. Brown, Four-parameter model of the sigmoidal relationship between parathyroid hormone release and extracellular calcium concentration in normal and abnormal parathyroid tissue, J. Clin. Endocrinol. Metab. 56:572 (1983).
35. E. Slatopolsky, C. Weerts, J. Thielan, K. Martin, and H. Harter, Marked suppression of secondary hyperparathyroidism by intravenous $1,25(OH)_2D_3$ in uremic patients, Program Abstracts, 15th Annual Meeting of The American Society of Nephrology, 69A (1982).

THE ROLE OF ABNORMAL VITAMIN D METABOLISM IN X-LINKED HYPOPHOSPHATEMIC RICKETS AND OSTEOMALACIA

Marc K. Drezner

Associate Professor of Medicine
Duke University Medical Center
Durham, North Carolina

INTRODUCTION

The contemporary theory for the pathogenesis of X-linked hypophosphatemic rickets/osteomalacia (XLH) has as its central tenet that a primary defect in transepithelial transport of phosphate in the kidney accounts for all of the biochemical and skeletal abnormalities characteristic of the disease. Consistent with this view phosphorus depleted animals develop abnormalities in bone morphology similar to those observed in XLH and treatment of affected subjects with orthophosphate promotes healing of the rickets and linear growth in childhood. Moreover, apparent localization of the proposed defect in renal phosphate wasting to the parathyroid hormone sensitive locus of the proximal renal tubule[1,2] lends further support to the primacy of a renal phosphate leak in the pathogenesis of XLH.

Renal phosphate wasting, however, does not account for all of the abnormalities integral to the syndrome. First, the weight of experimental evidence favors the view that the defect in phosphate transport is confined to the renal tubule and is not simultaneously expressed in the intestinal mucosal cell[3]. Thus, there is no explanation for the decreased intestinal absorption of calcium and phosphate in affected subjects, nor its normalization in response to small doses of $1,25(OH)_2D_3$. Secondly, there is no correlation between the magnitude of the hypophosphatemia and the severity of the expressed bone disease. Further, treatment of affected patients with phosphate alone, or in combination with vitamin D, although normalizing epiphyseal calcification, does not restore endochondral bone mineralization to normal[4]. These observations indicate that a primary abnormality of phosphate transport cannot solely account for the pathogenesis of XLH.

ABNORMAL VITAMIN D METABOLISM IN XLH

Recently several investigators have reported that abnormal vitamin D metabolism is an apparent ancillary defect in patients with XLH[5-8]. Untreated affected youths and adults have normal serum $1,25(OH)_2D$ levels in spite of hypophosphatemia and phosphate depletion, factors which should increase $1,25(OH)_2D$ production[5,9]. The paradoxical occurence of hypophosphatemia and normal serum $1,25(OH)_2D$ levels in affected subjects is consistent with a defect in $1,25(OH)_2D$ production, most likely due to diminished 25(OH)D-1-hydroxylase activity.

Recent studies of the X-linked hypophosphatemic (Hyp) mouse, the murine homologue of the human disease, have provided additional insights into the regulation of vitamin D metabolism. Lobaugh and Drezner[10] have confirmed that abnormal 25(OH)D-1-hydroxylase activity underlies the deranged metabolism of vitamin D in the hypophosphatemic syndrome. They measured enzyme activity in the kidneys of normal, phosphate depleted and Hyp mice (Figure 1). Renal homogenates from phosphate depleted mice repeatedly had profoundly increased (259%) activity compared to that of normals. In contrast, enzyme activity in the Hyp-mouse kidney was far below that in the kidneys of phosphate depleted mice, although significantly increased (65%) above that in normal kidneys. Moreover, further phosphate depletion of the Hyp-mouse reduced 25(OH)D-1-hydroxylase activity to significantly lower levels (Figure 1). The results of these investigations conclusively demonstrate that the Hyp-mouse kidney is not subject to normal homeostatic control of renal 25(OH)D-1-hydroxylase activity.

The extent of the defect in the regulation of vitamin D metabolism in the Hyp-mouse is not fully represented by these studies, however. The recent demonstration of inappropriately increased renal 25(OH)D-24R-hydroxylase activity and an increased circulating $24,25(OH)_2D$ concentration in the mutant mice suggests that a complex disturbance of vitamin D metabolism is present[11].

THE ROLE OF ABNORMAL VITAMIN D METABOLISM IN THE PHENOTYPIC EXPRESSION OF XLH

The recognition of abnormal vitamin D metabolism in patients with XLH has provided the basis for an unified hypothesis which can account for the multiple derangements which mark the phenotypic expression of this disease. Advocates of this hypothesis hold that the defects in renal phosphate transport and vitamin D metabolism are interrelated abnormalities which together produce the collective defects of the XLH syndrome. Several lines of evidence support this conclusion. Included among these is the observation that differences in the chemical manifestations of XLH and (the recently described syndrome[12]) Autosomal Recessive Hypophosphatemic Rickets (AHR), two

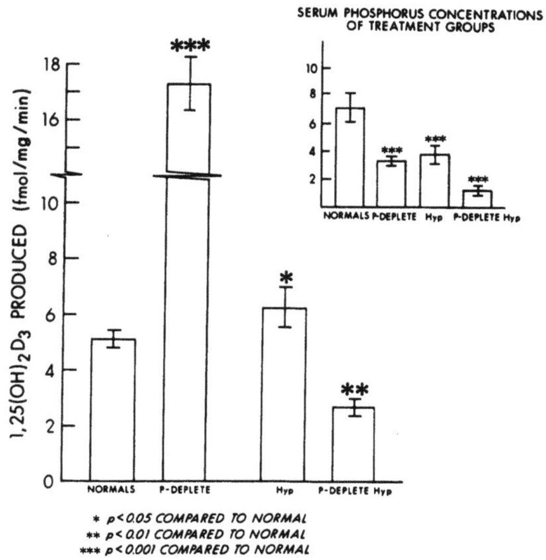

Fig. 1. Renal 25(OH)D-1α-Hydroxylase Activity In The Hyp-Mouse Kidney. Enzyme activity in the Hyp-mouse kidney, although significantly greater than normal, is far less than that in the kidneys of P-depleted mice, despite an equal degree of hypophosphatemia. Moreover, further P depletion of the Hyp-mice paradoxically decreases 1-hydroxylase activity.

rachitic/osteomalacic diseases marked by renal phosphate wasting, can be attributed to the normal vitamin D metabolism maintained in the latter disease (Table 1). Thus, the elevated serum $1,25(OH)_2D$ level observed in patients with AHR results in increased gastrointestinal absorption of calcium and phosphorus, as well as hypercalciuria. The normal regulation of vitamin D metabolism in AHR is also associated with therapeutic responsiveness to phosphate alone. In contrast, the defective vitamin D metabolism in patients with XLH abrogates the normal homeostatic response to phosphate depletion and alters the type of therapy required for healing of the bone disease. Indeed, successful treatment of XLH requires pharmacological amounts of $1,25(OH)_2D_3$ as well as oral phosphate supplementation. Such treatment results in complete healing of the bone disease as well as normalization of renal phosphate wasting. Moreover, in association with these changes, therapy results in an increase of the serum $1,25(OH)_2D$ levels from "relatively low" values to an appropriate elevated circulating concentration. These data support the hypothesis that abnormal vitamin D metabolism contributes to the clinical presentation of XLH.

Table 1. Comparison of Clinical and Biochemical Changes in XLH and AHR

	XLH	AHR
Serum		
Calcium	N	N
Phosphorus	↓	↓
Alkaline Phosphatase	↑	↑
25(OH)D	N	N
$1,25(OH)_2D$	N*	↑
iPTH	N	↓
Urine		
Calcium	↓	↑
Phosphorus	↑	↑
Gastrointestinal Absorption		
Calcium	↓	↑
Phosphorus	↓	↑
Response to Treatment		
Phosphorus	Ineffective	Heals
$1,25(OH)_2D$/Pi	Heals	?

* Relatively low in the presence of hypophosphatemia

RELATIONSHIP OF ABNORMAL VITAMIN D METABOLISM AND RENAL PHOSPHATE WASTING

While these observations indicate that abnormal vitamin D metabolism plays a role in the pathogenesis of XLH, the nature of the defect and its precise relationship to the renal phosphate wasting remain ill-defined. Although the coexistence of these defects appears certain, a single abnormality resulting in both is hypothetical. One explanation for their concurrence, however, is that an intrinsic defect of proximal renal tubular cells, resulting in abnormal phosphate transport, may also be reflected by altered $1,25(OH)_2D$ biosynthesis, a process occurring in the same cell. Abnormal phosphate transport may affect mitochondrial function and render the 25(OH)D-1-hydroxylase system unresponsive to normal stimuli. Alternately, a primary abnormality of mitochondrial function may alter vitamin D metabolism which in turn results in defective phosphate transport. We are presently investigating these possibilities in the Hyp-mouse model of the disease.

Regardless, it is certain that the pathogenesis of XLH involves a complex interrelationship between decreased renal phosphate transport and abnormal vitamin D metabolism. Indeed, variations in the severity of the disease, its heterogeneic clinical presentation and its responsiveness to therapeutic intervention may depend upon the relative contribution of each of its component defects.

REFERENCES

1. H. S. Tennenhouse, C. R. Scriver, R. R. McInnes, and F. H. Glorieux, Renal handling of phosphate in vivo and in vitro by the X-linked hypophosphatemic male mouse: evidence for a defect in the brush border membrane, Kidney Int. 14:236 (1978).
2. H. S. Tennenhouse and C. R. Scriver, Renal brush border membrane adaptation to phosphorus deprivation in the Hyp/y mouse, Nature 281:225 (1979).
3. F. H. Glorieux, C. L. Morin, R. Travers, E. E. Delvin, and R. Poirer, Intestinal phosphate transport in familial hypophosphatemic rickets, Pediatr. Res. 10:691 (1976).
4. K. W. Lyles, J. M. Harrelson, and M. K. Drezner, The efficiacy of vitamin D_2 and oral phosphorus therapy in X-linked hypophosphatemic rickets and osteomalacia, J. Clin. Endocrinol. Metab. 54:307 (1982).
5. K. W. Lyles, A. G. Clark, and M. K. Drezner, Serum 1,25-dihydroxyvitamin D levels in subjects with X-linked hypophosphatemic rickets and osteomalacia, Calc. Tissue Int. 34:125 (1982).
6. E. E. Delvin and F. H. Glorieux, Serum 1,25-dihydroxyvitamin D concentration in hypophosphatemic vitamin D resistant rickets, Calc. Tissue Int. 33:173 (1981).

7. C. R. Scriver, T. M. Reade, H. F. DeLuca, and A. J. Hamstra, Serum 1,25-dihydroxyvitamin D levels in normal subjects and in patients with hereditary rickets or bone disease, N. Engl. J. Med. 299:976 (1978).
8. R. W. Chesney, R. B. Mazess, P. Rose, A. J. Hamstra, and H. F. DeLuca, Supranormal 25-hydroxyvitamin D and subnormal 1,25-dihydroxyvitamin D: their role in X-linked hypophosphatemic rickets, Am. J. Dis. Child 134:140 (1980).
9. M. R. Haussler, M. Hughes, D. Baylink, E. T. Littledike, D. Cork, and M. Pitt, Influence of phosphate depletion on the biosynthesis and circulating level of 1,25-dihydroxyvitamin D, Adv. Exp. Med. Biol. 81:233 (1977).
10. B. Lobaugh and M. K. Drezner, Abnormal regulation of renal 25-hydroxyvitamin D-1α-hydroxylase activity in the X-linked hypophosphatemic mouse, J. Clin. Invest. 71:400 (1983).
11. J. Cunningham, H. Gomes, Y. Sieno, and L. R. Chase, Abnormal 24-hydroxylation of 25-hydroxyvitamin D in the X-linked hypophosphatemic mouse, Endocrinology 112:633 (1983).
12. M. Tieder, R. Samuel, A. Halabe, R. Arie, D. Modai, D. Gabizon, and U. A. Liberman, Autosomal recessive hypophosphatemic rickets, elevated 1,25-$(OH)_2$-D serum levels and hypercalciuria - a new syndrome, Calc. Tissue Int. (Abstr. Am. Soc. Bone and Mineral Res) In press (1983).

CALCIUM AND PHOSPHATE METABOLISM IN SARCOIDOSIS

C. Alberts, and H. van den Berg

Department of Pulmonology, University Hospital (AZUA)
Amsterdam, and Department of Clinical Biochemistry
Institute (CIVO) of Toxicology and Nutrition (TNO)
Zeist, The Netherlands

INTRODUCTION

Hypercalciuria with or without hypercalcemia is a well-known disorder in sarcoidosis. Recent reports have focused attention on 1,25 - dihydroxyvitamin D causing the abnormal calcium metabolism. (1,2,3,4) Most studies have looked at small numbers of patients with manifest calcium disturbances.

The present study concerns calcium and phosphate metabolism, related to vitamin D metabolism and parathyroid function, in an unselected group of patients with sarcoidosis.

PATIENTS AND METHODS

We studied 39 patients (16 women and 23 men, aged 21-67, mean 37 years), who were admitted with pulmonary symptoms and/or an abnormal chest radiograph. The diagnosis sarcoidosis was suggested by clinical, radiographic and laboratory findings, and was biopsy-proven in 33 patients. No patient was taking corticosteroids at the time of investigation and they were considered to have normal renal function. All patients underwent the following protocol. Fasting serum was analyzed for calcium, phosphate, creatinine, PTH and vitamin D metabolites. During a 6-day low-calcium (5-7 mmol) diet, 24-hour urinary calcium excretion (Ca 24) with calcium/creatinine ratios (Ca/Cr 24) were determined for the last 3 days and an average was made. From fasting 2-hour-urine and serum calcium, phosphate and creatinine values the calcium/creatinine ratio (FCa/CR 2) was calculated, and the renal phosphate threshold concentration ($TmPO_4/GFR$), was calculated, using the nomogram of Walton and Bijvoet (5). Hypercalcemia was defined as a serum calcium greater than 2.60 mmol/l,

and patients were considered hypercalciuric when urinary calcium excretion exceeded 4.5 mmol/day.
The serum concentration of parathyroid hormone (PTH) was measured by radioimmuno-assay using an antibody specific for the midregion (6). Reference values were from 0.2 to 12.0 pmol/l.
Serum 25-hydroxyvitamin D (25-OHD) was determined using a modified competitive protein-binding assay, according to Edelstein et al (7). The mean concentration of 25-OHD in serum of healthy subjects (n=45), sampled during the periods March through April and July through August, were 44 ± 17 nmol/l, and 85 ± 26 nmol/l, respectively.
Serum 24,25-dihydroxyvitamin D (24,25-$(OH)_2D$) and 1,25-dihydroxyvitamin D (1,25-$(OH)_2D$) were extracted and purified with liquid-chromatography on HPLC (8,9). The final quantification of serum 24,25-$(OH)_2D$ was similar to the procedure for 25-OHD. Sera of normal subjects (n=45), sampled in March through April and July through August, showed mean 24,25-$(OH)_2D$ values of 4.6 ± 2.0 nmol/l, and 7.5 ± 3.5 nmol/l, respectively. The serum 1,25-$(OH)_2D$ concentration was analyzed using a radioreceptor assay. In a group of normal subjects (n=39) the range for serum 1,25$(OH)_2D$ was 43-149 pmol/l (mean 89 ± 26 pmol/l).
Statistical analysis: calculation of mean and standard deviation, Student's t-test for comparison of mean values, and regression analysis with calculation of correlation coefficients (r).

RESULTS

This study provided a wide scatter in serum PTH levels (mean 6.2 ± 3.0 pmol/l, range 0.4 - 12.8 pmol/l), but they were on average normal.
Serum 25-OHD showed a tendency to lower values, but the mean value 41 ± 23 nmol/l also remained within the normal range. Serum 24,25-$(OH)_2D$ could be determined in 32 patients; the mean value was 2.8 ± 2.4 nmol/l. There was a significant positive correlation between these vitamin D metabolites. However, no correlation was found with the serum 1,25-$(OH)_2D$ concentrations.
Serum 1,25-$(OH)_2D$ varied greatly; the mean value 147 ± 68 pmol/l (n=34) was significantly ($p < 0.001$) higher than that obtained in normal subjects.
When evaluated for all patients, no correlations were observed between the vitamin D metabolites, PTH, serum calcium levels and the urinary calcium excretion.
With regard to the renal handling of phosphate and calcium, correlation could be established between $TmPO_4/GFR$ and serum phosphate ($r = 0.78$, $p < 0.001$), and either 24-hour urinary calcium excretion (Ca 24) and Ca/Cr 24 ratio ($r = 0.82$, $p < 0.001$) or FCa/Cr 2 ratio ($r = 0.66$, $p < 0.001$). As expected both urinary calcium/creatinine ratios also correlated ($r = 0.87$, $p < 0.001$).

The present study revealed an abnormal calcium metabolism in 18 (49%) patients: 10 showed only hypercalciuria, 4 were hypercalcemic with hypercalciuria, and 4 patients had slightly elevated serum calcium values and were normocalciuric.
The biochemical data of these patients are presented in Table 1. Serum 1,25-$(OH)_2D$ levels were elevated in 9 of 13 patients in whom this was measured. The 4 patients with hypercalciuric hypercalcemia showed a PTH level suppressed to values in the low-normal range. Only one patient had functional hypoparathyroidism resulting in an increased $TmPO_4/GFR$ of 1.43 mmol/l. The patients with normocalciuric hypercalcemia had serum PTH levels in the upper range of normal, probably due to an increased parathyroid gland activity. However, urinary phosphate excretion was normal in these patients.

Table 1. Biochemical data of patients with an abnormal calcium metabolism.

PARAMETER Mean ± SD	PATIENTS A (n=4)	B (n=4)	C (n=10)
BLOOD			
Ca, mmol/l	2.75 ± 0.23	2.67 ± 0.09	2.42 ± 0.10
PO_4, mmol/l	0.98 ± 0.17	1.01 ± 0.13	0.99 ± 0.13
PTH, pmol/l	3.2 ± 2.1	8.9 ± 2.5	7.5 ± 1.8
25-OHD, mmol/l	30 ± 17	34 ± 16	42 ± 11 (9)
24,25-$(OH)_2D$, mmol/l	0.3 - 3.1 (3)	0.8 - 2.3 (3)	3.2 ± 1.1 (7)
1,25-$(OH)_2D$, pmol/l	113 - 254 (3)	107 - 207 (3)	137 ± 51 (7)
URINE			
Ca 24, mmol/day	7.8 ± 2.3	2.0 ± 0.6	5.6 ± 1.5
Ca/Cr 24	0.94 ± 0.49	0.15 ± 0.03	0.45 ± 0.20
FCa/Cr 2	0.64 ± 0.51	0.16 ± 0.04	0.35 ± 0.10
$TmPO_4/GFR$, mmol/l	0.62 - 1.43	1.08 ± 0.08	0.95 ± 0.18

A) hypercalciuric hypercalcemia; B) normocalciuric hypercalcemia;
C) hypercalciuric normocalcemia.

In those patients (n=21) with normal calcium metabolism, 8 had a low $TmPO_4/GFR$ and 3 a raised $TmPO_4/GFR$. Serum PTH levels were within normal limits, and the mean values were similar to those obtained in the group of patients (n=10) with normal $TmPO_4/GFR$. No relationship was observed between serum 1,25-$(OH)_2D$ and serum phosphate or $TmPO_4/GFR$. In the whole group of patients with normal calcium metabolism, the mean serum 1,25-$(OH)_2D$ value of 156 ± 70 pmol/l was significantly ($p < 0.001$) increased, compared with the normal subjects. As shown in Table 2., an identical vitamin D status was observed in the 3 subgroups with respect to renal handling of phosphate.

Table 2. Biochemical data of patients with a normal calcium metabolism; subgroups with regard to renal handling of phosphate.

PARAMETER Mean ± SD	PATIENTS D (n=10)	E (n=8)	F (n=3)
BLOOD			
Ca, mmol/l	2.46 ± 0.09	2.43 ± 0.09	2.23 - 2.53
PO_4, mmol/l	0.96 ± 0.12	0.80 ± 0.10	1.12 - 1.24
PTH, pmol/l	5.7 ± 2.6	6.2 ± 3.7	1.1 - 7.7
25-OHD, nmol/l	43 ± 30	57 ± 21	15 - 35
24,25-$(OH)_2D$, nmol/l	3.6 ± 3.4 (9)	3.8 ± 2.5 (7)	0.8 - 1.7
1,25-$(OH)_2D$, pmol/l	168 ± 73	148 ± 76	83 - 198
URINE			
Ca 24, mmol/day	3.0 ± 1.2	3.2 ± 0.9	0.6 - 1.1
Ca/Cr 24	0.24 ± 0.10	0.20 ± 0.04	0.07 - 0.11
FCa/Cr 2	0.18 ± 0.10	0.18 ± 0.06	0.02 - 0.09
$TmPO_4$/GFR, mmol/l	0.92 ± 0.11(9)	0.71 ± 0.06	1.36 - 1.68

D) $TmPO_4$/GFR (N); E) $TmPO_4$/GFR (↓); F) $TmPO_4$/GFR (↑).

DISCUSSION

The results of this study provide further evidence of an abnormal regulation of the vitamin D metabolite 1,25-$(OH)_2D$ in sarcoidosis, which is not PTH mediated. In 22 (65%) of 34 patients we found an increased serum 1,25-$(OH)_2D$ whether or not an abnormal calcium metabolism had resulted. The mean serum 1,25-$(OH)_2D$ level was significantly increased in the whole population of patients (n=34). The question arises whether this metabolite reflects disease activity in sarcoidosis. At present, the factor or factors causing the elevation of 1,25-$(OH)_2D$ remain to be elucidated. The mechanism for the abnormal calcium metabolism seems to be very complex and may not result from increased serum levels of 1,25-$(OH)_2D$ alone. Increased or changed sensitivity of the target organs to 1,25-$(OH)_2D$ may be considered.

The cause of tubular dysfunction, resulting in disturbed renal handling of phosphate is unknown. We found no evidence for an abnormal parathyroid gland activity, as measured by serum PTH levels. On the other hand serum 1,25-$(OH)_2D$ and the abnormal renal handling of phosphate were not causally related. We therefore suggest that the tubular dysfunction may be due to sarcoid lesions in the kidney. This suggestion may be supported by the observation that during follow-up 6 patients showed a return to normal of the renal phosphate threshold concentration related to spontaneous remission of the disease.

Further investigation is required to clarify the exact mechanisms causing the disorders described in the metabolism of vitamin D and/or calcium and phosphate in sarcoidosis.

ACKNOWLEDGEMENTS

Serum PTH was assayed by W.H.L. Hackeng and W. Schopman, Endocrinological Laboratory, Bergweg-Hospital, Rotterdam. Miss C.H. von Freytag Drabbe and Mrs. A.M. Nahon provided secretarial assistance.

REFERENCES

1. S.E. Papapoulos, L.J. Fraher, L.M. Sandler, T.L. Clemens, I.G. Lewin and J.L.H. O'Riordan, 1,25-dihydroxycholecalciferol in the pathogenesis of the hypercalcaemia of sarcoidosis, Lancet 1: 627-630 (1979).
2. N.H. Bell, P.H. Stern, E. Pantzer, T.K. Sinha and H.F. DeLuca, Evidence that increased circulating 1α,25-dihydroxyvitamin D is the probable cause for abnormal calcium metabolism in sarcoidosis, J. Clin. Invest. 64 : 218-225 (1979).
3. P.H. Stern, J. de Olazabal and N.H. Bell, Evidence for abnormal regulation of circulating 1α,25-dihydroxyvitamin D in patients with sarcoidosis and normal calcium metabolism, J. Clin. Invest. 66 : 852-855 (1980).
4. Y. Koide, N. Kugai, S. Kimura, T. Fujita, N. Yamashita, T. Hiramoto, J. Sukegawa, E. Ogata and K. Yamashita, Increased 1,25-dihydroxycholecalciferol as a cause of abnormal calcium metabolism in sarcoidosis, J. Clin. Endocr. Met. 52 : 494-498 (1981).
5. R.J. Walton and O.L.M. Bijvoet, Nomogram for derivation of renal threshold phosphate concentration, Lancet 2 : 309 (1975).
6. P. Lips, W.H.L. Hackeng, M.J.M. Jongen, F.C. van Ginkel and J.C. Netelenbos, Seasonal variation in serum concentrations of parathyroid hormone in elderly people, J. Clin. Endocr. Met. 57 (1983 - in press).
7. S. Edelstein, M. Charman, D.E.M. Lawson and E. Kodicek, Competitive protein-binding assay for 25-hydroxycholecalciferol, Clin. Sci. and Mol. Med. 46 : 231-240 (1974).
8. M.J.M. Jongen, W.J.F. van der Vijgh, H.J.J. Willems, J.C. Netelenbos and P. Lips, Simultaneous determination of 25-hydroxyvitamin D, 24,25-dihydroxyvitamin D, and 1,25-dihydroxyvitamin D in plasma or serum, Clin. Chem. 27 : 1757-1760 (1981).
9. M.J.M. Jongen, W.J.F. van der Vijgh, H.J.J. Willems and J.C. Netelenbos, Analysis for 1,25-dihydroxyvitamin D in human plasma, after a liquid-chromatographic purification procedure, with a modified competitive protein-binding assay, Clin. Chem. 27 : 444-450 (1981).

EFFECT OF CALCITRIOL ON SERUM 1,25(OH)$_2$D$_3$ LEVELS AND ON RENAL PHOSPHOROUS THRESHOLD IN X-LINKED HYPOPHOSPHATEMIC RICKETS

O. Mehls, F. Manz, K. Kettenmann,
J.P. Bonjour, and U. Trechsel
Department of Pediatrics, University of Heidelberg, FRG and Dept. of Pathophysiology University of Bern, Switzerland

INTRODUCTION

Renal hypophosphatemic rickets is characterized by sustained hypophosphatemia due to a reduction in renal tubular reabsorption of phosphate which leads to severe growth retardation and ricketic bone disease. Normal (1) but also subnormal (2) calcitriol serum levels have been reported in X-linked hypophosphatemic rickets (XLH). Nevertheless one does not know from the literature, whether low 1,25(OH)$_2$D$_3$ levels are the consequence of pretreatment with vitamin D$_3$ and phosphorous or not.

There is consensus today that 1,25(OH)$_2$D$_3$ combined with oral phosphorous supplement is the treatment of choice for XLH. But it is uncertain whether 1,25(OH)$_2$D$_3$ is superior to D$_3$ because of the specific action of the active metabolite, or because of its pharmacokinetic characteristics, for example it has a short half life time which allows to prescribe higher than equally potent doses.

One specific effect of 1,25(OH)$_2$D$_3$ could be its influence of the renal threshold for phosphate. Drezner and coworkers (3) reported an increased renal phosphorous threshold with 1,25(OH)$_2$D$_3$ treatment, Glorieux et al. (4) and Scriver et al. (5) did not find such an increase. All three groups measured the renal phosphorous threshold by the method of Bijvoet using his nomogram. Direct measurements using inulin clearance techniques and phosphate loading have to the present never been performed.

EXPERIMENTAL PROTOCOL

8 children with X-linked hypophosphatemic rickets with a median age of 14 years were treated with 2 µg of 1,25(OH)$_2$D$_3$ per day for a minimum of 9 months (period A=treated state). When the 25(OH)D levels, which had been high in some patients because of the previous D$_3$ treatment had returned to a normal range, treatment with 1,25(OH)$_2$D$_3$ was stopped for 3 weeks (period B=non-treated state). Phosphate supplements were withheld one week prior to the end of periods A and B.

At the end of period A and period B, the following measurements were performed: fasting serum Ca, Pi, PTH and 1,25(OH)$_2$D$_3$; urinary cAMP excretion and the renal phosphorous threshold using the Bijvoet nomogram. In addition, the phosphorous threshold was also measured by the inulin clearance technique, without (TP/C_{inulin}) and with i.v. phosphate loading (TMP/C_{inulin}).

RESULTS

	with 1,25D (Period A)	*without 1,25D (Period B)*	*p* <
S Ca (mmol/l)	*2.3 ± 0.1*	*2.2 ± 0.1*	*NS*
S P (mmol/l)	*0.67 ± 0.21*	*0.86 ± 0.30*	*0.01*
*S iPTH (pmol/l)**	*15.0 ± 10.2*	*17.8 ± 7.9*	*NS*
*S 25(OH)D$_3$ (nmol/l)***	*168 ± 17*	*142 ± 15*	*NS*
*S 1,25(OH)$_2$D$_3$(pmol/l)****	*120.6 ± 72.2*	*40.7 ± 34.1*	*0.01*
UcAMP (µmol/g Cr)	*2.8 ± 0.8*	*3.6 ± 1.2*	*NS*
*TMP/GFR (mmol/l)*****	*0.64 ± 0.28*	*0.83 ± 0.30*	*0.01*
TP/C_{inulin} (mmol/l)	*0.56 ± 0.28*	*0.61 ± 0.24*	*0.01*
TMP/C_{inulin} (mmol/l)	*0.64 ± 0.26*	*1.04 ± 0.42*	*0.01*

Normal range:
** = 2-40 pmol/l*
*** = 50-240 µmol/l*
**** = 59-170 pmol/l*
***** = 1.2-2.5 mmol/l*

data are given as $\bar{x} \pm$ SD.

CONCLUSIONS

Serum 1,25(OH)$_2$D$_3$ levels are low in untreated patients with X-linked hypophosphatemic rickets. The levels remain low despite 1,25(OH)$_2$D$_3$ treatment.

Renal phosphorous threshold is slightly but significantly increased with $1,25(OH)_2D_3$ treatment; however, normalisation cannot be obtained. Suppression of PTH secretion should be discussed as a possible mechanism for the increase of the threshold, but this has to be clarified.

REFERENCES

1. Lyles, K.W., Clark, A.G., Drezner, M.K.: Serum 1,25-dihydroxyvitamin D levels in subjects with X-linked hypophosphatemic rickets and osteomalacia. Calcif. Tissue Int. 34, 125-130, 1982

2. Chesney, R.W., Mazess, R.B., Rose, P.: Supranormal 25-hydroxyvitamin D and subnormal 1,25-dihydroxyvitamin D: their role in X-linked hypophosphatemic rickets. Am. J. Dis. Child. 134, 140-143, 1980

3. Drezner, M.K., Lyles, K.W., Haussler, M.R.: Evaluation of a role for 1,25-dihydroxyvitamin D_3 in the pathogenesis and treatment of X-linked hypophosphatemic rickets and osteomalacia. J. Clin. Invest. 66, 1020, 1980

4. Glorieux, F.H., Marie, P.J., Pettifor, J.M.: Bone response to phosphate salts, ergocalciferol and calcitriol in hypophosphatemic vitamin D-resistant rickets. New Engl. J. Med. 303, 1023, 1980

5. Scriver, C.R., Reade, T.M., DeLuca, H.F.: Serum 1,25-dihydroxyvitamin D levels in normal subjects and in patients with hereditary rickets or bone disease. New Engl. J. Med. 299, 976-979, 1978

MISCELLANEOUS

IMPAIRED HORMONAL STIMULATION IN ISOLATED HEPATOCYTES OF PHOSPHOROUS DEPLETED RATS

Walter H. Hörl[1], Wilhelm Kreusser[2], Roland M. Schaefer[1], August Heidland[1], and Eberhard Ritz[2]
Departments Internal Medicine, Universities [1]Würzburg and [2]Heidelberg
D-8700 Würzburg and D-6900 Heidelberg

INTRODUCTION

Clinical evidence has been presented for disturbed liver function in patients with phosphorous depletion and hypophosphatemia[1]. Rajan et al.[2] emphasized that hypophosphatemic patients with cirrhosis tend to undergo greater hepatic decompensation than do patients with normal blood phosphorous. Furthermore, Klock et al.[3] found a defective hyperglycemic response to glucagon in alcoholic patients with hypophosphatemia. This abnormality was completely normalized after restoration of serum phosphorous levels. These observations were made in intact organism. Consequently, it cannot be decided whether hepatic cell function is altered or whether these changes are secondary to circulatory problems, altered tissue oxygenation[4] or altered hormone metabolism.

In the present investigation we used isolated hepatocytes of phosphate depleted rats to study generation of cAMP and gluconeogenesis under various conditions (basal state, in vitro phosphate repletion, hormonal stimulation).

METHODS

Male Sprague Dawley rats (Firma Ivanovas, Kisslegg/Allgäu) with an initial weight of 80 g were used. The rats were housed in single cages at constant temperature (24 °C) and humidity (70 %) with a 12 h light on - 12 h light off cycle. After an adaptation period of 3 days on control diet, the animals were randomly divided into two groups. The first was put on a low phosphorous (P_i) diet and the second received the control diet in a quantity adjusted to maintain the body weight equal to the phosphate depleted group; this group will be refered to as pairweight control (CO). The control diet (Altromin C 1000, Lage/Lippe, FRG) was identical with respect to all constituents except P_i (control diet: P_i 0.4 %; low P_i diet: P_i 0.02 %). The animals had free access to deionized water. After 4 weeks of phosphate depletion (PD) mean body weight was 155 g. A separate series of animals (PD: n = 9; CO: n = 9) received somatostatin (Serono, Freiburg, FRG; 0.25 ug/100 g body weight, i.p.) at 24 h, 18 h, 12 h, 6 h and one hour before hepatocyte isolation. To deplete the liver of glycogen, the animals were starved for 24 h before isolation of hepatocytes, but had free access to water.

In order to isolate hepatocytes, rats were anesthetized with pentobarbital (30 mg/kg b.w.), the abdomen was opened and blood was collected from the abdominal aorta. The liver was perfused with Krebs-Ringer-bicarbonate buffer (calcium and phosphorous free); cells were isolated with the method of Berry and Friend[5], using 0.05 % collagenase (type IV; Sigma Chemicals Comp., St. Louis, USA). The cells were counted with phase contrast microscopy.

Cell viability was evaluated with the trypan blue exclusion method. If more than 15 % of cells of an animal took up trypan blue cells were not used for incubation. In addition, electronmicroscopic studies were performed and showed a similar percentage of intact cells as the trypan blue method. Furthermore, LDH (test Kit Boehringer, Mannheim, FRG) was measured enzymatically in the medium to assess unspecific cell damage. At the end of incubation LDH activity was similar in media containing cells of CO (807 $\pm$ 212 U/l; n = 6) or PD animals (993 $\pm$ 175; n = 10). Protein in the incubation medium was measured according to Lowry et al.[6].

The hepatocytes were incubated in a buffer containing Na^+ 125 mM, K^+ 4.5 mM, Mg^{++} 1.25 mM, Ca 1.25 mM, Cl^- 96 mM, $HPO_4^{--}/H_2PO_4^-$ 0.96 mM, HCO_3^- 25 mM, SO_4^{--} 0.25 mM, BSA 0.2 %, Hepes 4.5 mM. The samples were incubated in siliconised Erlenmeyer flasks for 30 minutes at 37 °C in a 5 % CO_2/95 % O_2 atmosphere at pH 7.4 in a final volume of 1.5 ml which contained approximately 3 - 8 x 10^6 cells = 3 - 10 mg protein[7]. 10 mM pyruvate (Sigma Chemicals Comp., St. Louis, USA) was used as substrate. For hormonal stimulation, 28 nmol/l pork glucagon, 17 nmol/l pork insulin (both from Novo, Copenhagen, Denmark), 1 umol/l epinephrine as well as 1.94 umol/l or 0.194 umol/l (1.0 U/ml or 0.1 U/ml) 1-34 bPTH (Beckmann Instruments Inc., Fullerton, USA) were used. To control samples appropriate solvens was given. 1 mmol/l propranolol and 0.1 mmol/l phenoxybenzamine (Roehm-Pharma, Darmstadt, FRG) were added. Hormones and inhibitors were added at the time when incubation was started. Incubation was terminated after 30 min by addition of 300 µl of 30 % perchloric acid.

In separate experiments the effect of in vitro P_i repletion on hepatic gluconeogenesis was tested. Liver cells were incubated for 30 min as described above in an incubation medium containing 0.96 or 2.88 mM Na_2HPO_4/NaH_2PO_4. In addition, P_i repletion in vitro was also performed with permeabilized hepatocytes. Digitonin (Serva, Heidelberg, FRG) was added in final concentrations of 10^{-4}, 10^{-6} or 10^{-8}M.

After centrifugation for 5 minutes at 10.000 x g supernatant was neutralized with 4 M KOH and 0.5 M KH_2PO_4. Lactate was assayed enzymatically with the method according to Bergmeyer[8]. Glucose production was defined as the difference between glucose levels in hepatocytes at time 0 and after 30 minutes of incubation. In separate experiments, it was established that glucose production was linear with time during the incubation interval. Glucose was determined with the glucose oxidase method (Merckotest GOD-PAP; Merck, Darmstadt, FRG). Cell glycogen content did not exceed 5.5 nmol glucose equivalents per milligram of cell protein. For cAMP measurements cells were incubated for 30 min. Incubation was terminated by addition of 6 % trichloroacetic acid. After centrifugation, the supernatant was extracted with water saturated ether. For radioimmunoassay of cAMP, the procedure of Steiner et al.[9] was used. cAMP values represent the amount of cAMP per incubate, comprising both medium and cells.

Serum chemistry: Serum P_i was measured according to Fiske and Subbarow[10]. Serum glucose was measured using commercial kits (Merckotest, Merck, Darmstadt, FRG).

Results are expressed as mean ± SEM. The differences between groups were examined with the non-parametric Mann-Whitney U-test for random samples or for paired samples as appropriate.

RESULTS

An advanced degree of phosphorous depletion in the experimental animals is documented by severe fasting hypophosphatemia (2.79 ± 0.18 mg/dl) as compared to control rats (8.79 ± 0.16 mg/dl). Serum glucose in PD animals was significantly higher after overnight fasting (129 ± 4.5 vs. 97.5 ± 4.1 mg/dl, $p < 0.01$).

Glucose production from pyruvate by isolated hepatocytes of PD rats was markedly diminished (Table 1). Under basal conditions, glucose production was 61.3 % higher in CO than in PD animals. Glucagon caused a highly significant increase of glucose production (+ 30.1 %; $p < 0.01$) in CO, whereas no significant change was observed in PD rats. Glucose production from pyruvate by hepatocytes of somatostatin pretreated CO animals was significantly increased in the presence of glucagon (+ 21.5 %; $p < 0.05$), whereas no significant change was found in the presence of insulin. In contrast, no significant change of glucose synthesis was observed in somatostatin pretreated PD animals with glucagon or insulin. Epinephrine (10^{-6} M) caused a significant stimulation of glucose production in CO (16.5 %; $p < 0.01$). The percent increase of glucose production was significantly less in PD (8.4 %; $p < 0.01$). Epinephrine induced glucogenesis was inhibited by phenoxybenzamine (10^{-4}M) and propranolol (10^{-3} M). Phenoxybenzamine and propranolol had no effect on this preparation in the absence of epinephrine. However, in a separate series of experiments with more advanced PD (n = 8; 6 weeks of PD), the response to epinephrine was abolished (PD from 142 $\pm$ 27 to 149 $\pm$ 30 nmol x (mg protein)$^{-1}$ x (30 min)$^{-1}$; n.s.), but in contrast to all other series cell viability in this group was impaired (approx. 60 % viable cells) and results are not listed in the tables. Various concentrations of 1-34 bovine PTH (1 U/ml or 0.1 U/ml) failed to affect glucose production in control or PD rats.

Impaired basal and glucagon stimulated glucose synthesis with pyruvate as substrate in hepatocytes of PD animals was not reversed by incubation in a medium with 2.88 mM phosphate compared to 0.96 mM P_i of the standard medium. In an attempt to increase the efficiency of in vitro P_i repletion, hepatocytes were used which were permeabilized by digitonin (10^{-8}, 10^{-6}, 10^{-4}M). At 10^{-4}M in the presence of 2.88 mmol $HPO_4^{--}/H_2PO_4^{-}$ digitonin decreased glucose and lactate production both in control and P_i depleted hepatocytes to an equal extent (glucose production: control: -77.5 %; PD: -65.3%; lactate production: control: -48.5 %; PD -50.8 %). At lower concentrations, digitonin (10^{-6} or 10^{-8}M) increased glucose and lactate production to an equal extent both in control and P_i depleted hepatocytes (10^{-6}M digitonin; glucose: control 29.0 %; PD 32.5 %; lactate: control 110 %; PD 167 %) (Figure 1).

cAMP content was also markedly lower in hepatocytes of PD rats. Under basal conditions, cAMP content was 32.9 % higher in CO than in PD. Glucagon caused a highly significant increase of cAMP content in CO (+ 42.8 %; $p < 0.01$) and PD (+ 40.9 %; $p < 0.01$). No significant change was found in both groups in the presence of insulin (Table 2).

The epinephrine mediated increase of glucose production in hepatocytes of PD depleted animals was accompanied by a significant increase of hepatocyte cAMP content (basal conditions: 4.62 $\pm$ 0.25; + epinephrine: 5.61 $\pm$ 0.33 pmol x (mg protein)$^{-1}$; $p < 0.01$). In the presence of PTH (1 U/ml) cAMP concentration was significantly enhanced in controls, but unchanged in hepatocytes of PD animals.

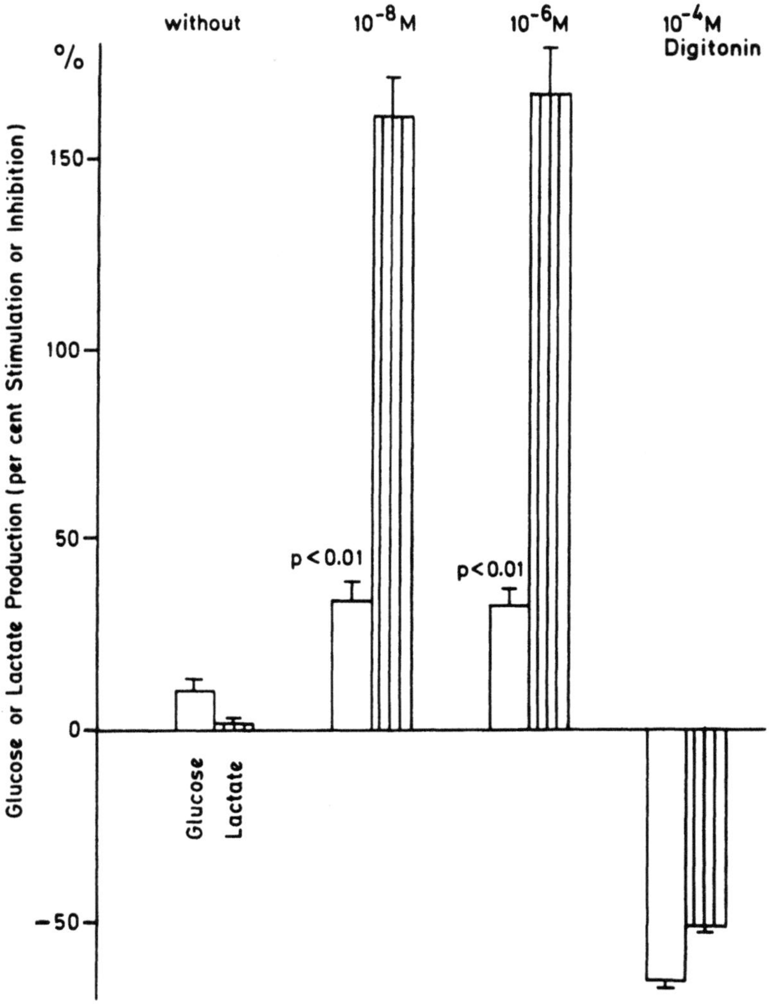

Figure 1: Effect of in vitro P_i-repletion on glucose and lactate production in permeabilized hepatocytes of PD rats.

Table 1

cAMP content and glucose or lactate production after glucagon, insulin and epinephrine stimulation of hepatocytes

		basal	glucagon	insulin	epinephrine
Glucose production nmol x (mg protein)$^{-1}$ x (30 min)$^{-1}$	CO	229 $\pm$20	298 §§ $\pm$25	239 $\pm$22	276 §§ $\pm$24
	PD	142^{x} $\pm$27	148^{xx} $\pm$24	134^{xx} $\pm$29	181^{xx} $\pm$21 §§
Lactate production nmol x (mg protein)$^{-1}$ x (30 min)$^{-1}$	CO	511 $\pm$58	389 § $\pm$41	516 $\pm$62	496 $\pm$62
	PD	459 $\pm$41	401 $\pm$33	448 $\pm$45	454 $\pm$47

Data are given as mean $\pm$ SEM $^{x}p < 0.05$, $^{xx}p < 0.01$ control vs. phosphorous depletion
§ $p < 0.05$, §§ $p < 0.01$ basal vs. hormonal stimulation (paired test).

Table 2

cAMP content after glucagon, insulin, epinephrine and PTH stimulation of hepatocytes

		basal	glucagon	insulin	epinephrine	1-34 b-PTH
cAMP content pmol x (mg protein)$^{-1}$	CO	6.14 $\pm$0.39	8.77 §§ $\pm$0.57	5.85 $\pm$0.43	7.56 §§ $\pm$0.37	6.54 §§ $\pm$0.31
	PD	4.62^{xx} $\pm$0.25	6.51^{xx} $\pm$0.40 §§	5.16 $\pm$0.24	5.61^{xx} $\pm$0.33 §§	4.93^{xx} $\pm$0.26

Data are given as mean $\pm$ SEM $^{x}p < 0.05$; $^{xx}p < 0.01$ control vs. phosphorous depletion
§§ $p < 0.01$ basal vs. hormonal stimulation (paired test).

DISCUSSION

The present study clearly establishes impaired gluconeogenesis in isolated hepatocytes of phosphorous depleted animals under basal conditions and after hormonal stimulation with glucagon and epinephrine. This finding is in agreement with previous observations of diminished basal gluconeogenesis in isolated renal cortical tubules of phosphate depleted animals[11].

Hepatocytes were incubated in a medium with a phosphate concentration which corresponded to the serum phosphate concentration of PD animals. The failure of normal P_i concentration in the medium (2.88 mmol/l) to correct abnormal gluconeogenesis is in agreement with our previous work in isolated tubuli of phosphorous depleted animals that abnormal glucogenesis was also not corrected by addition of P_i to the incubation medium[11]. Glucose and lactate production increased when P_i depleted hepatocytes, permeabilized by digitonin treatment, were incubated in high P_i medium (2.88 mM). However, a similar increase was also observed in control hepatocytes. Consequently the specificity of P_i induced glucose production remains in doubt.

Hormonal stimulation of gluconeogenesis could consistantly be demonstrated with great reproducibility. Since paired aliquots of hepatocytes from the same animal were used for basal and stimulated gluconeogenesis, the replicate error for repeat measurements was neglegible. In order to elucidate whether there was an abnormality at the level of the receptor of adenylate cyclase or of post-cAMP events, hormone mediated cAMP generation was measured. Unimpaired generation of cAMP after glucagon or epinephrine points to defective post-cAMP events.

Although, glucagon levels were not measured, it is unlikely that diminished response to glucagon was due to glucagon excess with receptor occupancy or receptor downregulation, since pretreatment with somatostatin did not alter the response in PD animals.

In contrast to glucagon, it cannot be safely excluded that high endogenous catecholamines are the cause of diminished epinephrine responsiveness of hepatocyte glucogenesis to epinephrine. Diminished cardiac glycogen content was found by us previously in phosphorous depleted rats and this was normalized by administration of nadolol[12]. Indeed, circulating norepinephrine levels were elevated in phosphorous depleted rats both under basal conditions and after stress (cold exposure)[13].

In previous studies, we demonstrated diminished hepatocyte nucleotides (ATP concentration and energy charge) in the liver and other organs of phosphate depleted rats[14]. Nucleotide concentrations were not measured in the present study but the present findings are compatible with diminished nucleotide generation in response to increased ATP requirements of gluconeogenesis.

REFERENCES

1. B. Frank, and F. Kern Jr., Serum inorganic phosphorus during hepatic coma, Arch. Int. Med. 110:865 (1962).
2. K. Rajan, R. Levinson, and C. Leevy, Hepatic anoxia secondary to hypophosphatemia, Clin. Res. 21:521 (1973).
3. J. Klock, H. Williams, and W. Mentzer, Hemolytic anemia and somatic cell dysfunction in severe hypophosphatemia, Arch. Int. Med. 134:360 (1974).
4. S. Travis, H. Sugermann, R. Tuberg, S. Dudrick, M. Delivoria-Papadopoulos, L. Miller, and F. Oski, Alterations of red-cell glycolytic intermediates and oxygen transport as a consequence of hypophosphatemia in patients receiving intravenous hyperalimentation, N. Engl. J. Med. 285:763 (1971).
5. M. Berry, and D. Friend, High yield preparation of isolated rat liver parenchymal cells, J. Cell. Biol. 43:506 (1969).
6. O. Lowry, N. Rosebrough, A. Farr, and R. Randall, Protein measurements with the folin phenol reagent, J. Biol. Chem. 193:265 (1951).
7. J. Stepinski, W. H. Hörl, and A. Heidland, The gluconeogenetic ability of hepatocytes in various types of acute uremia, Nephron 31:75 (1982).
8. H. Bergmeyer, Methoden der enzymatischen Analyse, p. 1510 (Verlag Chemie, Weinheim 1974).
9. A. Steiner, C. Parker, and D. Kipnis, Radioimmunoassay for cyclic nucleotides, J. Biol. Chem. 247:1106 (1973).
10. C. Fiske, and Y. Subbarow, The colorometric determination of phosphorous, J. Biol. Chem. 66:375 (1925).
11. W. Kreusser, C. Descoeudres, Y. Oda, and S. G. Massry, Effect of phosphate depletion on renal gluconeogenesis, Mineral Electrolyte Metab. 3:312 (1980).
12. W. H. Hörl, W. Kreusser, M. Rambausek, A. Heidland, and E. Ritz, Glycogen metabolism in phosphorous depleted rats, Mineral Electrolyte Metab. 9:113 (1983).
13. W. Rascher, W. Kreusser, H. Scholz, A. Schömig, R. Dietz, and E. Ritz, Dysfunction of adrenergic system in phosphate depleted rats, Pfluegers Arch. 395:71 (1982).
14. K. Kurokawa, W. Kreusser, and S. G. Massry, Phosphate depletion and adenine nucleotide metabolism in kidney and liver, in: "Homeostasis of Phosphate and other Minerals," S.G. Massry, E. Ritz, A. Rapado, eds., Plenum Press, New York-London (1978).

HYPERLIPOPROTEINEMIA IN PHOSPHATE DEPLETION

W. Kreusser, W. Haberbosch, A. Gnasso,

E. Ritz, and J. Augustin

Medizinische Univ.-Klinik Heidelberg, FRG

INTRODUCTION

Phosphate depletion is known to cause not only abnormalities of electrolyte metabolism (1, 2), but also disturbances of intermediary metabolism, e.g. abnormal insulin release (3), abnormal insulin responsiveness (4) and impaired hormonal stimulation of hepatic gluconeogenesis (5). The present communication describes another metabolic consequence of phosphate depletion, severe reversible hyperlipoproteinemia in the phosphate depleted dog.

MATERIAL AND METHODS

8 male foxhounds, 6 months of age, with initial weights of 14.0 ± 0.67 kg were used. After a preadaptation period of 2 weeks on control diet, the animals were switched to low phosphorous diet. In the low phosphorous diet, potassium phosphate was exchanged for potassium chloride to achieve a final phosphorous concentration of 0.03%; it was completely identical to the control diet with respect to carbohydrate and fat. The control diet contained 13.800 kJ/kg; 0.6% Ca, 0.4% phosphorous; 20% protein; 20% fat; 56% carbohydrate. Phosphate depletion caused only slight reduction of body weight (control: 14.0 ± 0.67 kg; phosphate depletion 13.0 ± 0.74 kg). After 21 days of phosphate depletion, 6 animals were switched to the original control diet and observed for another 21 days. In these animals, body weight rose by 1.20 ± 0.15 kg during the repletion period.

Blood was taken at the end of each period. Calcium was measured with atomic absorption spectrophotometry (Perkin Elmer, Frankfurt, FRG), phosphorous after Fiske and Subbarow (6); glucose, creatinine, cholesterol and triglycerides with Technicon autoanalyser, free fatty acids (FFA) after Novåk (7). Lipid electrophoresis was performed with a Lipidophor system (Immuno, Mannheim). Sequential separation of lipoproteins from EDTA-plasma into density classes < 1.006 g/ml (VLDL), 1.006-1.019 g/ml (IDL), 1.019-1.063 g/ml (LDL), 1.063-1.125 g/ml (HDL_2) and 1.125-1.21 g/ml (HDL_3) was achieved with a Beckman 70.1 Ti-rotor in a Beckman-L-8-centrifuge. Zonal ultracentrifugation was performed with a Beckman-40-Ti-rotor with a discontinuous NaBr-gradient. Apoprotein analysis was carried out by analytical isoelectric focusing in ultrathin flat bed gels (8). Postheparin lipolytic activities of lipoprotein lipase (LPL) and hepatic triglyceride lipase (HTGL) were determined in plasma obtained after intravenous injection of 100 U heparin/kg bw in an enzyme assay (9). Affinity chromatography of lipoprotein fractions was performed in heparin-sepharose gel with a continuous NaCl gradient from 0.05 to 0.5 M. All values are given as mean $\pm$ SEM. The significance of differences between the study periods was analyzed with Wilcoxon's test for paired samples.

RESULTS

Table 1 gives biochemical data for control (CO), P_i depletion (PD) and P_i repletion period. Besides marked hypophosphatemia, serum calcium considerably increased during phosphate depletion, whereas renal function, as measured by serum creatinine, glucose and free fatty acids remained unaltered. During P_i depletion, there was a moderate increase in triglycerides and a marked increase in cholesterol and phospholipids. Hypercholesterolemia after P_i depletion was mainly due to the elevation of LDL-cholesterol from 62 $\pm$ 5.3 mg% (CO), to 166 $\pm$ 11.4 mg% (PD). LDL-phospholipids increased significantly ($p < 0.01$) from 70.0 $\pm$ 9.4mg% (CO) to 199 $\pm$ 18.5 mg% (PD). Cholesterol of the HDL_2-fraction was also increased in PD from 66 $\pm$ 5.8 mg% (CO) to 88 $\pm$ 6.4 mg% (PD); $p < 0.01$, whereas HDL_3 cholesterol did not change significantly. When HDL-cholesterol was analyzed after precipitation of Apo-B-containing lipoproteins by phosphotungstic acid - Mn-precipitation it became evident that the elevation in plasma cholesterol after phosphate depletion is almost entirely due to an increase in lipoproteins lacking Apo-B but having flotation rates comparable to LDL. Lipid electrophoresis (fig. 1) confirmed this finding and demonstrated a lipoprotein which migrated in the prebeta-range comparable to alpha-2-globulins, which we called HDL_{PD}.

Table 1

Effect of phosphate depletion on serum chemistry

	control period n=8	depletion period n=8	repletion period n=6
Inorganic Phosphorous (mg/dl)	7.28±0.22	3.47±0.09**	6.72±0.25§§
Calcium (mg/dl)	9.48±0.16	10.7±0.09**	8.88±0.08§§
Creatinine (mg/dl)	0.69±0.03	0.63±0.06	0.48±0.01§
Glucose (mg/dl)	105±5.51	101±2.14	104±4.16
free fatty acids (μmol/l)	-----	424±49.7	364±34.7
Cholesterol (mg/dl)	140±8.71	301±20.7**	187±11.0§§
Triglycerides (mg/dl)	97.0±13.3	129±10.3*	110±8.04
Phospholipids (mg/dl)	453±24.2	595±284**	463±27.1§§

Values are given as mean ± SEM

* denotes significant difference between control and depletion period; $p<0.05$*; $p<0.01$**

§ denotes significant difference between depletion and repletion period; $p<0.05$ §; $p<0.01$ §

Similar results were obtained with zonal ultracentrifugation, which revealed a lipoprotein in the density range between HDL_2 and LDL with a migration in lipid electrophoresis in the $alpha_2$-position identical to HDL_{PD}. Apoprotein analysis of LDL showed a relatively high amount of Apo-E. Therefore, affinity chromatography on heparin-sepharose of this LDL fraction was performed in phosphate depletion; it revealed, that more than 40% of the material was bound to the column, when it was eluated in a buffer containing 0.05 M NaCl. The bound material could be eluted with 0.5 M NaCl. Chemical composition of the bound fraction (HDL_{PD}) was 10.5% triglycerides, 26.4% cholesterol, 38.1% phospholipids and

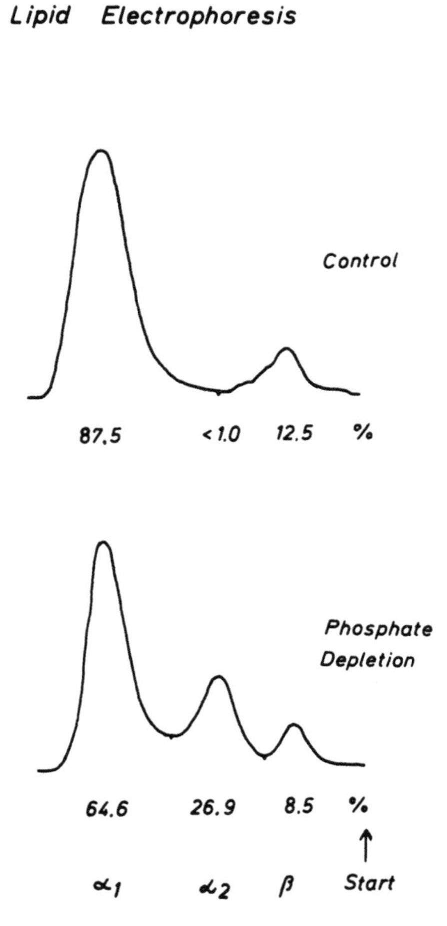

Figure 1: Lipidelectrophoresis in one dog during the control period (upper panel; triglycerides: 102 mg/dl; cholesterol: 124 mg/dl) and P_i depletion period (lower panel: triglycerides 125 mg/dl; cholesterol: 365 mg/dl).

25.0% proteins. Apoprotein analysis showed that nearly 30% of total protein in HDL_{PD} was Apo-E.
Determination of postheparin plasma lipolytic activities demonstrated a profound decrease in the enzyme of hepatic origin after phosphate depletion (CO: 27.9 ± 4.2 U; PD: 9.15 ± 1.1U; $p < 0.01$), whereas only minor changes in lipoprotein lipase were observed (CO: 24.0± 3.8U; PD: 19.0 ± 3.5 U, $p < 0.05$).

Pi-repletion

During P_i-repletion body weight rose by 1.0 ± 0.15 kg. During P_i-repletion all changes seen in P_i-depleted animals were completely normalized (table 1), including changes in serum electrolytes and serum lipids.

DISCUSSION

The present study demonstrates that chronic phosphate depletion causes marked hypercholesterolemia accompanied by slight hypertriglyceridemia, both of which almost completely disappeared after phosphate repletion in dogs. The increase of plasma cholesterol was due to extremely elevated LDL cholesterol, but only 60% of the PD-LDL had a chemical composition comparable to LDL from normal dogs. The remaining 40% of LDL material after PD contained high levels of Apo-E and resembled in size and structure HDL_C from cholesterol fed dogs. The appearance of HDL_{PD} may be the consequence of the threefold inhibition of HTGL activity. Kinnunen et al. (10-12) postulated the following LPL- and HTGL-reactions:

1. VLDL + HDL_3 $\xrightarrow{LPL}$ B-VLDL + HDL_1
2. B-VLDL $\xrightarrow{HTGL}$ LDL + apo E-rich particles
3. HDL_1 $\xrightarrow{HTGL}$ HDL_2 + apo E-rich particles

From these reactions (step 3) one would expect a negative correlation between HTGL-activity and HDL_1. Indeed, in PD HTGL-activity is decreased and HDL_{PD} (resembling HDL_1)-levels are increased. In addition, from step 2 of this reaction B-VLDL (remnants) should also be increased in the face of diminished HTGL-activity, but this could not be detected in PD. Another possibility is that inhibited synthesis of HTGL and the appearance of HDL_{PD} are two independent effects of chronic phosphate depletion. Our data favour the hypothesis that HTGL is not involved in the interconversion of HDL_2 to HDL_3 but, by an unknown mechanism, controls the disappearance of HDL_1 from the plasma compartment, possibly the uptake of HDL_1 into the liver.
Hyperlipoproteinemia of the phosphate depleted dog re-

veals another metabolic abnormality of phosphate depletion. Our studies for the first time demonstrate severe hyperlipoproteinemia caused by an electrolyte disturbance and this may provide an interesting experimental model for lipoprotein metabolism in general.
It is of note that abnormal lipid composition of erythrocyte (13) and subcellular membranes (14) have been described in phosphate depleted humans and rats. Whether this relates to the present abnormality of serum lipids is unknown.

Acknowledgement: The studies were carried out with the support of Deutsche Forschungsgemeinschaft (Kr 555/4-2)

REFERENCES

1. Knochel, J.P.: The pathophysiology and clinical characteristics of severe hypophosphatemia. Arch. Int. Med. 137, 203-220 (1977)
2. Kreusser, W., Kurokawa, K., Aznar, E., Massry, S.G.: Phosphate depletion, Mineral Electrolyte Metab. 5, 30-42 (1978)
3. Marshall, W.P., Banasiak, M.F., Kalkhoff, R.K.: Effects of phosphate deprivation on carbohydrate metabolism. Horm. Metab. Res. 10, 369-373 (1978)
4. De Fronzo, R.A., Lange, R.: Hypophosphatemia and glucose intolerance: Evidence for tissue insensitivity to insulin. J. Biol. Chem. 246, 4759-4763 (1971)
5. Hörl, W.H., Kreusser, W., Heidland, A., Stepinski,J., Ritz, E.: Defective hormonal stimulation of isolated hepatocytes in phosphorus depleted rats. Adv. Exp. Med. Biol. 151, 303-308 (1982)
6. Fiske, C.H., Subbarow, Y.: The colorimetric determination of phosphorus. J. Biol. Chem. 66, 375-381 (1925)
7. Novàk, M.: Colorimetric ultramicro method for the determination of free fatty acids. L. Lipid. Res. 6, 431-433 (1965)
8. Haberbosch, W., Poli, A., Marx, A., Augustin J.: Quantification of apoproteins - clinical significance. Inn.Med. 9, 99-103 (1982)
9. Augustin, J., Freeze, H., Teyada, P., Brown, W.V.: A comparison of molecular properties of hepatic triglyceride lipase and lipoprotein lipase from human post-heparin plasma. J. Biol. Chem. 253, 2912-2920 (1978)

10. Kinnunen, P.K.J., Vainio, P., Thurau, T.: Evidence against the role of hepatic endothelial lipase in the metabolism of plasma HDL_2. Atherosclerosis 40, 377-379 (1981)
11. Kinnunen, P.K.J., Virtanen, I.: Role of the hepatic endothelial lipase in the plasma lipoprotein metabolism. 22nd Intern. Conf. Biochem. Lipids, 24, 80 (1980)
12. Kinnunen, P.K.J., Virtanen, I.: Mode of action of the hepatic endothelial lipase - Recycling endocytosis via coted pits. In: A.H. Gotto, Jr., L.C. Smith, B.Allen (eds.), Atherosclerosis V, Springer-Verlag New York, Heidelberg, Berlin, 383-386 (1980)
13. Klock, J.C., Shohet, S.B.: Erythrocyte membrane lipid abnormalities in hypophosphatemic hemolysis. J. Clin. Invest. 52, 47A (1973)
14. Kreusser, W., Ritz, E., Boland, R., Brachmann, J.: Function of the sarcoplasmic reticulum in hypophosphatemic myopathy. Adv. Exp. Med. Biol. 128, 313-321 (1980)

STIMULATION OF CARDIAC CONTRACTILITY BY CATECHOLAMINES IS DIMINISHED IN EXPERIMENTAL UREMIA

W. Kreusser, M. Rambausek, P. Klooker,
U. Brückner, and E. Ritz

Depts. Internal Medicine and Experimental
Surgery, University of Heidelberg, FRG

Cardiovascular complications are common among uremic patients. Various factors such as hypertension, anemia, acidosis, overhydration and hyperkalemia may interfere with cardiac function and explain the high cardiovascular mortality of uremic patients. Therefore, much controversy exists as to whether these factors explain the cardiac dysfunction or whether some specific "uremic cardiomyopathy" exists (1, 2). To further clarify this issue, a model of acute uremia, in which all the above factors were absent, was chosen to study myocardial performance in uremia.

METHODS

8 female foxhounds, 6 months of age, with an initial weight of 18.1 ± 0.83 kg were used. Uremia was induced by subtotal ligation of renal arteries. For surgery, the dogs were premedicated with 0.6 mg/kg morphine sulphate and 0.15 mg/kg proprionyl-phenothiazine (Combelen[R]). Anaesthesia was induced with an intravenous injection of 15 mg/kg sodium pentobarbital (Nembutal[R]) and maintained with subsequent doses of 3 mg/kg/h. The animals were intubated and arteficially ventilated with O_2/N_2O mixture (1:3) with a respirator (Dräger, Kiel).

After hemodynamic measurements in the basal state, angiotensin II (Hypertensin[R], Ciba, Basel), was infused i.v. at 0.1 µg/kg/min., subsequently noradrenaline (Arterenol[R], Hoechst, Frankfurt/Main) at 0.9 µg/kg/min and finally orciprenaline (Alupent[R], Boehringer, Ingel-

heim) at 0.5 μg/kg/min. Hemodynamic measurements under angiotensin II or noradrenaline infusion were started when blood pressure had reached steady state. During orciprenaline infusion, hemodynamic measurements were started when dp/dt_{max} was in a steady state. Administration of pressor agents was not started before basal aortic pressure and dp/dt_{max} had been reached.
The following measurements were carried out: a Swan-Ganz catheter was inserted via the right jugular vein into the pulmonary artery for measurements of pulmonary arterial pressure. A Goodale-Lubin catheter was introduced via the left jugular vein into the coronary sinus to obtain coronary venous blood. A multipurpose catheter was inserted by Seldinger technique into the femoral artery for measurement of AOP. A catheter tip manometer (Millar) was inserted into a tributory of the contralateral femoral artery for measurement of left ventricular enddiastolic pressure and instantaneous left ventricular pressure. ECG was continuously monitored using surface needle electrodes.
Lactate and pyruvate were enzymatically measured (3) using modified microassays in 500 μg samples of deproteinized (6% PCA) whole blood; free fatty acids were determined after Novåk (4). Cyclic AMP was measured with a radioimmunoassay according to Steiner (5) using a double labeled antibody (NEN, Dreieichenhain, FRG). Statistics: All values are given as mean ± SEM. The significances of differences between the study periods were analyzed with Wilcoxon's test for paired samples.

RESULTS

Table 1 gives biochemical data for control and uremic period.

Table 1: Serum chemistry in uremic dogs

	Control	Uremia
K^+ mmol/l	4.04 ± 0.11	4.02 ± 0.16
Ca mmol/l	2.68 ± 0.16	2.52 ± 0.06
Creatinine mg/dl	0.66 ± 0.06	2.96 ± 0.42*
Hemoglobin mg/dl	11.1 ± 0.82	10.5 ± 1.1
pH	7.32 ± 0.01	7.35 ± 0.01
blood volume ml/kg	62.6 ± 9.8	76.7 ± 12.6*

Values are given as mean ± SEM; n=8 per group.
* denotes a significant difference between control and uremia; $p < 0.01$.

After 7 days of uremia (b.w. 16.5 ± 0.79 kg), serum creatinine averaged 2.96 ± 0.42 mg/dl; sodium, potassium, calcium, hemoglobin and blood gases were not different between the two groups. Blood volume was slightly, but significantly elevated in uremia (control 62.6 ± 9.1; uremia 76.7 ± 12.6, n=8 per group, $p < 0.05$). In the resting state, heart rate, left ventricular pressure and dp/dt_{max} were not different between control and uremic animals (table 2) (basal heart rate: control 140 ± 30 beats/min; uremia 150 ± 27).

Table 2: Hemodynamics under basal conditions and under infusion of angiotensin II (A II) and orciprenaline (ORC) in uremic dogs

		basal	A II	ORC
LVP	CO	125 ± 7.1	198 ± 9.2	173 ± 15.2
	U	135 ± 7.8	196 ±10.3	187 ± 11.3
dp/dt_{max}	CO	3250 ± 1207	2610± 511	7567± 2267
	U	3205 ± 1016	3445± 982	5657± 1874*

Values are given as mean ± SEM; n=8 per group.
* denotes significant differences between control (CO) and uremia (U), $p < 0.01$.
LVP = left ventricular pressure (mmHg)
dp/dt_{max} in mmHg/sec.

After infusion of angiotensin II or norepinephrine the rise in LVP was similar in both groups (table 2). However, maximal contractile response (dp/dt_{max}) was significantly ($p < 0.01$) less after infusion of noradrenaline (controls: 7360 ± 2106 mmHg/sec; uremia 5960 ± 2054) or orciprenaline (controls 7567 ± 2267 mmHg/sec; uremia 5657 ± 1874).

The substrate concentrations are illustrated in table 3. Under basal conditions, lactate and pyruvate concentrations were increased and FFA decreased in uremia, however, the arterial coronary venous difference (AVD_C) remained unchanged in uremia. Arterial cAMP concentrations were increased in uremia (CO: 19.0 ± 3.7 nmol/l; U: 37.0 ± 7.2; $p < 0.01$). After stimulation with norepinephrine and orciprenaline, AVD_C remained constant and cAMP rose to a similar extent in control and uremic animals (arterial cAMP under orciprenaline: CO: 29.2 ± 4.6 nmol/l; U: 60.5 ± 4.3; $p < 0.01$).

Table 3: Substrate concentrations in arterial (AB) and coronary venous blood (CVB) of uremic dogs

		Lactate µmol/l	Pyruvate µmol/l	FFA µmol/l
Control	AB	1127 ± 184	74.5 ± 11	200 ± 33
	CVB	1042 ± 164	78.1 ± 8.2	143 ± 29
Uremia	AB	2024 ± 586*	130 ± 2.8*	109 ± 28*
	CVB	1669 ± 648*	118 ± 29*	74 ± 28*

Values are given as mean ± SEM; n=8 per group.
*denotes significant difference between control and uremia ($p < 0.01$).

DISCUSSION

This study clearly demonstrates diminished myocardial contractile response to catecholamines in a model of acute uremia, in which other complicating factors were not present. Therefore, the uremic state itself may affect cardioadrenergic response of the myocardium. In the basal state, myocardial function is usually depressed in patients with chronic uremia (6). However, in acute experimental uremia, several indices of myocardial contractility have been found to be increased (7-10). We found also enhanced contractility, as measured by V_{max}, in dogs with short term moderate uremia.[9] However, in more severely uremic dogs with a longer duration of uremia, as in the present study, we observed no increase of dp/dt_{max} and no change of left ventricular enddiastolic pressure (LVEDP). Diminished myocardial contractile response to catecholamines in the face of elevated catecholamines in the blood (Rascher et al., 1982) may point to myocardial endorgan resistance to catecholamines. Attenuated response of the heart rate to isoproterenol in hemodialysis patients has previously been observed by Ulman et al. (11). Our findings on cardiac metabolism do not provide an immediate explanation for cardiac dysfunction, since AVD_C for various metabolic substrates remained unchanged in uremia. The decrease in FFA in uremia may be a consequence of catecholamine receptor downregulation in adipose tissue. Further studies are needed on the receptor status of myocardium and other tissues to clarify these points.

REFERENCES

1. Prosser, D., Parsons, V., 1975, The case for a specific uremic myocardiopathy, 15: 4.
2. Mason, M.F., Resnik, H.Jr., Minot, A.S., Rainey, J., Pilcher, C., Harrison, T.R., 1973, Mechanism of experimental uremia, Arch. Int. Med. 60: 312.
3. Bergmeyer, H.U., 1974, Methoden der enzymatischen Analyse; 3rd Ed. Acetoacetate, pp 1887-90; ß-hydroxybutyrate, pp. 1882-6; Oxyglutarate, pp. 1624-1627; citrate, pp 1607-11, lactate, pp 1510-4; pyruvate, pp 1491-96. Verlag Chemie, Weinheim.
4. Novàk, M., 1965, Colorimetric ultramicro method for the determination of free fatty acids, J. Lipid Res. 6: 431.
5. Steiner, A.L., Parker, C.W., Kipnis, D.M., 1972, Radioimmunoassay for cyclic nucleotides, J. Biol. Chem. 247: 1106.
6. Hung, J., Harris, P.J., Uren, R.F., Tiller, D.J., Kelly, D.T., 1980, Uremic cardiomyopathy - effect of hemodialysis on left ventricular function in end-stage renal failure, New Engl. J. Med. 302: 547.
7. Raab, W., 1944, Cardiotoxic substance in the blood and heart muscle in uremia (their nature and action). J. Lab. Clin. Med. 29: 715.
8. Nivatpumin, T., Yipintsoi, T., Penpargkul, S., Scheuer, J., 1975, Increased cardiac contractility in acute uraemia; Interrelationship with hypertension, Am. J. Physiol. 229: 501.
9. Zebe, H., 1977, Die kongestive Kardiomyopathie. Professoral thesis. University Heidelberg.
10. Hennemann, H., Hevendahl, G., Arnold, H., Kissling, G., 1976, Uremic cardiomyopathy, in Renal Insufficiency, ed. by Heidland A., Thieme, Stuttgart, pp 274-279.
11. Ulman, A., Drüeke, T., Zingraff, J., Crosnier, T., 1977, The response of heart rate to isoproterenol in hemodialysed patients before and after parathyroidectomy, Clin. Nephrol. 7: 58.
12. Rascher, W., Schömig, A., Kreye, V.A., Ritz, E., 1982, Diminished vascular response to noradrenaline in experimental chronic uremia, Kidney Int. 21: 20.

INFLUENCE OF CALCIUM AND CALCIUM REGULATING HORMONES ON RENAL COMPENSATORY GROWTH

J.P. Bonjour, J. Jobin, J. Caverzasio and C. Taylor

Department of Pathophysiology, University of Berne and Division of Pathophysiology, Department of Medicine, University of Geneva Switzerland

Reduction in the renal mass is followed by a compensatory hypertrophy of the remaining kidney (1, 2). The search for the mechanism which triggers renal compensatory hypertrophy (RCH) has been the object of numerous investigations (1, 2). Despite intense efforts, the exact nature of the signal or signals which is/are implicated in the renal compensatory response have not yet been identified. Nevertheless, there is convincing evidence that RCH is triggered by an organ-specific humoral substance which is present in the plasma but may originate from the kidney itself (2, 6). The rate of compensatory growth has been shown to be influenced by various factors such as age (8), protein intake (9), and several hormones including growth hormone (10, 11), testosterone (12), thyroid hormone (13) and adrenal steroids (14). All these factors influence not only the "compensatory" growth but also the normal or "obligatory" growth of the kidney. Therefore, these factors appear to be rather unspecific since evidence has been obtained that RCH after unilateral nephrectomy is a growth phenomenon different from normal growth (15). An important feature which distinguishes the two phenomena is the fact that RCH is reversible, whereas normal growth is irreversible (15).

Calcium (Ca) in partnership with cyclic AMP has been shown to control the proliferation of various non-tumorigenic cells in vitro and in vivo (16). Parathyroid hormone through its "calcemic" effect has also been shown to be a stimulatory regulator of cell proliferation in bone marrow, thymus and liver after subtotal hepatectomy (16-21). Despite this information there has been no report so far, indicating that the Ca status, or Ca regulating hormone could modulate the degree of the compensatory growth of the remaining kidney after reduction of the renal mass.

In the present work, the influence of calcium (Ca) supply, parathyroid hormone (PTH), calcitonin (CT) and 1,25-dihydroxyvitamin D3 (1,25(OH)2D3) on renal compensatory hypertrophy (RCH) has been studied in unilaterally nephrectomized (UNI-NX) rats. UNI-NX rats were pair fed diets with high (1.1 %, HCaD) or low (0.1 %, LCaD) Ca content for 3, 8 and 15 days. After UNI-NX the wet weight of the remaining kidneys increased much more in rats fed LCaD than HCaD. The increased wet weight of the remaining kidney under LCaD was associated with a highly significant augmentation in dry weight, total protein and DNA content. LCaD did not display such effects in sham-operated rats with intact renal mass. The amount of dietary Ca did not influence the progressive rise in glomerular filtration rate (clearance of inulin) of the remaining kidneys as assessed 3, 7 and 14 days after UNI-NX. The stimulatory effect of LCaD on RCG was associated with a slight decrease in plasma Ca and moderate augmentation in kidney Ca content/g d.w. In UNI-NX rats fed LCaD chronic administration of CT in doses which induced hypocalcemia did not inhibit the enhanced RCH induced by LCaD. In UNI-NX rats fed HCaD chronic administration of PTH mimicked the effect of LCaD. An increased RCH was also observed in UNI-NX rats fed HCaD and chronically treated with 1,25(OH)2D3.

In conclusion, dietary Ca restriction can enhance markedly the compensatory but not the normal growth of the kidney. The data suggest that among the Ca regulating hormones, PTH and may be 1,25(OH)2D3 could be involved in the stimulating action of Ca restriction on renal compensatory growth.

REFERENCES

1. Malt, R.A.: Compensatory growth of the kidney. N. Engl. J. Med. 280: 1446-1459 (1969).

2. Hayslett, J.P.: Functional adaptation to reduction in renal mass. Physiol. Rev. 59: 137-164 (1979)

3. Preuss, H.G., Terryl, E.F. and Keller, A.I.: Renotropic factor(s) in plasma from uninephrectomized rats. Nephron 7: 459-470 (1970).

4. Dicker, S.E. and Morris, C.A.: Presence of a renotropic factor in plasma of unilaterally nephrectomized rats. J. Physiol. 299: 13-27 (1980).

5. Hammond, G.L., Wieben, E. and Marker, C.C.: Molecular signals for initiating protein synthesis in organ hypertrophy. Proc. Natl. Acad. Sci USA 76: 2455-2459 (1979).

6. Dicker, S.E. and Morris, C.A.: Origin of the humoral factor responsible for compensatory renal hypertrophy. J. Physiol. 30: 1-5 (1980).

7. Galla, S.H., Klein-Robbenhaar, T. and Hayslett, J.P.: Influence of age on the compensatory response in growth and function to unilateral nephrectomy. Yale J. Biol. Med. 47: 218-226 (1974).

8. Ashinberg, L.C., Koskimies, O., Bernstein, J., Nash, M., Edelmann, C.M. and Spitzer, A.: The influence of age on the response to renal parenchymal loss. Yale J. Biol. Med. 51: 341-345 (1978).

9. Konishi, F.: Renal hyperplasia in young and old rats fed a high protein diet following unilateral nephrectomy. J. Gerontol. 17: 151-153 (1962).

10. Block, M.A., Wakim, K.G. and Mann, F.C.: Appraisal of certain factors influencing compensatory renal hypertrophy. Am. J. Physiol. 172: 60-66 (1953).

11. Astarabadim, T.: The effect of growth and lactogenic hormones on renal compensatory hypertrophy in hypophysectomized rats. Q. J. Exp. Physiol. 48: 85-91 (1963).

12. Schlondorff, D., Trizna, W., De Rosis, E. and Korth-Shutz, S.: Effect of testosterone on compensatory renal hypertrophy in the rat. Endocrinology 101: 1670-1675 (1977).

13. Reiter, R.J. In: The Endocrines and Compensatory Renal Enlargement in Compensatory Renal Hypertrophy. (W.W. Nowinski, ed.) New York, pp 183-204 (1969).

14. Goss, R.J.: Renal and adrenal relationships in compensatory hyperplasia. Proc.Soc.Exp.Biol.Med. 118: 342-346 (1965).

15. Silber, S. and Malvin, R.L.: Compensatory and obligatory renal growth in rats. Am.J.Physiol. 226: 114-117 (1974).

16. Whitfield, J.F., Boynton, J.P., MacManus, J.P., Sikorska, M. and Tsareg, B.K.: The regulation of cell proliferation by calcium and cyclic AMP. Mol. Cell. Biochem. 27: 155-179 (1979).

17. Whitfield, J.F., MacManus, J.P., Youdale, T. and Franks, D.J.: The roles of calcium and cyclic AMP in the stimulatory action of parathyroid hormone on thymic lymphocyte proliferation. J. Cell Physiol. 78: 355-368 (1971).

18. Rixon, R.H. and Whitfield, J.F.: Hypoplasia of the bone marrow in rats following removal of the parathyroid glands. J. Cell Physiol. 79: 348-352 (1972).

19. Rixon, R.H. and Whitfield, J.F.: Parathyroid hormone: A possible initiator of liver regeneration. Proc. Soc. Exp. Biol. Med. 141: 93-96 (1972).

20. Rixon, R.H. and Whitfield, J.F.: The control of liver regeneration by parathyroid hormone and calcium. J. Cell Physiol. 87: 147-155 (1976).

21. Rixon, R.H., MacManus, J.P. and Whitfield, J.F.: The control of liver regeneration by calcitonin, parathyroid hormone and 1,25-Dihydroxycholecalciferol. Mol. Cell Endocr. 15: 79-89 (1979).

ACKNOWLEDGMENTS

This work has been supported by the Swiss National Science Foundation (3.824.79 and 3.806.0.82), the Procter and Gamble Company, Cincinnati, USA, and the Ausbildungs- und Förderungsfonds der Arbeitsgemeinschaft für Osteosynthese (AO), Chur, Switzerland.

CHANGES IN TISSUE CALCIUM CONTENT DURING GENTAMICIN ACUTE RENAL FAILURE

Robert E. Cronin

Department of Internal Medicine
Veterans Administration Medical Center and
University of Texas Southwestern Medical School
Dallas, Texas

INTRODUCTION

Aminoglycoside nephrotoxicity is the most important clinical cause of nephrotoxic acute renal failure. The mode of action whereby the aminoglycoside antibiotics kill bacteria and cause nephrotoxicity is probably quite similar. In both cases, drug binding to membrane structures results in death or injury to the cell. In the kidney, aminoglycosides have important effects on plasma, lysozomal, and mitochondrial membranes (1). Studies from this laboratory have investigated the gentamicin model of acute renal failure by evaluating indices of renal cellular integrity that depend in a major way on the integrity of the plasma membrane, i.e. renal cortex ionic composition and renal cortex Na-K ATPase activity (2,3). These studies demonstrated that renal injury was consistently accompanied by a gain in the tissue content of calcium and sodium. Studies in renal and non-renal tissue using ischemic and toxic injuries indicate that accumulation of calcium in the cytosol may play a central role in irreversible cell death (4).

In gentamicin nephrotoxicity where tissue calcium may be an important factor in cell death, reducing the movement of calcium from the extracellular to intracellular fluid or decreasing the gradient for calcium movement between these two compartments might be expected to lessen nephrotoxicity and reduce tissue calcium accumulation. This paper reports the results of studies examining the link between cellular calcium and gentamicin induced injury.

METHODS

Studies were performed on 300-400 g Sprague-Dawley rats eating a standard laboratory diet. Study 1. Baseline studies: Six animals received a saline injection or gentamicin in a dose of 30 mg/kg by subcutaneous injection for 7 days. At the end of the experimental period the animals were anesthetized and the kidneys removed. Plasma creatinine was analyzed in a specimen of venous blood. The renal cortex of one kidney was analyzed for ionic composition and a homogenate was prepared from the renal cortex of the other kidney and analyzed for Na-K ATPase activity by previously described techniques (3). Study 2. Calcium channel blocker studies: Control and gentamicin groups were handled as in the above study. A third group received verapamil 4 mg/kg twice daily plus a sham saline injection. The fourth group received verapamil 4 mg/kg twice daily plus gentamicin 30 mg/kg twice daily. Renal function and renal cortex analyses were performed after 7 days of gentamicin administration.

Data were analyzed by one-way analysis of variance and the Student-Newman-Keuls multiple comparisons procedure.

RESULTS

Study 1 (Table 1, Figure 1). Nephrotoxicity was evidenced in the gentamicin group by a significantly higher plasma creatinine compared to control animals (2.3±0.4 vs 0.9±0.1 mg/dl, $p < .005$). Ionic composition was also altered in the rats receiving gentamicin compared with control with markedly higher sodium (29.8 ±1.1 vs 19.6±0.5 mEq/100 g FFDS, $p<.001$), chloride (14.5±0.5 vs 8.9±0.3 mEq/100 g FFDS, $p<.001$), and calcium (1.7±0.3 vs 0.7±.01 mM/100 g FFDS, $p<.001$). Smaller but significant increases also occurred in potassium (31.8±0.6 vs 28.6±0.3 mEq/100 g FFDS, $p < .001$) and magnesium (3.8±0.1 vs 3.3±0.4 mM/100 g FFDS, $p<.001$). Phosphorus was unchanged. Figure 1 shows the relative changes in renal cortex electrolyte and mineral composition following gentamicin administration plotted as the percentage change from control. The most striking changes were noted in the ions primarily located in the extracellular compartment, calcium (143%), sodium (52%), and chloride (63%).

Study 2 (Table 2). The purpose of this study was to determine whether a slow channel calcium blocker, verapamil, given at the same time as gentamicin would prevent or reduce gentamicin nephrotoxicity. Table 2 demonstrates that gentamicin had a small but similar nephrotoxic effect in both normal and verapamil treated animals. Specifically, verapamil did not afford protection against gentamicin nephrotoxicity.

DISCUSSION

These studies demonstrate that a sharp rise in cellular calcium and sodium content is a feature of gentamicin nephrotoxicity in the rat. Similar changes have been recorded in dogs exposed to nephrotoxic doses of gentamicin (2). However, in the dog the changes in sodium and calcium are preceded by a fall in cellular potassium, magnesium, and phosphorus. Why this sequence of changes was not demonstrable in the rat is unclear, but the standard rat diet (Wayne Lab Blox) is substantially higher in potassium compared with the dog diet (Wayne Dog Diet). Thus cellular potassium stores may have been better protected in the rat because of dietary factors. The present data are compatible with an increase in tissue calcium being a contributing cause to cell death, but it might be argued that the changes rather represent calcification of dead cells. Against the latter possibility is the fact that tissue calcium rose at a time when tissue phosphorus, the usual ion accompanying calcium with tissue calcification, fell.

Schanne and associates (4) have offered evidence that a rise in cytosolic calcium concentration in a number of tissues exposed to ischemic as well as toxic injuries represents the final common pathway to cell death. Thus, a drug known to impede the movement of calcium across the plasma membrane might be expected to afford protection against a nephrotoxic insult. However, administration of verapamil in this study did not protect against gentamicin-induced acute renal failure and failed to block the rise in tissue calcium. The possible reasons for this lack of effect include 1) a systemic hypotensive effect of verapamil that offset any protective effect on calcium entry, and 2) calcium entry into the cells occurred over pathways or channels not blocked by verapamil. For example, gentamicin may have altered plasma membrane phospholipids in a non-specific way such that they were more permeable to several ionic species, including calcium and sodium. In another study from this laboratory, a reduction of the extracellular calcium available to enter the cell was produced by selective parathyroidectomy (6). This approach also failed to protect against gentamicin nephrotoxicity.

Thus, tissue calcium accumulation is a predictable component of gentamicin nephrotoxicity, but the pathway by which the additional calcium enters renal cortical cells is still unknown. Cytosolic calcium concentration represents the net result of passive inward calcium movement and active calcium extrusion by energy requiring membrane pumps, (e.g. Ca^{++} - ATPase and calcium-sodium exchange dependent on the sodium gradient established by Na-K ATPase). Future studies will probe where among these pathways and pumps gentamicin might cause its toxic effects.

Table 1, Study 1: Effect of gentamicin (60 mg/day) on renal function and renal cortex ion composition.

	PCr	Na	Cl	K	Ca	Mg	Pi
	mg/dl	- mEq/100 g FFDS -			- mM/100 g FFDS -		
C	0.9±0.1	19.6±0.5	8.9±0.3	28.6±0.3	0.7±.01	3.3±.04	38.1±0.6
p value	<.005	<.001	<.001	<.001	<.001	<.001	<.001
G	2.3±0.4	29.8±1.1	14.5±0.5	31.8±0.6	1.7±0.3	3.8±0.1	36.7±0.7

Table 2, Study 2: Effect of gentamicin (30 mg/kg twice daily) on plasma creatinine and renal cortex electrolyte and mineral composition in normal and verapamil (4 mg/kg twice daily) treated animals.

	PCr mg/dl	Na	Cl	K	Ca	Mg	Pi
		- mEq/100 g FFDS -			- mM/100 g FFDS -		
C	0.7±.04	16.9±0.4	10.6±0.3	33.2±0.3	1.18±0.05	3.7±0.03	38.5±0.3
p value	NS	<.001	<.01	NS	NS	NS	NS
G	1.1±0.1	20.4±1	14.3±0.7	33.3±0.5	1.36±0.07	3.6±0.08	37.5±0.7
V	0.6±0.04	20.8±0.5	12.4±0.3	33.6±0.2	1.01±0.03	3.84±0.02	38.2±0.2
p value	<.025	<.001	<.005	NS	<.05	NS	NS
VG	1.22±0.3	29.3±2.1	17.0±1.4	34.8±0.5	1.72±0.23	3.77±0.06	38.9±0.2

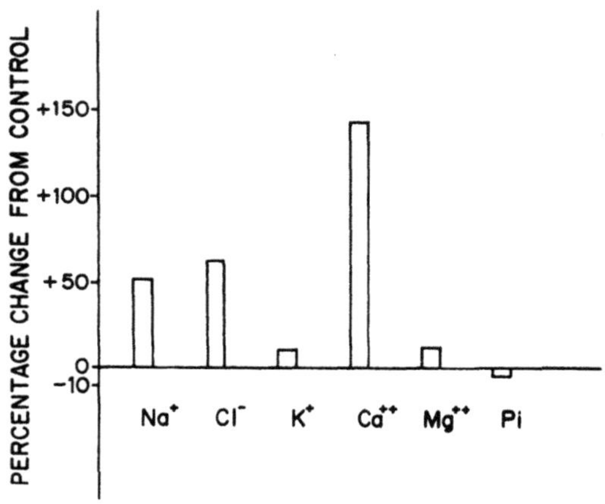

Figure 1, Study 1: Changes in renal cortex ion composition after 7 days of gentamicin administration. The data are plotted as percentage change from control.

REFERENCES

1. Humes, D.H., Weinberg, J.M., and Knauss, T.C.: Clinical and pathophysiologic aspects of aminoglycoside nephrotoxicity. Am. J. Kidney Dis. 2:5-29, 1982.

2. Cronin, R.E., Nix, K.L., Ferguson, E.R., Southern, P.M., and Henrich, W.L.: Renal cortex ion composition and Na-K-ATPase activity in gentamicin nephrotoxicity. Am. J. Physiol. 242:F477-F483, 1982.

3. Cronin, R.E., Splinter, K.L., Ferguson, E.R., and Henrich, W.L.: Gentamicin nephrotoxicity: protective effects of diabetes on cell injury. Min. Elect. Metab. 9:38-44, 1983.

4. Schanne, F.A.X., Kane, A.B., Young, E.E., and Farber, J.L.: Calcium dependence of toxic cell death: a final common pathway. Science 206:206-208, 1979.

5. Nayler, W.G.: The role of calcium in the ischemic myocardium. Am. J. Pathol. 102:262-270, 1981.

6. Cronin, R.: Role of PTH and Throxine in gentamicin-induced acute renal failure. Clin. Res. 31:549A, 1983.

NUCLEAR MAGNETIC RESONANCE

PHOSPHORUS METABOLITES BY NMR

B.D. Ross, D.M. Freeman and L. Chan

Nuffield Dept Clinical Medicine, John Radcliffe Hospital
Clinical Magnetic Resonance Laboratory, Radcliffe
Infirmary and Biochemistry Dept, University of Oxford

INTRODUCTION

^{31}Phosphorus NMR has been applied to intact biological systems for almost 10 years (1) and it is opportune to review what has been learned from this technique over this period. The first observation of NMR signals from intact living tissues were in red cells, E. Coli and in cooled frog muscle, but has progressed rapidly to isolated perfused organs of poikilotherms, intact animals, and to man (2). Major technical developments have aided this progress with larger magnets and not least the invention of the "surface-coil" (3). This development obviated the necessity to envelop the entire sample in a transmitter (receiver) coil, and opened the way to the use of ^{31}P NMR in the diagnosis of muscle disease, in the intact human subject (4). This technique will now be used in Oxford, to examine the brain and other organs of human subjects, non-invasively, in a high field magnet of 60 cm internal diameter. Much of what has so far been achieved with ^{31}P NMR can be classed as confirmatory when viewed from the standpoint of the metabolic biochemist or clinical investigator. Presumably this will change markedly when the metabolic measurements are made upon inaccessible internal organs and the brain in man, since then only ^{31}P NMR is applicable in the acquisition of biochemical information.

The present paper is concerned to examine the new insights which ^{31}P NMR has given into phosphate metabolism. There are several discoveries which must be considered as significantly altering views on intermediary metabolism.

TABLE 1 LESSONS FROM ^{31}P NMR

1. Phosphorus metabolites are in two forms: free and bound
2. [ADP] is significantly different from previous estimates
3. [Pi] is significantly lower than previous estimates
4. $[Pi]_{cyt}$ may control cellular respiration
5. ΔG_{ATP} (free energy per ATP hydrolysed) in vivo is at least = 61.5 kJ/Mol

   equivalent to the maximum for isolated mitochondria
6. Cytoplasmic pH = 7.04 Human muscle
7. Cytoplasmic pH = 7.10 Rat kidney
8. Glycolysis is active at pH <5.9
9. Oxidative phosphorylation and glycogenolysis contribute disproportionately to phosphocreatine synthesis in muscle

TABLE 2 OBSERVABLE INORGANIC PHOSPHATE (Pi) BY NMR

Tissue	NMR	Chemical Assay	NMR/Chemical assay	Reference
Cat biceps (fast twitch)	0.9	5.6	15%	Meyer et al
Cat soleus (slow twitch)	6.1	9.2	76%	Meyer et al
Mouse Liver*	4.5	4.5	100%	McLaughlin et al
Rat Liver*	4.0	4.25	100%	Iles et al
Human muscle (resting)	4.3	10.0	43%	Edwards et al Ross et al
Rat Kidney	0.6	2.2	27%	Freeman et al

References*

Meyer R A, Kushmerick M J, Brown T R (1982) Am J Physiol 242, C1-C11

McLaughlin A C, Takeda H, Chance B (1979) Proc Natl Acad Sci 76, 5445-5449

Iles R A et al (1980) Biochem J 192, 191-202

Edwards R H T et al (1982) Lancet i, 725-731

PRINCIPLES OF NMR

Applying a radiofrequency pulse to a population of nuclei, "aligned" in a powerful, homogeneous magnetic field induces a new orientation of nuclei, which can be observed as a nuclear magnetic resonance signal, itself of radiofrequency (5). The frequency used to excite is specific for the molecular species - say phosphorus; the frequency of emission, that is the signal observed, is measurably different for each phosphorus nucleus (chemical shift), and hence distinguishes Pi, PCr, ATP (α, β and γ). This chemical shift information is the basis of chemical analysis by NMR (2). Two novel examples in biology may be cited. The renal ^{31}phosphorus spectrum contains very little phosphocreatine, but has instead two unusual peaks. One is confined to the renal papilla, and is glycerophosphoryl choline (6) the putative waterproofing substance of collecting duct cells. The other is unidentified still, but is of interest for its negative property. Thought to be AMP (7), this was readily excluded by progressive enzymic destruction of AMP in perchloric acid extracts of kidney, leaving some 3 μmoles/g of a stable, mobile phosphate compound of the same chemical shift as AMP but confined to renal cortex (8, 9).

Quantification of ^{31}P NMR signals is itself inherently straightforward but involves determination of another magnetic property, the spin-lattice relaxation time T_1. T_1 is a property of great biological interest, as it is greatly prolonged in tumour tissue. In proton (H^1) NMR tomography, this property which is shared by ^{31}P has been exploited extensively in identifying and localising tumours in man. This application of T_1 information is outside the scope of the present discussion. However, knowledge of T_1 for Pi and its metabolites permits accurate quantification and furthermore opens the way to measurement of reaction-rates. Comparison of quantitative ^{31}P NMR with standard total chemical or enzymatic analysis after extraction has been of striking interest and has important lessons for many branches of biochemistry. Using an internal standard of methylenediphosphate, ADP observed by ^{31}P NMR is a small fraction of that determined chemically. This has been a controversial issue since the first NMR spectra of muscle were observed (2), and is now demonstrated directly for the kidney (3, 9). Careful comparison of the values obtained on the same sample shows 27% of ADP to be "visible" in perfused kidney (10). This figure falls to below 10% for the kidney in vivo (see below). The most probable explanation is that NMR detects "free" ADP; the corollary is that a large proportion of ADP is bound in all cells (an exception are the erythrocytes lacking mitochondria (11)). A similar division has been suspected from indirect comparisons for inorganic phosphate (Table 2). When directly assayed in the intact perfused kidney, 75% of Pi is bound and only 25% is free (10). Indirect evidence, some of which is discussed below, suggests that the NMR signal for Pi is derived principally from cytoplasmic free-phosphate. This has important consequences.

(i) The NMR-observed or free-[Pi] might be the determinant of cellular respiration: Evidence for this possibility comes from three different observations in muscle and kidney. In a single patient with twice-the-normal oxygen consumption(12), resting [Pi] is between 2 and 3 times normal. During exercise, progressive increase in [Pi] in muscle to a new-steady state occurs. Finally, in thyrotoxicosis, the isolated perfused kidney continues to demonstrate increased respiratory rate, and [Pi] observed by NMR is about twice the control (13).

(ii) pH determinations which are an important capability of ^{31}P NMR probably reflect the cytoplasmic compartment alone (14). This follows from the use of chemical shift of Pi in pH determinations. Normal and pathological responses of intracellular pH have now been observed with NMR. In the kidney, respiratory acidosis results in a parallel fall in intracellular pH (8), which is similar to that observed in metabolic acidosis (7). This in turn has important consequences for our understanding of urinary acidification; respiratory acidosis occurs with an elevated intracellular bicarbonate concentration, 50% above control and some 4 to 5 times higher than that seen in metabolic acidosis. Very much lower urine pH, at least in the isolated kidney, is achieved in metabolic acidosis than respiratory acidosis for this reason.

In hypoxia, ischaemia and the early stages of all forms of experimental ischaemic acute renal failure, cytoplasmic pH of the kidney falls to very low levels (15). The extent and duration of acidosis may determine the outcome of the ischaemic insult, since irreversible damage to renal function follows after more than 30 minutes at an extracellular pH of 6.5 (16).

In skeletal muscle, ^{31}P NMR demonstrates the small but significant intracellular acidosis which accompanies generalised metabolic acidosis (12), and the intracellular alkalosis which accompanies respiratory alkalosis (17). Pathological changes in intracellular pH were observed in human muscle in a variety of diseases; in phosphorylase, or amyloglycosidase deficiency (18) during exercise, pH rises, as a reflection of H^+ consumed during breakdown of phosphocreatine, and in Duchenne's and Becker type muscular dystrophy at rest pH is abnormally high (19). In the latter case, a possibility that abnormal pH represents an underlying abnormality of muscle membrane potential has been raised.

TURNOVER OF PHOSPHORUS METABOLITES BY NMR

Two methods of determining phosphate turnover of living cells by NMR have been explored. The first derives from the rapid and

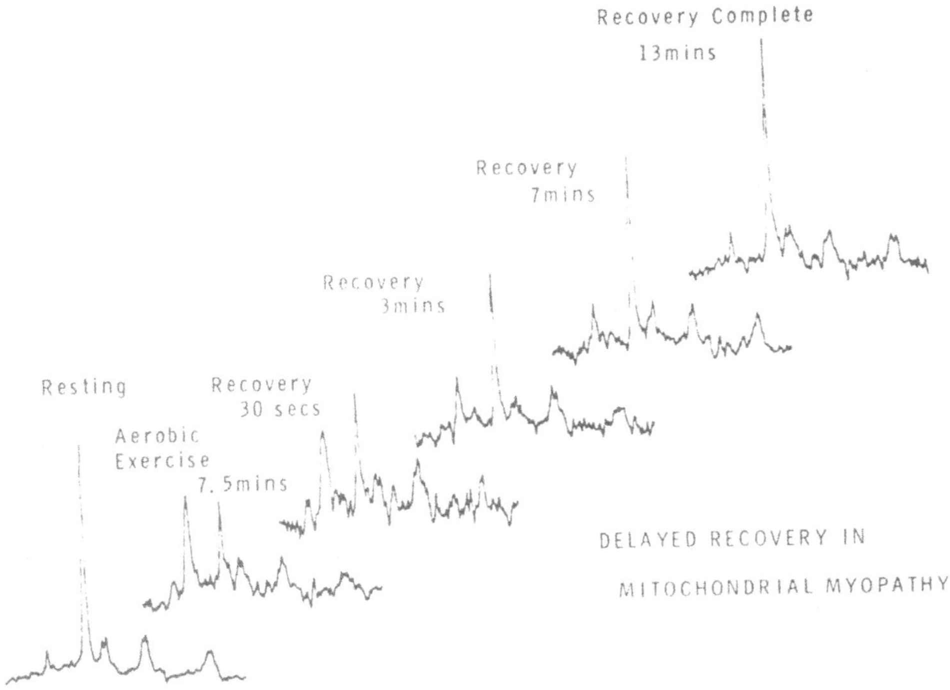

FIGURE 1

TABLE 3 PHOSPHORUS METABOLITES BY NMR - values in µmoles/g wet wt(rat)

	Perfused kidney (n = 11)	In vivo (n = 5)
ATP	2.42	2.75
ADP	0.27	0.07*
Pi	0.92	0.71
Glycerophosphorylcholine	1.42	1.74
AMP/Unknown (at +12 ppm)	3.1	1.93

* undetected by NMR difference spectrum

QUANTITATIVE ^{31}PHOSPHORUS NMR SPECTRUM OF IN VIVO ANAESTHETISED RAT KIDNEY.

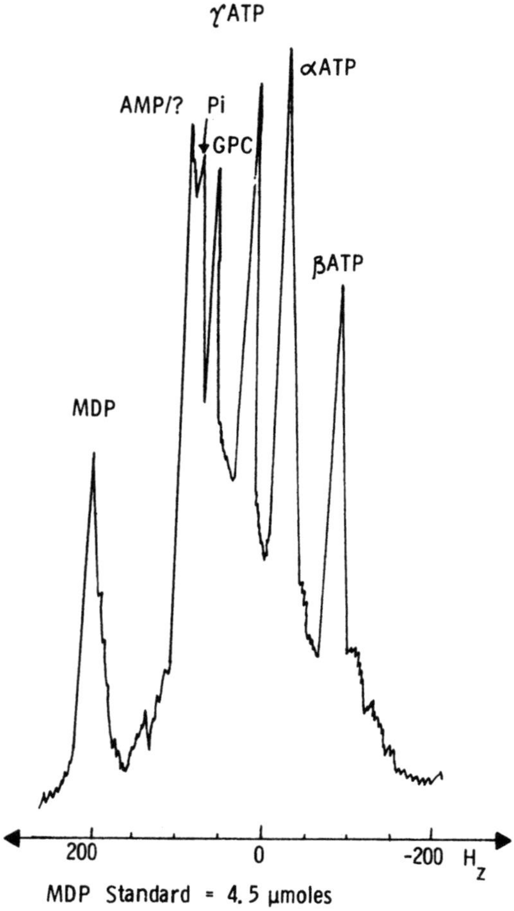

MDP Standard = 4.5 μmoles

Mean weight of three kidneys = 1.2 g

6,400 scans, 4 sec. delay

FIGURE 2

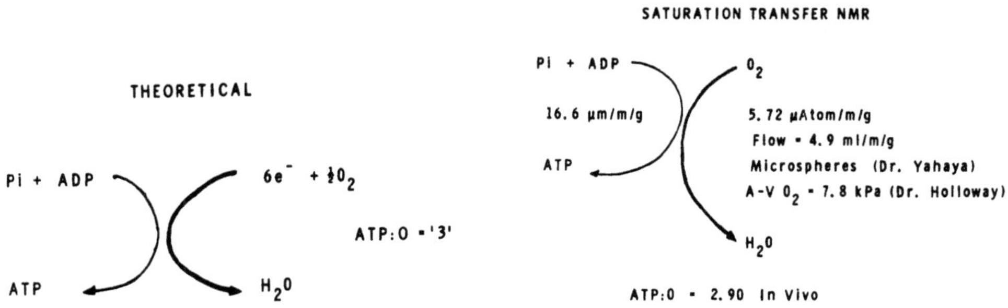

FIGURE 3

TABLE 4 METABOLIC RATE IN VIVO BY ^{31}P NMR

1. F = K Pi (F = ADP + Pi $\xrightarrow{K}$ ATP)
2. K from saturation transfer = Ma/Mo
   Pi = 0.6 mM/g wet weight
   Ma/Mo = 0.49 (n = 2)
   Assume the T_1 for saturation in vivo
3. ATP synthesis = 16.6 µmoles/m/g wet weight
4. Oxygen consumption = 2.86 µmoles/m/g wet weight
5. ATP : O = 16.6/5.72 = 2.9

non-destructive nature of the technique and is most readily illustrated by reference to an unusual muscle disease. Accumulation of a spectrum of between 30 and 60 scans permits metabolite quantitation so that the time course of the metabolic response to exercise can be followed with a resolution of about 30 seconds. As shown in Figure 1, during muscle contraction PCr is consumed, with formation of inorganic phosphate, while pH falls. Recovery from these changes depends upon efficient oxidative phosphorylation (20), and is normally conplete within $1\frac{1}{2}$ minutes. In the patient illustrated this recovery is prolonged, and both Pi and PCr remained abnormal 8 minutes after cessation of exercise. This is the characteristic finding in mitochondrial myopathy.

An exciting application of NMR to measurement of metabolite turnover, allows the rate of creatine kinase to be followed in vivo (21), and more recently the rate of ATP synthesis has been determined in the intact perfused kidney (10). The technique is that of saturation transfer, proposed originally by Forsen and Hoffman (22). Irradiation at the frequency of one phosphate atom can abolish the NMR signal from that atom due to "saturation". Exchange during metabolism leads to transfer of "saturated" phosphorus nuclei to another pool; the extent of the exchange is observed as a reduction in intensity of the second phosphate pool (23). The power of this technique can be illustrated by our recent studies (in Press) in which both the rate of oxidative phosphorylation and the degree of coupling to respiration (ATP:O) for the in vivo rat kidney have been measured.

Quantitative NMR spectra from perfused kidneys (10) and in vivo kidneys are closely comparable (Table 3; Figure 2). Saturation of γ ATP was achieved regularly in the perfused kidney experiments, and now in the kidney in vivo. Transfer of "saturation" to inorganic phosphate was readily and reproducibly demonstrated, indicating that ^{31}P NMR can be used to measure the rate of oxidative phosphorylation in vivo. Following the method described in detail elsewhere (10), the rate of ATP synthesis was calculated to be 16.6 µmoles/min/g of kidney. This value is entirely new, and its validity is best assessed by comparison with renal oxygen uptake. Thus, in theory 3 ATP are synthesised for each pair of electrons as it passes down the electron transport chain from NAD to cytochrome a_3 and oxygen. An ATP:O ratio of 2.9 has been calculated for the experiments described here (Table 4; Figure 3). Oxygen consumption was determined in parallel experiments, and flow rate for the rat kidney in animals under nembutal anaesthesia determined using microspheres (Dr Halleyru Yahaya; unpublished work in this Laboratory).

The good agreement between these findings and the value for ATP:O of isolated mitochondria in vitro permits the following conclusions to be drawn:

i) Saturation transfer measures the rate of ATP synthesis in a heterogeneous tissue such as kidney.

ii) Free reversibility of ATP synthesis and breakdown is a reflection of an active Na-K-ATP'ase, at least as great as the rate of oxidative phosphorylation.

iii) Mitochondria in kidney are "well-coupled".

iv) Finally, and most important for any discussion of intracellular [Pi]: the [Pi] determined in fully relaxed spectra by NMR is a pool which is totally and exclusively involved in metabolic turnover in the renal cell. Were this not the case, and for example the NMR-invisible [Pi] was involved in oxidative phosphorylation, a quite meaningless result would obtain in the saturation-transfer calculation.

It remains to be seen whether other metabolic and physiological manipulations in the kidney or in other tissues bear out this conclusion.

REFERENCES

1. Hoult D I, Busby S J, Gadian D G, Radda G K, Richards R E, Seeley P J (1974) Nature (Lond) 252, 285-287
2. Gadian D G, Radda G K (1981) Ann Rev Biochem 50, 69-83
3. Ackerman J J H, Grove T H, Wong G G, Gadian D G, Radda G K (1980) Nature 283, 167-170
4. Ross B D, Radda G K, Gadian D G, Rocker G, Esiri M, Falconer-Smith J (1981) New Eng J of Medicine 304, 1338-1342
5. Block F (1946) Physical Review 70, 460-473
6. Balaban R S (1982)"Biochemistry in Kidney Function" ed Morel F, Elsevier Biomedical Press, Amsterdam
7. Ackerman J J H, Lowry M, Radda G K, Ross B D, Wong G G (1981) J Physiol 319, 65-79
8. Freeman D M, Lowry M, Radda G K, Ross B D (1982) Biochem Transact 10, 399
9. Wong G G, Ross B D (1983) NMR in renal physiology and biochemistry. Mineral and salt metabolism (in Press)
10. Freeman D M, Bartlett S, Radda G K, Ross B D (1983) Biochim Biophys Acta 762, 325-336
11. Wong G G (1981) DPhil Thesis, Oxford
12. Gadian D G, Radda G K, Ross B D, Hockaday J, Bore P J, Taylor D J, Styles P (1981) Lancet ii, 774-775
13. Ross B D, Radda G K, Bartlett S B, Freeman D M (1983) Clin Sci 64, 37
14. Bailey I A, Williams S R, Radda G K, Gadian D G (1981) Biochem J 196(1), 171-178

15. Chan L, Ledingham J G G, Dixon J A, Thulborn K R, Waterton J C, Radda G K, Ross B D (1982)"Acute renal failure" ed Eliahou, John Libbey, London pp 35-41
16. Chan L C (1983) D Phil Thesis, Oxford
17. Ross B D, Radda G K, Taylor D J, Bore P J, Styles P (1981b) ed Alberti G G M, CIBA Symposium: Metabolic acidosis 87, 145-152
18. Ross B D (1983) Biochem Soc Transact Cambridge (in Press)
19. Newman R J, Bore P J, Chan L, Gadian D G, Styles P, Taylor D J, Radda G K (1982) B M J 284, 1072-1074
20. Radda G K, Bore P J, Gadian D G, Ross B D, Styles P, Taylor D J, Morgan-Hughes J (1982) Nature 295, 608-609
21. Shoubridge E A, Briggs R W, Radda G K (1982) FEBS Lett 140, 288-292
22. Forsen S, Hoffman R A (1963) J Chem Phys 39, 2892-2901
23. Gadian D G (1982) "NMR and its application of living systems", Clarendon Press, Oxford

Acknowledgements: BDR was supported in this work, and in attending the 6th International Workshop on Phosphate and other Minerals, by the Wellcome Trust. The Authors are particularly grateful to Dr G K Radda, FRS, and members of his Laboratory, for facilities and important contributions to this work. In addition, we are grateful to Dr Haliru Yahaya for permitting us to use his data on renal blood flow, and to Dr Paul Holloway for determining oxygen consumption. The spectra for Fig. 1 were produced with the help of Dr. G. Arnold and Ms. Judith Harley.

APPLICATIONS OF NUCLEAR MAGNETIC RESONANCE (NMR) IN NEPHROLOGY

Juha Kokko

The University of Texas Health Science Center
at Dallas, Southwestern Medical School
Dallas, Texas

INTRODUCTION

Nuclear magnetic resonance techniques (NMR) were developed in the mid-1940's[1,2]. Initially the technology was applicable in different branches of chemistry to determine the fine structure of various small molecular weight molecules and to examine the effect of perturbation of ambient media on the structure of these compounds. In spite of the explosive growth of NMR literature, application of NMR technology to physiological issues is relatively new. This has only become possible with development of superconductive magnets, pulse technology with Fourier transformation, and large-bore magnets.

The salient theoretical concepts of NMR spectroscopy are not difficult to understand. In general it can be considered that many nuclei are magnetic dipoles and thus behave as if they are small magnets. Of importance to the physiologist is the realization that ^{31}P, the predominant naturally-occurring phosphorous, can be described by quantum mechanic laws as if it were a small magnet. When these nuclei are placed in a magnetic field (Figure 1), the majority of them orient themselves in a low energy state with the south pole of the nuclide oriented toward the north pole of the applied magnetic field. The laws of physical chemistry dictate that ^{31}P can exist only at two energy levels and that the transition from the lower energy level to the higher one can occur only when the magnetic field strength and resonance frequency of the nucleus have unique values where energy absorption can occur. When these conditions are met, the ^{31}P nuclide will absorb energy and "flip" to a higher energy level. As a magnetic dipole returns to its low energy state, it re-emits radiofrequency energy which

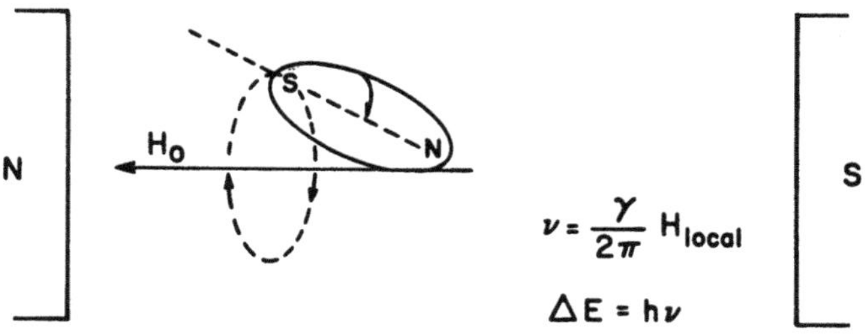

Figure 1. Schematic to illustrate the orientation and precession of a nuclide (I.e., ^{31}P with a magnetic moment) in a magnetic field, H_0. The frequency of precession (P) is unique to a given nuclide in a known magnetic field and is a direct function of the magnetogyric ratio (r). ^{31}P can exist in only two energy levels. The lower of the two is depicted above. The change in energy level occurs only when frequency of precession is equal to the externally imposed radio frequency.

can be detected by appropriate receiver components of the NMR spectrometer. Since each nuclide has a unique resonance frequency, it is obvious that the energy level transitions can be used to identify specific nuclides.

There are two parameters in NMR spectroscopy which are of interest to the physiologist. The first is the measurement of the area under a given peak, while the second is the magnetic field strength at which the energy level transitions occur.

The greater the number of nuclides absorbing energy in a given magnetic field, the larger the resultant spectral signal. Thus, the relative areas under the given spectral lines (Recorded as broadened peaks) are directly related to the relative concentration of molecules giving rise to those signals. Thus NMR can be used advantageously to obtain concentrations of various intra- and extracellular ^{31}P-containing constituents.

The second NMR parameter of interest to the physiologist is the "chemical shift" of the signal. Chemical shift refers to the specific magnetic field in which a signal will occur. Commonly, chemical shifts of spectral lines are expressed as displacement from some known standard. It is important to realize that a local magnetic field around a nuclide is different from the applied magnetic field because of various molecular environmental factors which screen the nuclide from the applied field. The most important of these screening effects is due to electron density about the nuclide. The higher the electron density around a given ^{31}P nuclide, the higher must be the applied magnetic field to get the same local magnetic field as is around the ^{31}P nuclide with lower ambient electron density. The chemical shifts are exceedingly sensitive to small variations in chemical environment of a given nuclide and therefore chemical shifts of spectral lines are used to identify the nature of compound in question. Thus NMR spectroscopy can be used to identify rapidly and noninvasively the presence of various compounds and their respective concentrations.

The remainder of this manuscript will examine the potential applications of NMR spectroscopy to four general areas of nephrology: 1) epithelial transport, 2) whole kidney metabolism, 3) dialysis, and 4) transplantation.

EPITHELIAL TRANSPORT

Thus far NMR has not been applied to examine biochemical events in homogeneous cell lines from specific segments of the nephron. This has not been feasible because of the large quantities (About 1 gram net weight) of tissue required by most available instrumentation. However, two studies have recorded spectra from either toad urinary bladder[3] or from frog skin[4,5]. These studies are relevant since both of these tissues are transport models of the mammalian collecting duct.

Figure 2 is a typical NMR spectrum of frog skin epithelial ducts (Connective tissue separated), obtained at room temperature, in Cl Ringers[5]. These skins were bubbled with 100% oxygen. Several interesting points emerge: The ADP concentration is only 8.9 ± 2.0% of the ATP concentration; the phosphocreatine concentration is quite low; and the inorganic concentration of phosphate is low[5]. While NMR determinations allow for accurate estimation of relative concentrations of compounds it is difficult to obtain absolute concentrations by this technique unless all of the tissue is within the detector coils. Nevertheless, the estimates from our studies suggest that both the inorganic phosphate and ATP/ADP concentrations are certainly below 5 mM--a far cry from the chemically determined total intracellular phosphate concentration of roughly 100 mEq/l. Thus it is clear that most of the intracellular phosphate is in bound form: Phospholipids, nucleic acid, proteins and intermediary carbohydrates. Therefore, unlike the

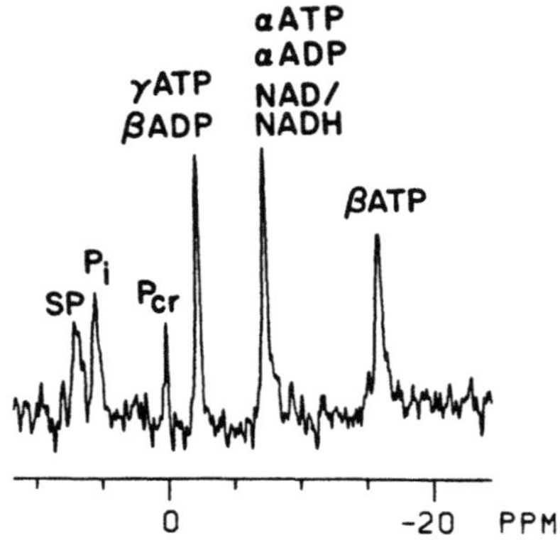

Figure 2. ^{31}P NMR spectrum of frog skin epithelia at room temperature[5]. Epithelia were bubbled with 100% O_2.

major intracellular cation (Potassium), the major intracellular anion (Phosphate) is not readily exchangeable.

Our studies also demonstrate that the ATP concentrations are quite sensitive to oxygen tensions. Figure 3 illustrates the complete disappearance of the ATP after 15 minutes of hypoxia (100% oxygen replaced by 100% nitrogen bubbling). These values return to pre-hypoxic controls within five minutes of return of oxygen bubbling[5]. Thus adequate oxygenation of tissue must be assured during NMR experiments.

WHOLE KIDNEY METABOLISM

The recent development of surface coils now makes it possible to examine metabolic events of in situ kidneys in intact animals[6,7]. This technique has been called topical magnetic resonance and has the tremendous potential advantage that renal metabolic events may be examined noninvasively. Figure 4 represents a NMR spectrum of kidney from an anesthetized rat[7]. The signal-to-noise ratio demonstrates the feasibility of using NMR to design pathophysiologically important studies. Indeed, recent studies

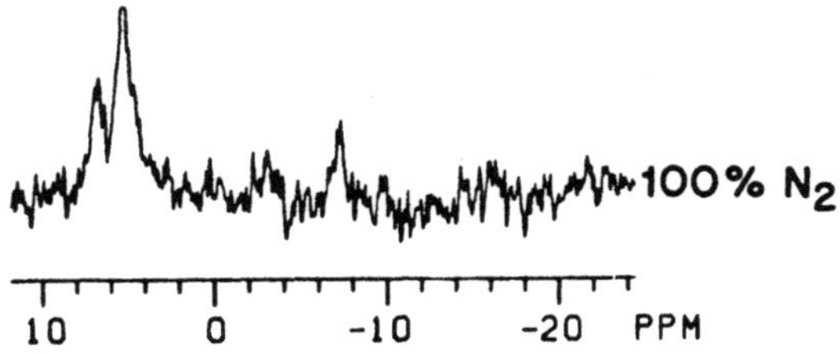

Figure 3. ^{31}P NMR spectrum of same frog skin epithelia as in Fig. 2 but obtained 15 minutes after change of 100% O_2 to 100% N_2.

using topical magnetic resonance techniques have examined the role of Mg-ATP infusions for prevention of ischemic acute renal failure in rats[8].

DIALYSIS

It is now possible to study phosphorous-containing metabolites in human beings with NMR since the construction of large-bore superconducting magnets[9]. The possible utility of NMR in clinical medicine was demonstrated in a patient with McArdle's syndrome when it was shown that this patient failed to decrease his intracellular pH in response to ischemic exercise[9].

We wanted to use these same general techniques to determine the concentrations of ATP, ADP, phosphocreatine, inorganic phosphate, and intracellular pH in dialysis patients. In these studies we questioned whether acute hemodialysis causes a change in the metabolic profile of muscle of uremic patients and the effect of dialysis on intracellular pH. Our ultimate aim was to determine whether NMR can be used to determine an index of adequacy of hemodialysis in a select group of patients. While our studies are preliminary, they do describe a rise in phosphocreatine to ATP ratio and a slight alkalinization of intracellular pH[10]. Unfortunately, we have not noted any specific changes which would allow us to use the NMR techniques effectively to determine adequate end points for dialysis. This area of research requires further investigation.

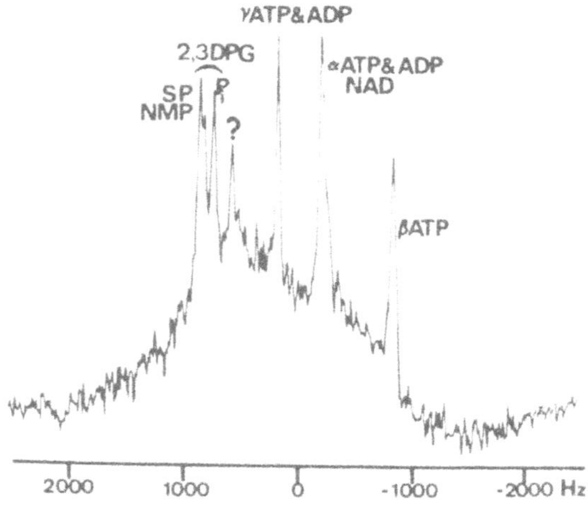

Figure 4. ^{31}P NMR spectrum of in situ rat kidney[7].

TRANSPLANTATION

The combination of newly developed NMR imaging techniques with simultaneous evaluation of metabolic profile of transplanted kidney should aid in differential diagnosis of acute tubular necrosis from immunological rejection. While no studies have been published in this area, a preliminary report[11] has appeared which used NMR imaging to evaluate potential differences in acute tubular necrosis as contrasted to transplant rejection in dogs. These studies are not complete but they do show promise and offer hope that NMR can be developed as a noninvasive and a safe technique to differentiate between various forms of renal disease in the post-transplant period.

SUMMARY

The ^{31}P NMR techniques can be applied in different areas of nephrology. Particularly advantageous is the ability to detect metabolic events occurring in vivo by safe and noninvasive techniques. It will be interesting to see how clinically relevant these new applications will be.

REFERENCES

1. E. M. Purcell, H. C. Torrey, R. V. Pound, Resonance absorption by nuclear magnetic moments in a solid, Phys. Rev., 69:37, 1946
2. F. Bloch, W. W. Hansen, M. E. Packard, Nuclear induction, Phys. Rev., 69:127, 1946
3. M. Bond, M. Shporer, K. Peterson, M. M. Civan, ^{31}P Nuclear magnetic resonance analysis of toad urinary bladder, Mol. Physiol., 1:243-263, 1981
4. L. E. Lin, M. Shporer, M. M. Civan, ^{31}P nuclear magnetic resonance analysis of frog skin, Am. J. Physiol., 243(Cell Physiol. 12):C74-C80, 1982
5. R. L. Nunnally, J. S. Stoddard, S. I. Helman, J. P. Kokko, The response of ^{31}P nuclear resonance (NMR) spectra of frog skin to variations in pCO_2 and hypoxia, Am. J. Physiol., in press
6. G. K. Radda, J. J. H. Ackerman, P. Bore, P. Sehr, G. G. Wong, ^{31}P NMR studies on kidney intracellular pH in acute renal acidosis, Int. J. Biochem., 12:277-281, 1980
7. R. S. Balaban, Nuclear magnetic resonance studies of epithelial metabolism and function, Federation Proc., 41:42-47, 1982
8. N. J. Siegel, M. J. Avison, H. Reilly, R. G. Shulman, Accelerated recovery of cellular ATP by the postischemic infusion of ATP-$MgCl_2$ (Abstract), Clin. Res., 31:441A, 1983
9. B. D. Ross, G. K. Radda, D. G. Gadian, G. Rocker, M. Esiri, J. Falconer-Smith, Examination of a case of suspected McArdle's syndrome by ^{31}P nuclear magnetic resonance, N. Engl. J. Med., 304:1338-1342, 1981
10. J. P. Kokko, S. R. Hayes, R. L. Nunnally, Nuclear magnetic resonance study of chronic hemodialysis patients, (Submitted for publication)
11. T. M. Slemmer, K. L. Moon, Jr., C. E. Alpers, H. Hricak, Nuclear magnetic resonance imaging of the kidney in acute tubular necrosis and rejection, Proc. Am. Soc. Transplant Physicians, 2:39A, 1983

INDEX

www.ingramcontent.com/pod-product-compliance
Ingram Content Group UK Ltd.
Pitfield, Milton Keynes, MK11 3LW, UK
UKHW051451290926
15471UKWH00008B/1135
* 9 7 8 1 4 6 8 4 4 8 0 9 2 *